Developments in
Cardiovascular Medicine

Developments in Cardiovascular Medicine

Edited by C. J. Dickinson

Professor of Medicine, St Bartholomew's Hospital Medical School, London

and J. Marks

Director of Medical Studies, Girton College, Cambridge

The Proceedings of the special symposium,
organised by the Royal College of Physicians,
to celebrate the 400th Anniversary of the birth
of William Harvey.

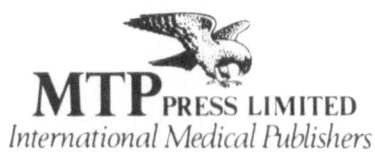

MTPPRESS LIMITED
International Medical Publishers

Published in UK by
MTP Press Limited
Falcon House
Cable Street
Lancaster, England.

Copyright © 1978 MTP Press Limited

Softcover reprint of the hardcover 1st edition 1978

ISBN 978-94-015-7343-6   ISBN 978-94-015-7341-2 (eBook)
DOI 10.1007/978-94-015-7341-2

REDWOOD BURN LIMITED
Trowbridge & Esher

Contents

CONTENTS

List of Contributors

N. BOM
Department of Medical Engineering,
University Hospital,
Rotterdam,
Holland

E. BRAUNWALD
Hersey Professor of the Theory and Practice
of Physic,
Harvard Medical School,
Boston, Massachusetts, USA

Hilary BROWN
Laboratory of Physiology,
University of Oxford

Frans J. L. van CAPELLE
University of Amsterdam,
Wilhelmina Gasthius,
Amsterdam, Holland

H. E. DE WARDENER
Department of Medicine,
Charing Cross Hospital Medical School,
London

D. DURRER
Department of Cardiology and Clinical
Physiology,
University of Amsterdam,
Wilhelmina Gasthuis,
Amsterdam, Holland

M. A. FLOYER
Department of Medicine,
The London Hospital Medical College,
London

D. G. GRAHAME-SMITH
Department of Clinical Pharmacology,
Radcliffe Infirmary, Oxford

A. C. GUYTON
Department of Physiology and Biophysics,
School of Medicine,
University of Mississippi,
Mississippi, USA

A. GUZ
Department of Medicine,
Charing Cross Hospital Medical School,
London

P. G. HUGENHOLTZ
Department of Cardiology,
Thoraxcenter,
University Hospital,
Rotterdam, Holland

Michiel J. JANSE
University of Amsterdam,
Wilhelmina Gasthius,
Amsterdam, Holland

B. R. JEWELL
Department of Physiology,
University College, London

L. KREEL
Department of Radiology,
Northwick Park Hospital,
Harrow, Middlesex

D. M. KRIKLER
Royal Postgraduate Medical School,
London

C. Th. LANCEE
Department of Medical Engineering,
University Hospital,
Rotterdam, Holland

DEVELOPMENTS IN CARDIOVASCULAR MEDICINE

Part I
Non-invasive techniques for the study of the cardiovascular systems

1
Computed tomography and the cardiovascular system

L. KREEL

In computed tomography tissue attenuation values are measured by transmitted X-ray photons. Radiation from both the interlinked X-ray tube and scintillation detectors is measured and by arithmetic multiplication/addition and back-projection tissue attenuation values are computed in axial body sections approximately 13 mm thick[1].

The first whole-body scanner with a scan time of 18–20 s, which allowed examinations during breath-holding, used a rotate/translate system. Each pass of the interlinked tube and detectors across the body records 18 000 readings and after 10° rotations to cover 180° some 32 000 readings are recorded to give a 320 × 320 matrix[2].

With this scanner considerable detail is visible in the thoracic-wall soft tissues, in bone and in the lung fields, although there are some streak artefacts adjacent to the heart[3]. However, no detail is visible in the ventricular region, although some chamber definition is possible in the atrial region and the major vessels are easily visible. The ascending aorta, main pulmonary and major branch arteries are visible as well as the descending aorta. Heart valves are only visible when calcified and then show marked radiating streak artefacts (Figure 1). Where sufficient sub-pericardial fat is present the pericardium can be distinguished, but it is difficult to diagnose even large pericardial effusions, although pericardial calcification is well shown. Even after intravenous contrast medium there is little further information from the cardiac chambers or the myocardium. With a scan time of 20 s there is thus very little useful information obtained from the heart itself, although the major vessels are well shown.

The situation is quite different with major vessels of the thorax and abdomen. The size, shape and position of the aorta is well shown on axial sections allowing accurate assessment of the diameter of aneurysms. For diagnosing dissection and the position of the channel, contrast enhancement

3

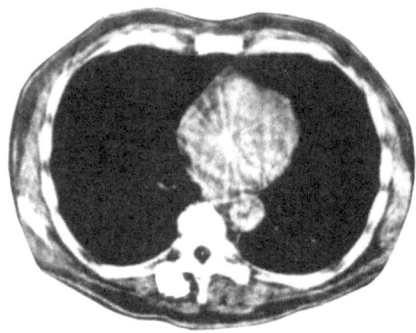

Figure 1 Calcification of aortic valve. With a 20 s scan considerable streak artefacts are produced

must be used because there is no difference in tissue attenuation values between lumen and blood clot. Malrotation of the aorta with a right aortic arch is easily recognized, as is the degree and extent of aortic calcification.

In a known case of Takayashu's disease the area of obstruction in the descending aorta was markedly narrowed and contained marked intraluminal calcification. A sliver of calcification was also visible in the right main pulmonary artery.

Angiomatous malformations in the lung are shown as a leash of vessels, usually seen end-on, together with a large feeding vessel. Similarly, cerebral angiomatous malformations can be shown, but then contrast enhancement is needed.

In the abdomen, where aneurysms are common, any enlargement of the aorta in cross-section is readily documented and easily distinguished from other retroperitoneal masses, especially lymphadenopathy, and is especially important in lymphoma. Aortic aneurysm and lymph node enlargement may, of course, co-exist. As in the thorax, dissecting aneurysms enlarge the aorta, the outer margin becomes ill-defined when there is perivascular leak of blood but, to show the channel, intravenous contrast enhancement is needed.

While the cross-sectional display of aortic aneurysms is clear (Figure 2) and unequivocal, the cranio-caudal display is problematical. It is unusual to display renal arteries in relationship to the aneurysm with any degree of accuracy, although the left renal vein is easily identified and it is usually possible to show whether the aortic bifurcation is involved.

Computed tomography has been successfully used in diagnosing post-operative complications after aortic resection with prosthetic replacement, particularly surrounding abscess and gas formation. An estimation of the length of aneurysms requires careful localization in terms of the lumbar vertebrae on a 'scanogram', which is a radiograph of the area taken with a slit-beam diaphragm to eliminate parallax. Without contrast enhancement

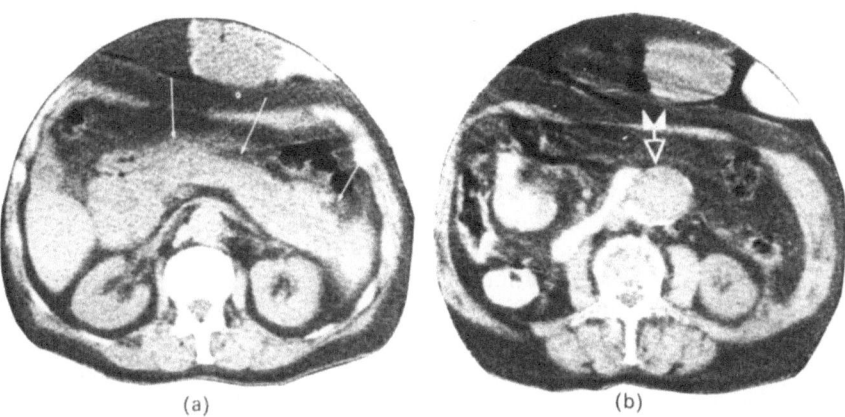

Figure 2 A palpable mass was present after an attack of pancreatitis: (*A*) very early pseudocyst formation around pancreas (arrows); but also (*B*) aortic aneurysm (arrow)

the lumen is not visible and thrombus cannot be distinguished. It is clear, therefore, that ultrasonography is better suited to diagnosis of aortic aneurysms because the channel is visible and the aorta can be shown longitudinally.

While inferior vena caval obstruction with calcification is uncommon (Figure 3), it must be distinguished from other types of calcification, particularly in its transhepatic portion. The position of the calcification in axial sections is so definite that its anatomical localization becomes unequivocal. Collateral vessels also become visible.

In abdominal haemorrhage, blood usually has higher attenuation values than surrounding tissue although blood around the liver may appear isodense.

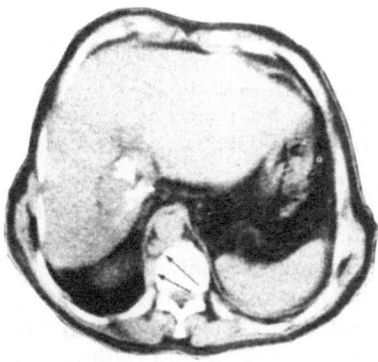

Figure 3 Calcification of inferior vena cava (white arrow) associated with enlarged hemi-azygos system (black arrows)

The main value of computed tomography lies in being able to localize the bleed to the abdominal wall, to the mesocolic compartment, to perirenal area or as free blood within the peritoneal cavity.

Carotid body tumours are highly vascular and can be shown after contrast enhancement, while in hypertension associated with raised catecholamines, phaeochromocytomas can be localized, especially if in the suprarenals.

Thus, with a scan time of 20 s, computed tomography is of very limited value in cardiovascular diagnosis compared with its role in neuroradiology or oncology. The obvious reason is that, while a 20 s scan time does not interfere with the demonstration of neurological lesions or mass lesions in the abdomen or thorax, it is far too long for visualization of cardiac structures[4].

In third- and fourth-generation scanners the scan time has been reduced to 2–5 s. These scanners have a circular motion taking readings through 360°. By using two superimposed scans during a single breath-holding episode and a gated programme to use only the readings during diastole, a 'stop action' picture of the heart can be obtained[5]. After intravenous contrast injection cardiac cavities and myocardial wall thickness are clearly shown. Without intravenous contrast medium ventricular cavities cannot be differentiated from myocardium. Furthermore, repeated single-section scans are inadequate for accurate reconstruction programmes to determine myocardial mass and left ventricular volumes because of the changing position of the heart and respiration, and the impossibility of accurately aligning 13 mm sections in the axial plane of the heart during successive episodes of breath-holding.

It therefore seems most unlikely that any further advance in cardiac diagnosis will become available with 2–5 s scanners, particularly if the currently available information from cardiac ultrasonography and dynamic isotope scanning is borne in mind. Furthermore, experimental evidence indicates that, even with perfect 'stop action' views of the heart myocardium cannot be distinguished from cardiac cavities without contrast medium[6].

It is, however, of considerable interest that a research group at the Mayo Clinic are at present engaged in developing a cardiac scanner. Ritman[7], in an extensive review, has defined the requirements for such a device and indicated its structure. He argues that for an accurate evaluation of cardiac status the heart must be displayed in full in 'dynamic three-dimensional geometry' and there must be exact evaluation of regional perfusion distribution. Although ideally a measure of cardiac functional reserve is the most important requirement, this is at present beyond the capability even of modern technology. He emphasizes dynamic three-dimensional geometry because he considers that cardiac status is dependent on left ventricular volume and that chamber volume is a poor substitute. Conventional indices, such as left ventricular myocardial mass, chamber volume and ejection fraction, are workable in practice only because they represent the closest available approximations to left ventricular geometry and its rate of change.

Ritman maintains that theoretically computed tomography can provide this evidence by direct observation and without interfering with cardiac structure or function by manipulation, sedation or anaesthetic. Computed tomography was for the first time the potential of anatomical and functional evaluation of cardiac status without interfering with the heart or the rest of the patient.

Because it should be possible to accurately characterize cardiac geometry and regional myocardial perfusion as well as intracardiac blood flow patterns and synchronous rate of change of the myocardium, it then becomes a matter of computation to establish regional myocardial length and tension, force velocity variables, stroke volumes, flow in major vessels, abnormal intracardiac flows and to analyse their functional relationships.

Ritman goes even further by outlining the possibility of very exact location of coronary artery narrowing and fractional lumenal narrowing to calculate regional perfusion and myocardial shape and its dimensions.

All this is now within the bounds of possibility, and the degree of accuracy of computed tomography in securing this data depends on the complexity of the scanning device and its computational capability[8] as well as on the radiation. The group at the Mayo have planned such a 'versatile, general purpose, reconstruction imaging system', but they point out that it must be able to vary spatial density and temporal resolution to tailor the examination to particular requirements. Specifically then it must be multi-purpose, electronic, view the whole heart in a synchronous cylindrical manner as well as having a scanning and reconstruction facility. This then would be the dynamic spatial reconstructor (DSR).

With these specifications it would be possible to have a variety of scanning configurations. At the one extreme there would be a high temporal resolution, but having the least density resolution, this would use an all-electronic scanning mode; at the other extreme it could produce highest-density resolution with a reduced temporal resolution which would use a combined electronic and mechanical scanning mode.

This device would then be able to show coronary arteries of 2–3 mm after coronary angiography, but would only need a single injection in each artery. The size and position of moderate-sized transmural infarcts could be measured to within 5% accuracy, and left ventricular wall thickness and total muscle mass could be measured to within 5% accuracy. To do this it would have to have a spatial resolution of 0.01 s in systole and 0.1 s in diastole during the slow-filling phase, a scan repetition rate of at least 50/s for cylindrical scans of the entire three-dimensional extent of the heart in systole and 5/s in diastole with less than 1 mm of movement of structure during each scan. Each full set of multi-planer scans would be recorded in 0.01 s.

Acknowledgments

Grateful acknowledgment is made to the Department of Health and Social Security, whose farsighted and generous help has assisted greatly in the development of this project.

The assistance and considerable help from all the staff associated with the whole body scanner is also gratefully acknowledged and, in particular, Steven Henman and Malcolm Brooker who have been managing the equipment.

References

1. Hounsfield, G. N. (1978). In *Medical Imaging – C.T., U/S, I.S. and N.M.R.* (Aylesbury: H.M. & M. Publishers Ltd). (In publication)
2. Hill, K. R. (1976). E.M.I. total body scanner: technical aspects. *Br. J. Clin. Equip.*, **1**, 207
3. Kreel, L. (1978). Computed tomography of the thorax, seminars in roentgenology. (In press)
4. Alfidi, R. J., Haaga, J. R., MacIntyre, W. J., Bacon, K. T. and Ferrario, C. M. (1977). Gated computed tomography of the heart. *Computed Axial Tomography*, **1**, 51
5. Harell, G. S., Guthaner, D. F., Breiman, R. S., Morehouse, C. C., Seppi, E. J., Marshall, Jr., W. H. and Wexler, L. (1977). Stop-action cardiac computed tomography. *Radiology*, **123**, 515
6. Adams, D. F., Hessel, S. J., Judy, P. F., Stein, J. A. and Abrams, H. L. (1976). Computed tomography of the normal and infarcted myocardium. *Computed Tomography*, **126**, 786
7. Ritman, E. L. (1977). Quantitative transaxial imaging of the heart. *Eur. J. Cardiol.*, **5**, 203
8. Gilbert, B. K., Storma, M. T., James, C. E., Hobrock, L. W., Yang, E. S., Ballard, K. C. and Wood, E. H. (1976). A real-time hardware system for digital processing of wide-band video images. *IEEE Trans. Computers*, **25**, 1089

2
Study of local cerebral blood flow

N. A. LASSEN

Before 1945, i.e. before Seymour S. Kety, who then worked in Schmidt's laboratory in Philadelphia, devised the nitrous oxide method[1], the cerebral circulation in man was essentially an unknown territory. Many animal experiments had been reported. In particular, Forbes[2] had observed changes in diameter of pial arteries, through a small skull window. But their relevance to the completely intact human cerebral circulation was not necessarily so obvious. We now know, however, that much of what was then seen in experimental animals was indeed pertinent to man.

Kety's method is based on observing the *rate* of saturation of the brain by nitrous oxide inhaled at constant concentration of 15%. By sampling arterial blood the input concentration curve is ascertained. Cerebral venous blood collected from the internal jugular vein gives the *output* concentration curve. Mass balance (difference between cumulative input and cumulative output equals the amount retained in the organ) shows that the cerebral blood flow in millilitres per gram and per minute is inversely proportional to *the area between the arterial and cerebral venous N_2O curves*. Kety's method remains the standard for comparison to other methods. It was one of the very first observations that an increase in carbon dioxide tension—hypercapnia—augments cerebral blood flow sharply, while hypocapnia reduces it. A multitude of other physiological and pathophysiological observations soon followed—including studies in essential hypertension, tumours, stroke, and drug effects.

Kety's nitrous oxide method does not permit measurement of blood flow in discrete *regions* of the human brain. This first became possible when Lassen and Ingvar in 1961 introduced the use of radioactive inert gases instead of 'cold' nitrous oxide[3]. In man, in particular, the use of [133]Xenon combined with counting over the brain by externally placed scintillation detectors, is widely used[4,5,6]. Among the prominent centres in the United Kingdom using this technique it is appropriate to mention the Jennett–Harper group in Glasgow and the Symon–Marshall group from the National

Hospital of Neurological Diseases at Queen Square, in London. The field constitutes one of truly international collaboration demonstrated in a series of eight international meetings. At the most recent one (in 1977, in Copenhagen), there were more than 400 active participants from many countries.

In our laboratory in Copenhagen ^{133}Xenon dissolved in saline is injected via the internal carotid artery. This limits our studies to neurological patients who are having cerebral angiography. Because we inject the isotope as a bolus directly into the main inflow to the brain, a large amount of it reaches the brain without interference from other tissues. The arrival and subsequent wash-out is followed by a battery of 254 small scintillation detectors, each of which 'sees' about 2 cm^2 of brain surface. The wash-out is recorded for about 1 min, the slope of this curve segment giving a measure of flow in the fast-flow tissues, i.e. in the cortex. After 10–15 min a new injection can be made so as to study the effect of changes in arterial carbon dioxide tension, in arterial blood pressure or in brain function. We routinely make a total of four or five injections during a single session.

We confirm that carbon dioxide is indeed a strong cerebral vasodilator. This is so except in cases of stroke and cerebral tumour. It is particularly in such cases that even a small improvement of tissue perfusion might be very helpful, but unfortunately the damaged vessels do not react to carbon dioxide, and sometimes flow even decreases further in the critically perfused area. This is called the *intra-cerebral steal* effect and it reflects a deviation of flow towards more normal brain regions, where the vessels can still vasodilate.

When the blood pressure is moderately elevated by angiotensin infusion, the blood flow does not change in normal, intact brain tissue. Evidently an active cerebral vasoconstrictor response has counteracted the rise in perfusion pressure. But angiotensin does not act directly on the cerebral vessels— it is without cerebral vasoconstrictor effect if infused directly into the carotid artery. Hence the constriction appears to be the brain vessels' autonomous response to the increased wall tension. This so-called *autoregulation of the cerebral circulation* was in particular studied by Strandgaard[7,8], who showed the adaptation to a higher pressure level in chronic hypertension. The autoregulatory cerebral vasoconstriction is broken, if the pressure is made to rise suddenly to very high levels[9]. In this situation the flow suddenly increases sharply. The small arterioles balloon up, they over-distend, and the blood–brain barrier to protein breaks. This acute response of hyperperfusion (not ischaemic) is now thought to be the initiating event in acute hypertensive encephalopathy.

In acute cerebral diseases, in trauma, tumours or after a stroke, cerebral autoregulation is typically abolished. This can be used to localize the disease. A peculiar finding in severe cases is what is called 'false autoregulation': an induced hypertension has no effect on cerebral blood flow, which may be unchanged or even decreased[10]. Perhaps local variations in tissue pressure explain these paradoxical responses.

Having now mentioned two of the brain's major vasoactive responses—the chemical control by CO_2 and the autoregulation by blood pressure—let us turn to the third one: metabolic control. When cerebral metabolism increases, as in an epileptic seizure, the blood flow follows suit. (See Figures 1a and 1b.)

We can use this observation to localize the trigger zone in focal epilepsy[11] more precisely than by using the scalp electroencephalogram. But even within strictly physiological limits the same coupling of neuronal activity, metabolism and blood flow is seen. Simply clenching the hand augments cerebral oxygen uptake and blood flow in the contralateral sensori-motor hand area[12,13]. If a complex *sequence* of movements are made, like typing on a typewriter, then the supplementary motor area also shows augmented flow on both sides. Visual, auditory and tactile stimuli cause increases in flow to appropriate areas of the brain. With more complex tasks a specific pattern of regions show up—for example reading a text activates seven distinct areas in each hemisphere.

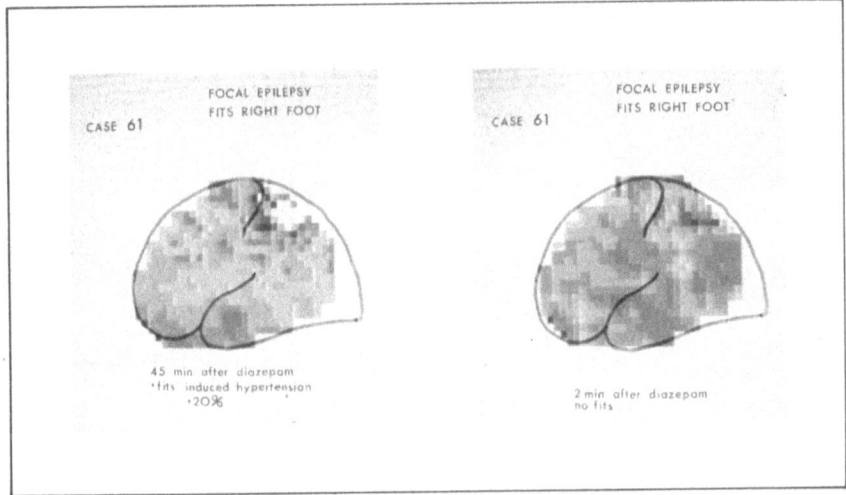

Figure 1 (*a*) Regional cerebral blood flow by [133]Xenon injection in focal epilepsy, left side of head, abnormal area, very high blood flow in upper posterior region (parietal lobe). After anti-epileptic drug treatment (Figure 1(*b*)) the area decreases in size and no longer corresponds to the motor cortex, so the jerks in the opposite foot stop temporarily. This smaller area must be assumed to contain the trigger zone. The electroencephalogram was normal in this case of continuous epileptic discharge

Such studies of metabolic control of cerebral circulation can be extended to patients with brain lesions, where lack of cortical activation (no focal increase in flow) can be analysed in the context of the neurological deficit. It should be stressed that the inactivity of an area *is not evidence of a physical destruction of that same area*: deafferentiation in the form of a disruption or dysfunction of fibre tracts may be sufficient to silence an area. Hence by mapping tissue metabolism variations (with deoxyglucose[14]) or its accompanying blood flow responses, the functional anatomy can be studied.

How is cerebral blood flow regulated to follow the metabolic needs of the tissue? This problem was posed by Roy and Sherrington in their classical paper in 1890, and they proposed that acid vasodilator metabolites might accumulate with enhanced activity. Certainly carbon dioxide, the end product of cerebral metabolism, forms hydrogen ions when hydrated. Yet current evidence suggests that due to the very rapid onset of functional hyperaemia (starting within few seconds) CO_2 cannot be responsible. Currently other 'candidates' for coupling flow to metabolism appear more likely. In particular a local accumulation of potassium ions (released from the cells) or of adenosine (produced from ATP-ADP-AMP) are being considered (Figure 2).

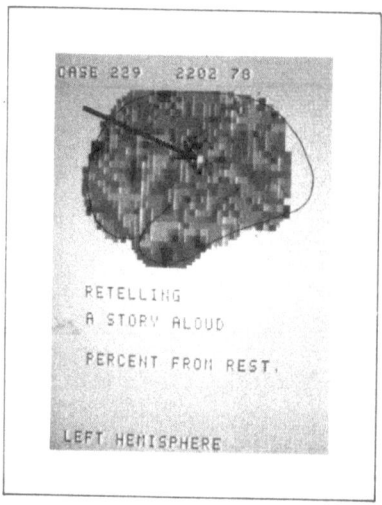

Figure 2 Changes in regional cerebral blood flow during normal activity. The changes are expressed as *percentage* changes from a control study made 15 min before. During retelling a story the flow increases by 30% in the mouth motor area (central arrowed area), in the auditory cortex (below mouth area) and in the supplementary motor cortex (upper part of frontal cortex). The picture is taken from a healthy left hemisphere, but the changes are essentially the same in both hemispheres

Regardless of the detailed mechanism, however, the coupling between tissue metabolism and blood flow can be used to reveal changes in metabolism. Actually, as is seen particularly well in epilepsy, the flow changes tend to rise proportionally more than metabolism. This overshoot implies that the local capillary oxygen tension *rises* during enhanced metabolic activity. Since oxygen must reach the cells by diffusion an enhanced oxidative metabolism must imply steeper oxygen diffusion gradients. Hence the increased capillary oxygen tension during functional activity means that the diffusional flux can go up without tissue Po_2 decreasing. In other words during normal physiological states of enhanced functional activity, there is no decrease of tissue oxygen tension, no impending oxygen lack.

The disproportionate increase in local flow during enhanced metabolic and functional activity implies that measurement of the flow response is a sensitive indicator of the metabolic level.

TRAUMATIC VERSUS ATRAUMATIC METHODS

Both Kety's nitrous oxide method and the intra-arterial [133]Xenon injection method must be termed traumatic or 'invasive' in that they involve cannulation or catheterization of arteries and veins. This has limited their applicability.

Currently a group of completely atraumatic methods are being developed that promises to extend vastly the clinical usefulness of the principles just outlined. Inhalation of [133]Xenon combined with external counting is being tried in several centres[15,16], but the spatial resolution is rather poor. In our laboratory we are currently trying the same approach using a computerized tomographic radioisotope scanner, much like the computerized tomographic X-ray scanner developed by Hounsfield[17]. Positron emitting isotopes such as [15]O$_2$ or ^{18}F offer other possibilities. This field, pioneered by the Postgraduate Medical School in London[18], is currently developing dramatically. Despite almost forbiddingly high costs, several computerized positron tomographs are currently being developed. Their application to the study of regional cerebral metabolism and flow is most promising. One approach suggested by the positron tomograph's chief inventor (M. M. Ter-Pogossian in Saint Louis[19]) is to use [15]O$_2$-labelled nitrous oxide, i.e. a radioactive variant of the same inert gas as used by Kety 34 years ago, when he started the whole field of cerebral blood flow measurements in man.

SUMMARY

The topic of how to measure cerebral blood flow in man has been reviewed with special emphasis on the coupling between functional activity, metabolism and blood flow. As in skeletal muscle this coupling exists *at a local level*, even down to brain areas of millimetre size. Hence by measuring the regional blood flow or metabolism one can gain much insight into the function of the brain. Specifically the technique can localize various functions in the intact brain cortex, and examine how different areas collaborate in more complex types of brain activity. This would appear to constitute a most powerful tool for the exploration of the brain in health and disease. A new type of neurophysiology is in sight, supplementing the classical one—electroneurophysiology. There are also promising new atraumatic techniques based on radioisotopes and on the 3-dimensional reconstruction of their internal distribution in the brain.

References

1. Kety, S. S. and Schmidt, C. F. (1945). The determination of cerebral blood flow in man by the use of nitrous oxide in low concentrations. *Am. J. Physiol.*, **143**, 53
2. Forbes, H. S. and Wolff, H. G. (1928). Cerebral circulation. III. The vasomotor control of the cerebral vessels. *Arch. Neurol. Psychiat.*, **19**, 1057
3. Lassen, N. A. and Ingvar, D. H. (1961). The blood flow of the cerebral cortex determined by radioactive Krypton-85. *Experientia*, **17**, 42

4. Lassen, N. A. and Ingvar, D. H. (1963). Regional cerebral blood flow in man. *Arch. Neurol.*, **9**, 615

5. Olesen, J., Paulson, O. B. and Lassen, N. A. (1971). Regional cerebral blood flow in man determined by the initial slope of the clearance of intra-arterially injected ^{133}Xenon. *Stroke*, **2**, 519

6. Sveinsdottir, E., Larsen, B., Rommer, P. and Lassen, N. A. (1977). A multi-detector scintillation camera with 254 channels. *J. Nucl. Med.*, **18**, 168

7. Strandgaard, S., Olesen, J., Skinhøj, E. and Lassen, N. A. (1973). Autoregulation of brain circulation in severe arterial hypertension. *Br. Med. J.*, **1**, 507

8. Strandgaard, S. (1976). Autoregulation of cerebral blood flow in hypertensive patients. The modifying influence of prolonged antihypertensive treatment on the tolerance to acute, drug-induced hypotension. *Circulation*, **53**, 720

9. Strandgaard, S., MacKenzie, E. T., Sengupta, D., Rowan, J. O., Lassen, N. A. and Harper, A. M. (1974). Upper limit of autoregulation of cerebral blood flow in the baboon. *Circ. Res.*, **34**, 435

10. Pàlvölgyi, R. (1969). Regional cerebral blood flow in patients with intracranial tumors. *J. Neurosurg.*, **31**, 149

11. Hougaard, K., Oikawa, T., Sveinsdottir, E., Skinhoj, E., Ingvar, D. H. and Lassen, N. A. (1976). Regional cerebral blood flow in focal cortical epilepsy. *Arch. Neurol.*, **33**, 527

12. Olesen, J. (1971). Contralateral focal increase of cerebral blood flow in man during arm work. *Brain*, **94**, 635

13. Raichle, M. E., Grubb, R. L., Mokhtar, H. G., Eichling, J. O. and Ter-Pogossian, M. M. (1976). Correlation between regional cerebral blood flow and oxidative metabolism. *Acta Neurol.*, **33**, 523

14. Sokoloff, L. (1976). Chapter III: [1-^{14}C]-2-deoxy-D-glucose method for measuring local cerebral glucose utilization. Mathematical analysis and determination of the 'lumped' constants. *Neurosciences Res. Prog. Bull.*, **14**, 466

15. Mallett, B. L. and Veal, N. (1965). The measurement of regional cerebral clearance rates in man using Xenon-133 inhalation and extracranial recording. *Clin. Sci.*, **29**, 179

16. Risberg, J., Ali, Z., Wilson, E. M., Wills, E. L. and Halsey, J. H., Jr. (1975). Regional cerebral blood flow by ^{133}Xenon inhalation. Preliminary evaluation of an initial slope index in patients with unstable flow compartments. *Stroke*, **6**, 142

17. Hounsfield, G. N. (1973). Computerized transverse axial scanning (tomography). Part I: Description of system. (Ambrose, J. Part II: Clinical application). *Br. J. Radiol.*, **46**, 1016

18. Pinching, A. J., Travers, R. L., Hughes, G. R. V., Jones, T. and Moss, S. (1978). Oxygen-15 brain scanning for detection of cerebral involvement in systemic lupus erythematosus. *Lancet*, **1**, 898

19. Ter-Pogossian, M. M., Mallinckrodt Institute of Radiology, St. Louis, Minnesota, U.S.A. (Personal communication to the author, May 1978)

3
Current status of echocardiology

P. G. HUGENHOLTZ, J. R. T. ROELANDT,
N. BOM AND C. Th. LANCEE

As we all know, echocardiography uses the echo principle, which is as old as Methuselah, although his sound was not 'ultra' high. It is therefore a fair question to ask when scientists began to use this method. The original initiative to use short sound pulses for the measurement of distance seems to stem from the great catastrophe of the ocean liner *Titanic* which in 1912 collided with an iceberg on her way to America with a loss of 1500 lives as a result. This disaster attracted much attention throughout the world and considerable thought was given to methods which might prevent similar accidents in the near future. Among other ideas, it was proposed to use a sound transducer in the bow of the ship to search the waters in the sailing direction for solid objects by the echo principle. However, at that time no transducer existed which could generate or receive the necessary short sound pulses and so the idea was not realized.

During the First World War, German submarines became an acute danger to supplies to the British Isles. This again made the detection of objects under the surface of the water a very urgent problem and investigations were started to develop necessary equipment. However, the First World War ended before any practical apparatus had been contrived but the intensified research during the war years had led to the discovery of the piezoelectric and magnetostrictive transducers for the generation of ultrasound. As a result of this research the first applications of the echo principle materialized in the field of peaceful uses, since the earlier war work allowed the construction of echo-sounding equipment for depth measurements and the detection of fish shoals.

During the years between the two world wars much fundamental research was done in physics laboratories investigating the properties of ultrasound. Thus on the eve of the Second World War an immense amount of knowledge had been amassed from studies in the animal kingdom (dolphins, whales, bats) and by experimentation about the generation, detection and properties of ultrasound such as the fact that ultrasound travelled at 1600 m/s through muscle, but only at 1450 m/s in fat, thus allowing the detection of boundaries even within the human body. Practical applications of ultrasound to technological or medical problems, however, were still comparatively few, and no ultrasound reflectoscope had yet been built on either side of the Atlantic. The reason for this was mainly that the development of the electronics necessary for such an instrument had not been carried forward far enough.

The Second World War provided an immense stimulus to the development of electronics and electronic instrumentation for use in many fields. Radar techniques, especially, required advanced pulse techniques and the measurement of very short transit times. As a result of this, the oscilloscope was developed from being an apparatus for the demonstration of the properties of an electronic beam into the most important and versatile instrument for the measurement of short electric events. The abundant use of sonar for the detection of submarines also increased our knowledge of the technology of ultrasonic transducers. Because of these advances it was quite logical that in 1945 Firestone in the USA, and shortly after that Sproule in England, could develop the first flaw-detector for non-destructive testing of materials. In this reflectoscope they made use of the electronic art evolved during the war years mainly for radar equipment. In fact, 2 years earlier Dussik in Austria had tried to map the liquid-filled ventricles in the brain but failed in his effort, presumably for lack of adequate instrumentation.

From this survey it is clear that the necessary engineering prerequisites for the application of the echo principle in medicine existed shortly after 1945, and it is not surprising that this opportunity was grasped by several medical groups in the USA. Thus about 1950 Wild and Reid, Howry, Bliss and Holmes and others applied the ultrasound reflectoscope to medical diagnosis. Using 'sophisticated' apparatus, they tried to visualize cross-sections of different parts of the human body showing inner structures, such as cancer of the breast, muscles, blood vessels and inner organs which could not easily be depicted by X-rays. In Europe, too, experiments were made on applying ultrasound to medical diagnosis by several groups such as Dussik in 1948 and Keidel in 1950. However, since they did not have access to the advanced reflectoscope techniques existing in America, no practical results were obtained.

Now let us turn our attention for a moment to Lund in Sweden, where Dr Inge Edler at the University Hospital was responsible for diagnosis preceding cardiac surgery. Quite accidentally Hertz, the Harvey of the cardiac ultrasound world, met Dr Edler in 1953 and in the course of their discussion the latter expressed his deep concern about the delicate task of making the right diagnosis in mitral valve diseases before major cardiac operations. He therefore asked Hertz if something like radar could not be used to help him in this decision. Luckily, at that time (and I quote Hertz):

> I knew that the first ultrasonic reflectoscope for flaw detection had been delivered to the Tekniska Röntegencentralen, a company in Malmö which was responsible for the non-destructive material testing at the large shipyards in that city. After consulting my medical student friends

about the position of the heart, I went to Malmö to see if any echoes could be obtained from my heart with that equipment. Because of the positive result of that experiment Dr Edler and I contacted the company who kindly agreed to let us have the reflectoscope for a weekend in the hospital in Lund. An intensive study during those two days convinced us that the ultrasonic reflectoscope method could become a valuable tool for heart diagnosis and we decided to carry out further studies[1]. However, at that time neither Dr Edler nor I had such an academic status that we were able to raise the necessary funds to acquire a reflectoscope. Thanks to certain connections in Germany I managed to persuade Mr R. Gellinek, vice-president of the medical branch of the Siemens Company, to send us a reflectoscope as a loan for one year for our experiments.

And so the technique for cardiac ultrasound was really introduced in Sweden by Edler and Hertz in the early 1950s and its rapid clinical application since remains a striking example of productive interaction between cardiologists, physicists and industry today[2].

The method, however, did not immediately find widespread acceptance by cardiologists. Reasons for this were mainly technical, especially the insensitivity of the transducers and the lack of appropriate recorders. I remember vividly while training at the cardiology division of the Thorndike Memorial Laboratory at the Boston City Hospital in 1957 that my chiefs Larry Ellis and Walter Abelmann laughed at me when I presented them with a research protocol aimed at reproducing in Boston the work of Edler and Hertz and of the German group in Aachen. In fact, they scoffed at the idea and told me rather to concentrate on the measurement of cardiac output in mitral stenosis.

I wonder what would have happened if I had persisted? There certainly were enough electronic firms on Route 128 and money seemed no object in those days. At any rate my curiosity made me return to the field when taking my post in Rotterdam in 1968 where I met Ir. Bom who has developed most of our instruments. The situation changed dramatically in the late 1960s when more sensitive instruments and, more importantly, strip-chart recorders became available while at the same time the physicians' attitudes had changed. These developments stimulated improvements in examination techniques and allowed a more accurate interpretation of the recordings and hence a more reliable diagnosis of a surprisingly wide variety of cardiac diseases. This resulted in an explosive interest in the method and the real acceptance of M-mode echocardiography as an effective technique for cardiac diagnosis. From Germany (Effert), England (Gibson), America (Feigenbaum, Henry, Popp) and many other centres a veritable deluge of papers, largely employing the M-mode display, filled the literature. Yet, the M-mode display proved unable to provide detailed information about spatial geometry. Indeed, the apparent lateral distances between the intracardiac structures often reflect the speed of transducer motion rather than true anatomical dimensions. In addition, the observed amplitude of motion is diminished by angular relationships and only the vectors of motion parallel to the sound beam are correctly displayed. It took a number of years, however, before investigators allowed for these limitations. In an attempt to solve some of the problems, imaging systems yielding a correct anatomical representation of an entire cardiac cross-section were developed.

REAL-TIME IMAGING SYSTEMS

The first ultra-sonotomograph was described by Ebina et al. in 1967[3] and used a waterbath B-scanner and (by rapidly angling the transducer), produced real-time images, in addition to compound B-scan images. A cinematographic technique, described in 1967 by Äsberg[4], with a reciprocating mirror system containing two reflectors and two transducers, provided cross-sectional images at a rate of seven frames per second. About the same time, Flaherty et al.[5] developed an ultrasonic scanner which worked in conjunction with a fluoroscopic image to locate both the ultrasonic transducer and the cross-section being explored. With this instrument, sectors from 10 to 30 degrees at rates up to 40 frames per second could be obtained. Patzold et al.[6] used a rotating sound source around the focal lines of a cylindrical parabolic mirror so that the sound beam would make rectangular scan (Vidoson system).

Images at a speed of 15 per second were obtained. Hertz and Lindstrom[7] also employed a waterbath contact for their scanner. Fast sweeping of the sound beam across a cardiac cross-section resulted in images at a speed of 16 frames per second. Eggleton et al.[8,9] originally devised a catheter with four small transducers at its tip for intraoesophageal and later, precordial examination of the heart. Their experience obtained with these techniques finally resulted in the design of a mechanical hand-held sector scanner[10]. The practical clinical use of the earlier mechanical sector scanners was limited by difficulties resulting from their complexity for routine application (large size transducers, waterbath contact) and technical problems (gear wear, limited scanning rates). Most of these problems are partially overcome with a recently introduced ultrasonocardiotomograph and the hand-held mechanical sector scanners[11,12].

Meanwhile, at the Thoraxcenter in Rotterdam, Bom et al.[13,14] developed the multi-element linear array scanner (Figures 1 and 2) and Roelandt et al. published clinical results with this instrument in 1973[15,16]. This approach undoubtedly stimulated much of the subsequent interest in dynamic cardiac imaging. Similar approaches for cardiac imaging have been used since, by other investigators[17,18].

ADVANTAGES OF REAL-TIME CARDIAC IMAGING

Real-time cardiac imaging provides both the pictorial image and a record of the motion of each echo signal. This allows identification of cardiac structures from their specific motion patterns, which proved particularly helpful when studying unfamiliar cross-sections. Cross-sectional cardiac images look more familiar to the cardiologist than M-mode echocardiograms. In addition, real-time images yield an immediate visual feedback which allows the examiner to change gain setting controls and adjust the transducer until the image quality is optimized.

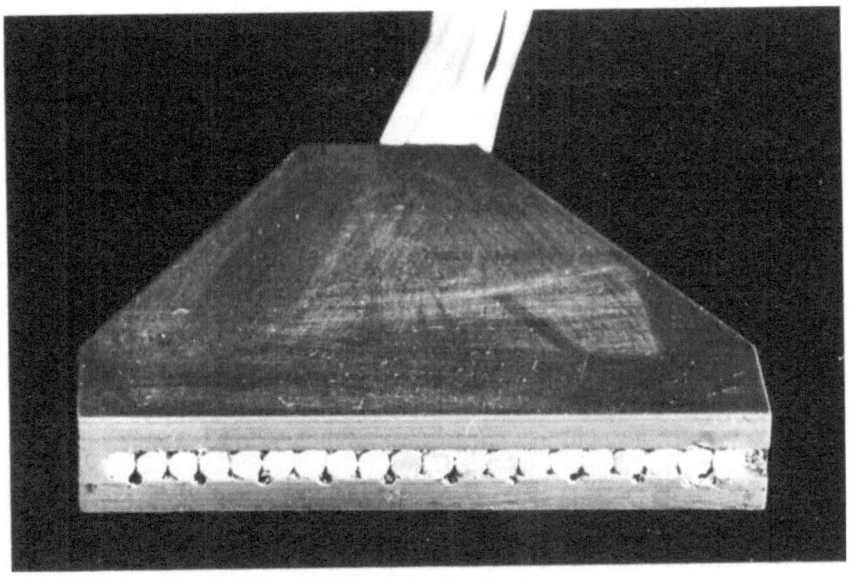

Figure 1   One of the first linear array transducers used in cardiology

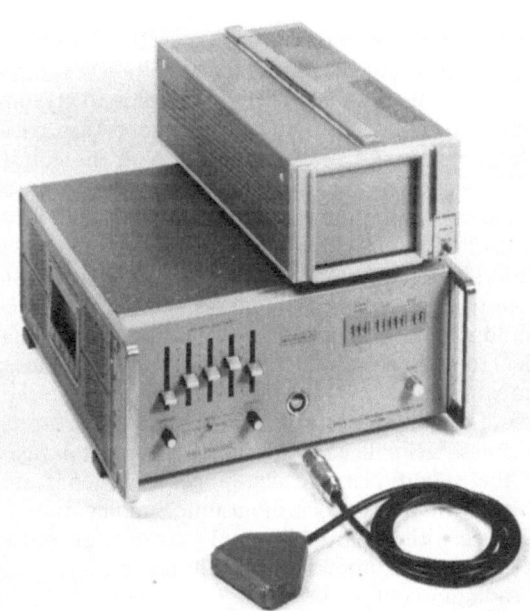

Figure 2   Prototype of the first available multiscan system

The technique considerably shortens the duration of the examination period when compared to B-scanning and M-mode echocardiography. For these methods the exact location of the cardiac scanning plane remains the most time-consuming part of the examination and is one of the major hurdles. Another advantage of real-time imaging, particularly when rectangular images are available, is its direct compatibility with video systems which have the advantage of image storage, immediate playback and low cost.

CLINICAL USEFULNESS OF REAL-TIME IMAGING

Two-dimensional real-time imaging provides a considerable amount of information for motion analysis of cardiac valves since the whole valve is visualized at the same time and perpendicular motion is also recorded. As a result, the dynamic events of the mitral valve, for example, can be demonstrated over its whole length rather than a limited area at a time. Real-time images give direct qualitative information about the thickness and mobility of the valve in rheumatic aortic and mitral stenosis. The mitral valve orifice area has been calculated from transverse cross-sectional images in mitral valve stenosis with the use of both electronic and mechanical sector scanners, and the method found to be highly accurate even in the presence of mitral regurgitation[19]. In mitral valve prolapse syndrome, the flailing exaggerated motion of the anterior mitral valve is strikingly demonstrated on real-time cross-sectional images. Arching of the leaflets into the left atrium has only been reliably demonstrated in patients with symptomatic mitral valve prolapse syndrome.

In a recent study with a phased array sector scanner, Gilbert et al.[20] in fact suggested that the cross-sectional ultrasonic method could be more sensitive than angiocardiography in detecting mild mitral valve prolapse.

Sahn et al.[21] have used the output of individual crystals of the multi-crystal transducer array to help elucidate some of the confusing M-mode patterns which are commonly seen in patients with the mitral valve prolapse syndrome. Cross-sectional imaging was also used to assess intracardiac morphological abnormalities as their size, shape and location are more readily appreciated with this technique than from M-mode echocardiograms. This is particularly useful for the demonstration of vegetations on cardiac valves[22] and intracardiac masses (Figure 3). Direct visualization of the tumour mass and its relationships allows its diagnosis and makes its location and size easier to appreciate than with M-mode echocardiography. An intracardiac moving mass can be followed throughout the cardiac cycle, whereas it may disappear during some period of the cardiac cycle on the M-mode recordings[23]. Smaller tumours with a long stalk may intermittently pass through the sound beam which appears as confusing 'echo burst' patterns on the M-mode echocardiogram. Smaller tumours are usually difficult to visualize with angiocardiography as they do not leave a negative shadow in the contrast medium. The capabilities of diagnostic ultrasound for studying the right and left ventricles are extended by a real-time cross-sectional imaging system. The cardiac walls are visualized in their correct spatial relationships at any specific moment within the cardiac cycle in the

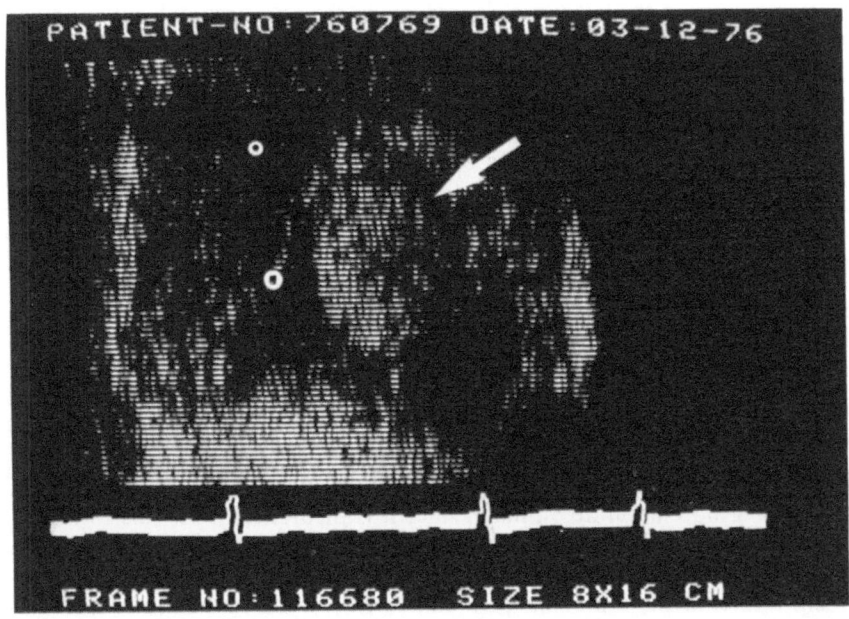

Figure 3 Transverse cardiac cross-section showing the huge mass (see arrow) appearing in the left ventricular cavity

ultrasonic plane. This allows one to obtain information about ventricular size, shape and, to some extent, of wall dynamics and hence from both a qualitative appreciation of left ventricular function.

A unique advantage of ultrasonic cross-sectional imaging over X-ray techniques is that one can study sections of the ventricles which are perpendicular to the left ventricle long axis. Large areas of the left ventricle become accessible for study. This possibility has helped in the understanding of motion patterns of the interventricular septum in normal and volume-overloaded right ventricles[24]. It also makes the method attractive for the study of patients in whom left ventricular shape abnormalities are present or likely to be present, such as in mitral stenosis, dilated and hypertrophic cardiomyopathy, congenital heart disease and coronary artery disease[25]. The method allows for a more accurate study of the left ventricular areas between the papillary muscles and the apex, since it avoids the deformation of the spatial relationships and the reduced motion amplitudes on M-mode recordings as a result of reduced beam angulation. Here the electronic sector scanner placed over the apex of the left ventricle and viewing cranially has come into its own. The versatility in angulation makes these sector scanners particularly useful for the study of these left ventricular areas. It must be pointed out, however, that the interpretation of the images at present remains subjective and must only be attempted by experienced investigators. Qualitative assessment of size and shape of the ventricles is usually not a major problem, but analysis of normal and abnormal wall motion is fraught with several potential pitfalls.

Some parts of the left ventricle, especially the apex, are difficult to image at all and the endocardium may not be visualized as it is a rather poor reflector over most of the areas of the left ventricular cavity in about one-half of the patients studied. Furthermore, with a fixed transducer position, the cardiac cross-section studied moves in and out of the explored ultrasonic cross-section during the cardiac cycle and evaluation of the same cardiac section is not always possible. This limits the analysis of wall motion for a specific area of the left ventricle. Even so, remarkable visualization of early cardiac dysfunction after myocardial ischaemia has been achieved[26].

SOME LIMITATIONS TO CROSS-SECTIONAL CARDIAC IMAGING

Since the major limitation of M-mode echocardiography in the assessment of left ventricular volumes is that only a one-dimensional cavity view is obtained, long axis cross-sectional images of the left ventricular cavity seemed to allow a more accurate estimate, since it is theoretically possible to obtain a measurement of both the long axis and surface area of the left ventricle which allows correction for variations in left ventricle geometry. This would seem to permit the use of the formulae largely tested in quantitative single-plane angiocardiography. The results, using this approach with the earlier imaging systems, although initially promising were not found to be reproducible[27,28].

These studies will certainly be repeated with the newer instruments which have better resolution and more appropriate display facilities for data processing. The most common cause of failure to obtain adequate cross-sectional images is the small ultrasonic 'window' which is present in many patients with obstructive airway disease or anterior chest wall deformity. Intervening dense tissues such as calcified ribs may obscure strips of the image, especially in the older age group. However, considerable detail may still be visible between the obscured areas, similar to looking at a chest X-ray or a landscape through venetian blinds. Differences in ultrasound transmission between cartilaginous rib tissue and the other chest wall tissues never cause appreciable distortions on the images. Surprisingly, it is uncommon to have incomplete images of cardiac structures at greater depth as a result of a large anteroposterior chest diameter. Only the left atrial posterior wall in patients with giant left atrium in mitral stenosis, and the posterior pericardium in patients with large pericardial effusion, may occasionally be beyond the 16 cm viewing depth. The size of the transducer and the fixed position of the crystals limits the possibility of directing the sound beam through different structures simultaneously. In particular, the interventricular septum and the posterior wall are not always favourably aligned to the sound beams in the ultrasonic cross-section. This results in dropouts of parts of these structures on the display.

Furthermore, the larger viewing area with the multiscan, accentuates this problem in comparison to the sector scanners where this problem is less apparent since a smaller area is visualized at a time. Proper angulation of the transducer to visualize cardiac areas that are eccentrically located in relation

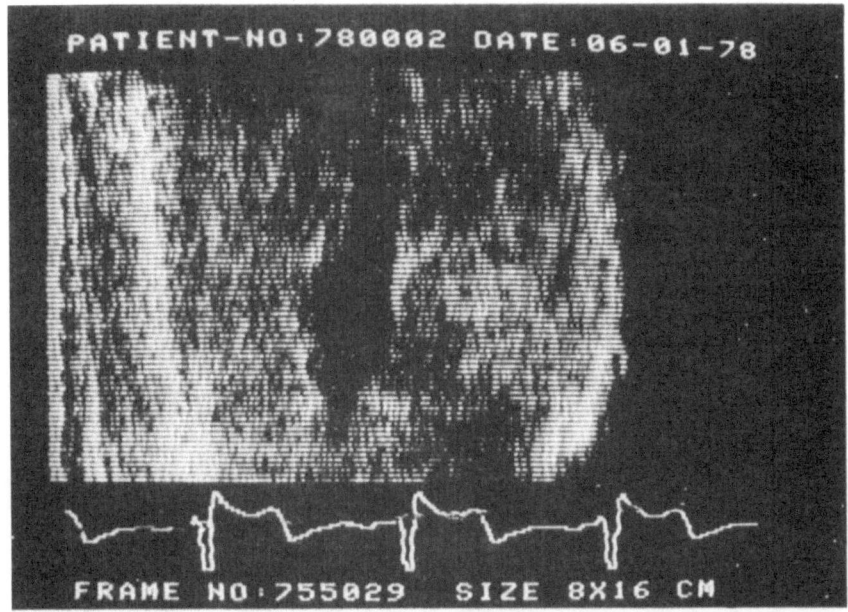

Figure 4 Diastolic transverse cross-section of a hypertrophic heart

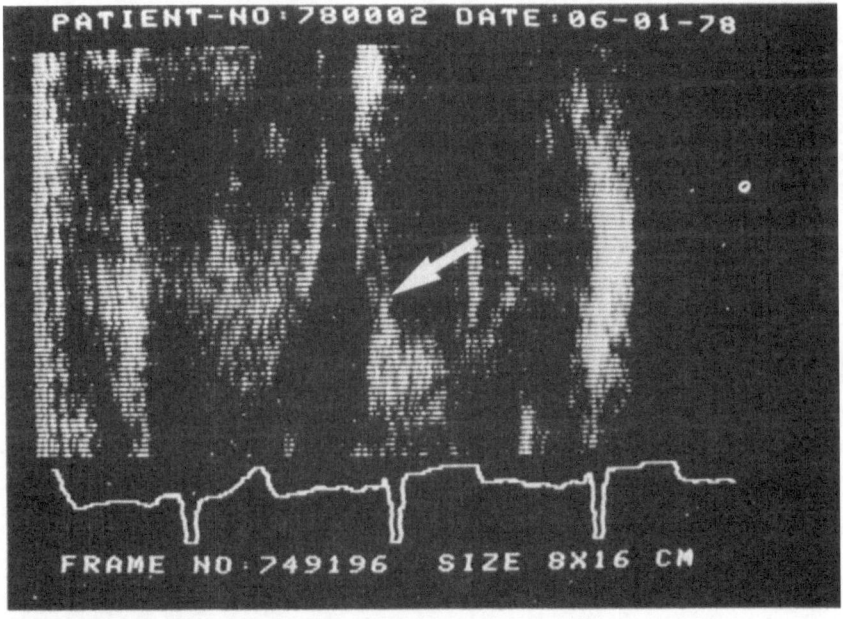

Figure 5 Diastolic longitudinal cross-section in the same patient as in Figure 4. Note the thick septum; the perpendicular cross-section shown in Figure 4 was obtained at a level below the anterior mitral leaflet (see arrow)

23

to the acoustic window, such as the apex of the left ventricle, may pose a problem. The most serious limitation of the presently used cross-sectional imaging systems is their limited lateral resolution caused by the finite width of the sound beam which may result in non-structural or spurious echoes on the display, and distortion of structures and cavities. The resulting problems for clinical interpretation are extensively discussed elsewhere[29]. The published instrument resolutions in the literature are difficult to compare because there is usually no indication of how, at what distance and in what direction beam-width measurements were made. The experienced echocardiographer, however, often makes a fairly reliable estimation of the resolving power of a particular instrument by viewing clinical results. The best acoustic resolution presently available for cross-sectional imaging is probably obtained with the dynamically focused multiscan system[30]* as is evident from the movie film, out of which illustrations are taken (Figures 4, 5 and 6).

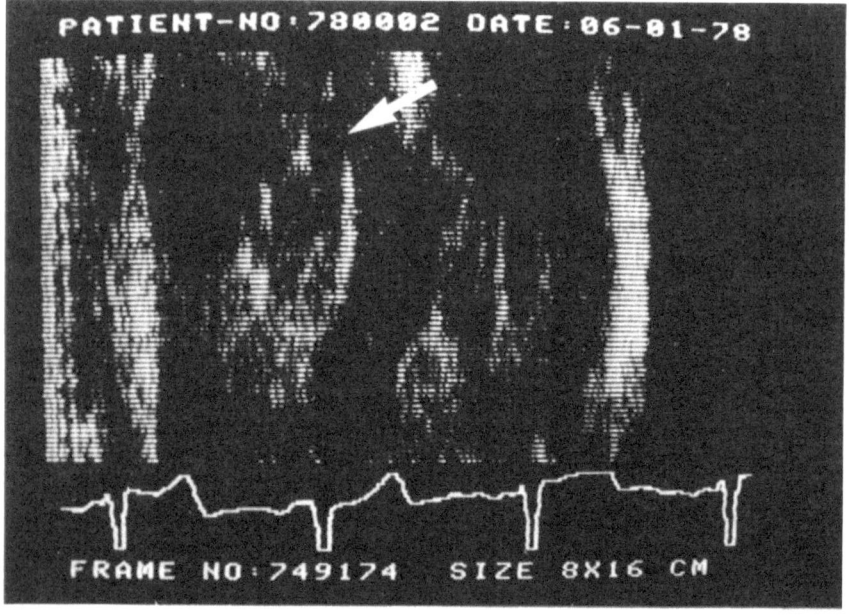

Figure 6 A systolic longitudinal frame shows clearly the obstruction (see arrow) in the left ventricular outflow area which is caused by the thick septum

ANALYSIS OF REAL-TIME CROSS-SECTIONAL IMAGES

A significant problem for real-time two-dimensional imaging analysis results from the enormous amount of data that becomes available per unit of time. It is clear that, compared to each moment when a complete cardiac cross-section is visualized at a frame speed of 100–150 per second, the information

* The images were obtained with the Fociscan from Organon Teknika.

obtained by the M-mode display is scanty. Adding the dimension of time allows one to accurately track the motion pattern of the structures in a single sound beam pathway but results in further increases in data and hence difficulties for analysis. To cope with this problem, the digital processor proved useful since the moving image can be directly recorded on video tape and analysed later at actual speed, slow motion or still frame. Photographs can then be made from a slave TV monitor display for documentation purposes.

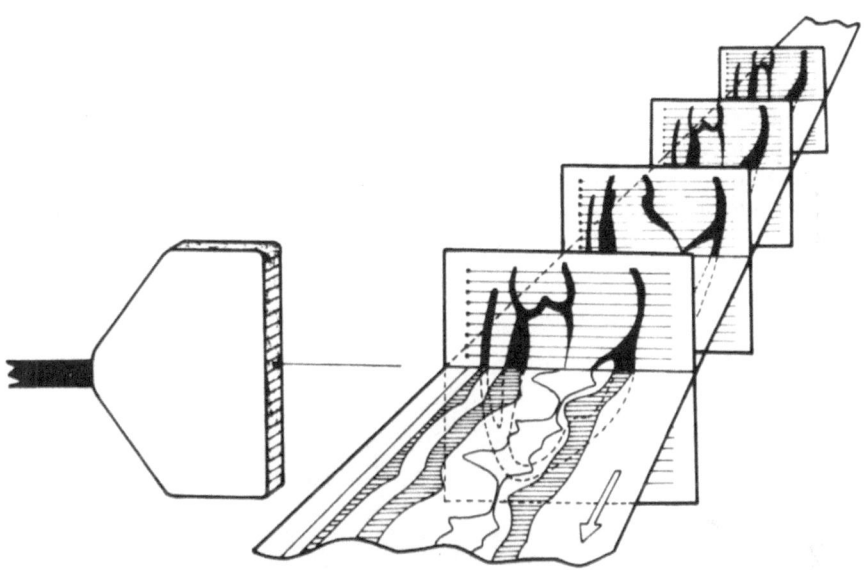

Figure 7 This figure indicates the principle where each line from a linear array transducer may yield the well-known M-mode

An additional facility allows one to select any individual element or two elements simultaneously (i.e. dual M-mode) and to record the basic echo data, being in the B-mode on the images in the M-mode (Figure 7). The principle is exactly the same as recently used in quantitative angiocardiography where analysis of video lines is used rather than the complete images to track motion patterns of specific parts of the left ventricular walls. The additional advantage of this approach is that the sound beam pathway through the cardiac structures is easily identified.

FUTURE DEVELOPMENTS

There are two major directions discernible for the next 5 years:

1. Increased use of digital processing techniques both for data acquisition and for data display and interpretation. Quantitative information will

become available for cardiac dimensions, in cardiovascular monitoring and in a host of related fields such as Doppler flow measurements. Combinations with pressure measurements will make further inroads on cardiac catheterization techniques. All of these require immediate data processing, which the current generation of microprocessors make economically feasible.

2. Increased technical sophistication in the sense of better transducers and electronic miniaturization. The former, perhaps in combination with contrast agents, will lead to actual tissue recognition, i.e. the differences between healthy and ischaemic cardiac tissue while the latter will bring us small portable devices. One of these is developed at our laboratory[31,32]. Properly it should be called the 'ultrasonic stethoscope' or perhaps just stethoscope since, unlike the current stethoscope, the ultrasonic one actually can look inside. The device employs (Figure 8) a linear array of twenty transducers and has a frame rate of 25 per second. The display screen on the device as well as the electronics are powered by a battery. Preliminary experience has shown its usefulness on ward rounds, as a teaching device, and as a complement to cardiac auscultation. Other organs such as the uterus, liver and kidney, are readily visualized as well.

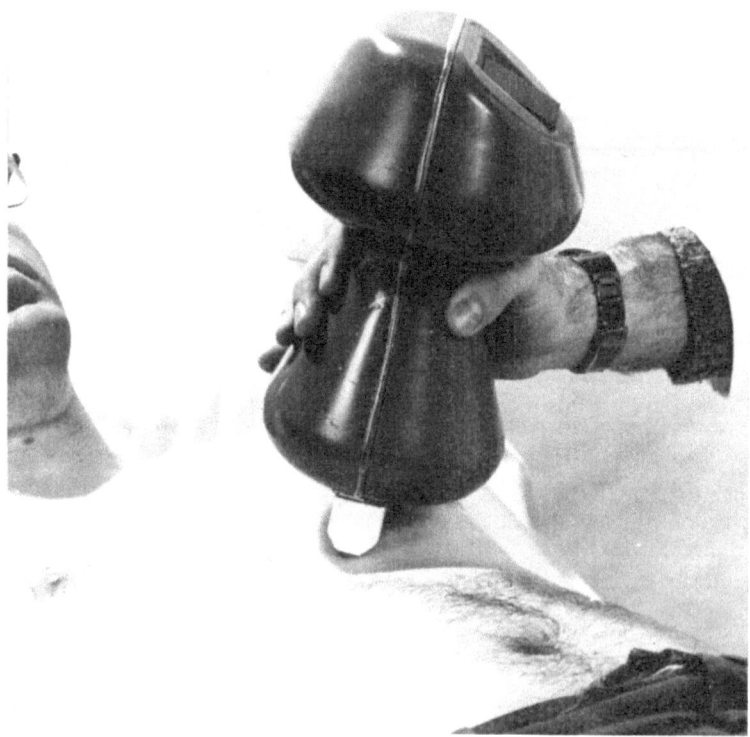

Figure 8 The minivisor; a new, miniaturized, hand-held real-time imager

CONCLUSION

Real-time cross-sectional imaging will probably become the principal method for imaging intracardiac anatomy and its abnormalities. As the M-mode is better able to demonstrate certain functional abnormalities, the methods may be used to advantage in combination. Further developments in miniaturization will give increased accuracy and versatility. Harvey would have enjoyed working with these tools since they permit on-line visualization of cardiac motion without any damage to the tissues.

References

1. Edler, I. and Hertz, C. H., (1954) Use of ultrasonic reflectoscope for continuous recording of movements of heart walls. *Kungl. Fysiogr. Sällsk. Forhandl.* (Lund), **24**, 5
2. Hertz, C. H. (1973). The interaction of physicians, physicists and industry in the development of echocardiography. *Ultrasound Med. Biol.*, **1**, 3
3. Ebina, T., Oka, S. and Tanaka, M. (1967). The ultrasono-tomography of the heart and great vessels in living human subjects by means of the ultrasonic reflection technique. *Jap. Heart J.*, **8**, 331
4. Äsberg, A. (1967). Ultrasonic cinematography of the living heart. *Ultrasonics*, **6**, 113
5. Flaherty, J. J., Clark, J. W. and Walgren, H. N. (1967). Simultaneous fluoroscopic and rapid scan ultrasonic imaging. *Dig. Int. Conf. Med. Biol. Engng.*, **7**, 221
6. Pätzold, J., Krause, W. and Kresse, H. (1970). Present state of an ultrasonic cross section procedure with rapid image rate. *IEEE Trans. Biomed. Engng. BME*, **17**, 263
7. Hertz, C. H. and Lindstrom, K. (1972). A fast ultrasonic scanning system for heart investigation. In *Proc. 3rd Int. Conf. Med. Physics (Gothenburg)*, **35**, 6
8. Eggleton, R. C., Townsend, C. and Herrick, J. (1970). Ultrasonic visualization of left ventricular dynamics. *IEEE Trans. Sonics and Ultrasonics*, SU-17
9. Eggleton, R. C. (1973). Ultrasonic visualization of the dynamic geometry of the heart. In: Proc. 2nd World Congr. Ultrasonics in Med., *Excerpta Medica*, **10**
10. Eggleton, R. C., Feigenbaum, H. and Johnston, K. W. (1975). Visualization of cardiac dynamics with real time B-mode ultrasonic scanner. In Dennis White (ed.). *Ultrasound in Medicine*, vol. 1, p. 385. (New York: Plenum Press)
11. Griffith, J. M. and Henry, W. L. (1974). A sector scanner for real time two-dimensional echocardiography. *Circulation*, **49**, 1147
12. Shaw, A., Paton, J. S., Gregory, N. L., *et al.* (1976). A real time two-dimensional ultrasonic scanner for clinical use. *Ultrasonics*, **14**, 35
13. Bom, N., Lancee, C. T. and Honkoop, J. (1971). Ultrasonic viewer for cross-sectional analysis of moving cardiac structures. *Bio-Med Engng.*, **6**, 500
14. Bom, N., Lancee, C. T. and van Zwieten, G. (1973). Multiscan echocardiography. I: Technical description. *Circulation*, **48**, 1066
15. Roelandt, J., Kloster, F. E. and ten Cate, F. J. (1973). Multiscan echocardiography; description of the system and initial results in 100 patients. *Heart Bull.* **4**, 51
16. Roelandt, J., Kloster, F. E. and ten Cate, F. J. (1974). Multi-dimensional echocardiography: an appraisal of its clinical usefulness. *Br. Heart J.*, **36**, 29

17. King, D. L. (1973). Real time cross-sectional ultrasonic imaging of the heart using a linear array multi-element transducer. *J. Clin. Ultrasound*, **3**, 196

18. Whittingham, T. A. (1976). A hand-held electronically switched array for rapid ultrasonic scanning. *Ultrasonics*, **14**

19. Henry, W. L., Griffith, J. M. and Michaelis, L. L. (1975). Measurement of mitral orifice area in patients with mitral valve disease by real time echocardiography. *Circulation*, **51**, 827

20. Gilbert, B. W., Schatz, R. A. and Von Ramm, O. T. (1976). Mitral valve prolapse: two-dimensional echocardiographic and angiographic correlation. *Circulation*, **54**, 716

21. Sahn, D. J., Allen, H. D. and Goldberg, S. J. (1976). Mitral valve prolapse in children. A problem defined by real time cross-sectional echocardiography. *Circulation*, **53**, 651

22. Gilbert, B. W., Haney, R. S. and Crawford F. (1977). Two-dimensional assessment of vegative endocarditis. *Circulation*, **55**, 346

23. Roelandt, J., Vletter, W. B. and Leuftink, E. W. (1977). Ultrasonic demonstration of right ventricular myxoma. *J. Clin. Ultrasound*, **5**

24. Weyman, A. E., Wann, S. and Feigenbaum, H. (1976). Mechanism of abnormal septal motion in patients with right ventricular volume overload: a cross-sectional echocardiographic study. *Circulation*, **54**, 179

25. Weyman, A. E., Peskoe, S. M. and Williams, E. S. (1976). Detection of left ventricular aneurysms by cross-sectional echocardiography. *Circulation*, **54**, 936

26. Meltzer, R. S., Woythaler, J. N. and Buda, A. J. (1978). Non-invasive quantification of infarct size by two-dimensional wide-angle echocardiography. (Personal communication)

27. Roelandt, J., ten Cate, F. J. and Van Dorp, W. G. (1974). Limitations of quantitative determination of left ventricular volume by multiscan echocardiography. *Circulation* (Suppl. iii), **50**, 28

28. Roelandt, J., Van Dorp, W. G. and Bom, N. (1976), Resolution problems in echocardiology: A source of interpretation errors. *Am. J. Cardiol.*, **37**, 256

29. Roelandt, J. (1977). *Practical Echocardiology* (1st edn.). (Forest Grove: Research Studies Press)

30. Ligtvoet, C. M., Ridder, J., Lancee, C. T., Hagemeijer, F., Vletter, W. B. and Gussenhoven, W. J. (1978). A dynamically focused multiscan system. In: N. Bom, (ed.). *Echocardiology* (The Hague: M. Nijhoff)

31. Ligtvoet, C. M., Rijsterborgh, F. R., Kappen, L. and Bom, N. (1978). Real time ultrasonic imaging with a hand-held scanner. Part I—Technical description. *Ultrasound in Med. and Biol.* (in press)

32. Roelandt, J., Wladimiroff, J. W. and Baars, A. M. (1978). Real time ultrasonic imaging with a hand-held scanner. Part II — Initial clinical experience. *Ultrasound in Med. and Biol.* (in press)

Part II
The myocardium – aspects of conduction

4
The initiation of the heartbeat and its control by autonomic transmitters

H. BROWN, D. NOBLE AND S. NOBLE

'The heart of an eel and of certain other fish and animals, being taken out of the body, beats without auricles. Furthermore, if you cut it in pieces, you will see the separate pieces each contract and relax, so that in them the very body of the heart beats and leaps after the auricles have ceased to move.' (W. Harvey, *De motu cordis*, ch. 4, trans. G. Whitteridge).

INTRODUCTION

Harvey would not have been the first to observe that the heart continues to beat when taken out of the body. That fact was known to the ancient Greeks, and it was explicitly noted by Leonardo da Vinci ('The heart moves by itself', see Bottazzi[1]).

However, Harvey may have been the first to think of cutting pacemaker tissue into small pieces and observing that each of the pieces continues to beat. His experiment was carried out on the pacemaking *ventricular* tissue of eels and certain fish, and he was well aware that he was dealing here with unusual pacemaker activity, for the passage quoted from *De motu cordis* refers to an exception to what he himself had shown was the normal state of affairs in which the auricular tissue is required to excite the ventricle. We must not therefore read too much into Harvey's interpretation of this particular experiment. His experiment does however establish that pacemaker activity originates in small pieces of cardiac tissue.

In the nineteenth century, Gaskell[2] used a similar approach involving dissection to establish the myogenic origin of the heartbeat. By then, the question whether nervous or muscular tissue was primary in generating pacemaker activity was a major one. In Harvey's time, however, it is unlikely that this question was even formulated. The relative 'primacy' of the heart and the blood was a live issue[3-5], but throughout *De motu cordis* the nervous system is hardly mentioned.

Since the introduction of microelectrode techniques, and more recently of voltage clamp techniques, it has been a major aim of cardiac electrophysiology to provide an ionic explanation for pacemaker activity and of its control by the autonomic nervous system.

POTASSIUM CURRENTS INVOLVED IN PACEMAKER ACTIVITY

In all the regions of the heart that show pacemaker activity it is found that its origin lies in an instability of the cell membrane potential. Before each contraction, the cardiac cell is excited by an action potential. In non-pace-making regions, the potential then simply returns to its resting (negative) level until the next excitation arrives. However, in pacemaker regions, the potential slowly declines during diastole until the threshold for action potential initiation is reached. This slow depolarization was first observed by Arvanitaki[6] and Bozler[7] using external electrodes. It is now called the pacemaker potential.

One of the first attempts to analyse the mechanism of the pacemaker potential was made by Weidmann in 1951[8]. He recorded the pacemaker potential in sheep Purkinje fibres using a microelectrode. At the same time he used a second intracellular microelectrode to inject small current pulses and so measure the membrane conductance. His result is shown in Figure 1.

The conductance was found to be relatively high at the beginning of the pacemaker potential and to fall progressively as the depolarization proceeds.

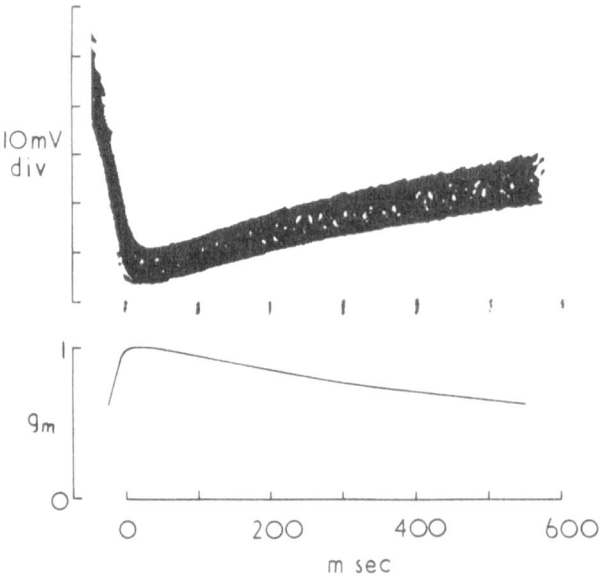

Figure 1 Variation of membrane conductance, g_m, during small current pulses applied repetitively during the pacemaker potential in cardiac Purkinje fibres. *Top:* voltage deflections. A series of pacemaker potentials have been superimposed to produce a 'band' of voltage deflections whose width is dependent on the membrane resistance. *Bottom:* calculated variation of g_m during pacemaker depolarization (based on Weidmann[8])

This result is consistent with the view that the membrane permeability falls during the pacemaker potential. One obvious possibility is that the potassium permeability is involved. If this permeability were high at the end of the action potential it would drive the membrane potential in a negative direction as positive potassium ions leave the cell. As the permeability declines, this hyperpolarizing effect would become weaker, and the cell might then depolarize as positive charge is transferred back into the cell, either by sodium or calcium ions.

However, Weidmann's experiment, though highly suggestive, is not uniquely explained by this hypothesis. The change in membrane conductance measured by this technique bears a fairly complex relation to the individual ionic membrane conductances and to the way in which they change with potential (Noble and Tsien[9], p. 136). Moreover, it is not possible to distinguish changes in permeability that are primarily *responsible* for the depolarization from changes that are secondarily *produced* by the depolarization: a decrease in potassium conductance is in fact produced by depolarization[10]. Furthermore, some theories of the pacemaker potential suggest that such secondary changes (including also increases in sodium or calcium conductance) may in turn enhance the depolarization. It is impossible to 'dissect' the contributions of the various changes in ionic permeability without controlling the variable that is involved in mediating such self-reinforcing cycles, i.e. the membrane potential itself. It is the purpose of 'voltage clamp' techniques to introduce this control. Indeed, they might equally well be called 'voltage control' techniques.

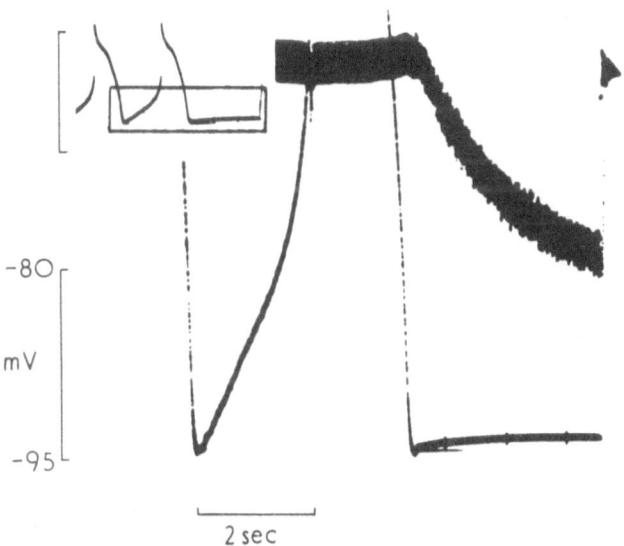

-80

mV

-95

2 sec

Figure 2 Change in membrane current with time on holding potential constant at its maximum diastolic level. *Left:* pacemaker potential before voltage clamping. *Right:* voltage clamp applied at beginning of pacemaker potential. Outward current is represented as an upward deflection (Vassalle[16])

33

Deck et al.[11] first introduced the voltage clamp technique in cardiac physiology using microelectrodes in Purkinje fibres. Rougier et al.[12] and Brown and Noble[13] started the use of sucrose gap methods that enabled voltage control to be achieved where the use of microelectrodes was difficult or impossible. Morad and Trautwein[14] and Beeler and Reuter[15] first used hybrid techniques using sucrose gaps and microelectrodes.

One of the first important applications of voltage clamping to the study of the pacemaker depolarization was made by Vassalle in 1966[16] (see Figure 2). He controlled the membrane potential at the beginning of the pacemaker potential in a Purkinje fibre. The net membrane current required to prevent the pacemaker depolarization was found to change exponentially with time. It slowly became more inward. This experiment was important in showing that, even when the membrane potential is controlled, the membrane current changes spontaneously in the direction required to depolarize the cell. Thus, not all the changes in permeability during the pacemaker potential are secondary consequences of the potential change itself. Are they then independent of the membrane potential? Perhaps the oscillation in membrane potential is a secondary consequence of some intracellular oscillatory mechanism. Indeed, it has recently been found that the oscillatory activity induced by toxic levels of cardiac glycosides may be of this kind, part of the experimental evidence being that oscillations of membrane current continue to occur during voltage clamp conditions[17]. In the case of the normal pacemaker mechanism, no such oscillations occur. On applying the voltage clamp the current simply changes monotonically to a steady level, determined by the potential applied.

Figure 3A shows the results of an experiment similar in concept to Vassalle's

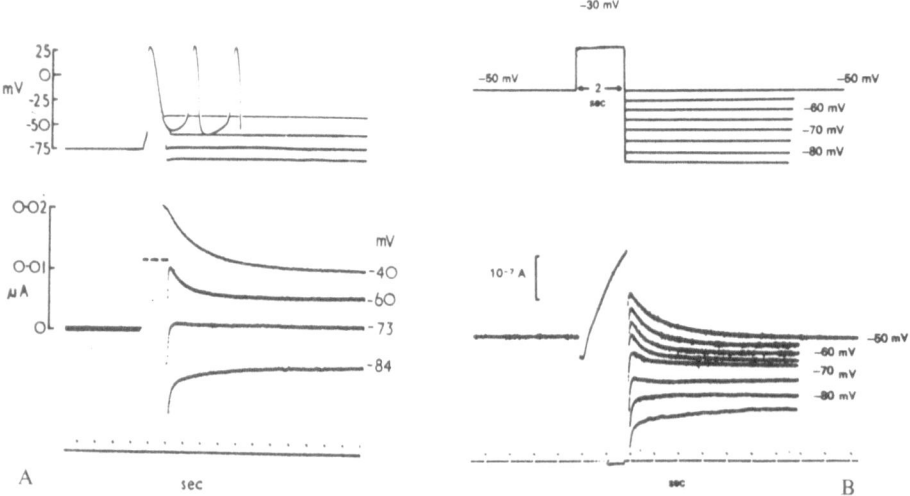

Figure 3 A: a series of voltage clamps applied at various levels during induced pacemaker activity in frog atrial muscle. *Top:* voltage records. *Bottom:* current records. Note that current change reverses sign at -73 mV[61]. B: series of current records obtained following repolarization to various potentials in frog sinus venosus. A 2 s depolarization to -30 mV was used to activate the current. Current reverses sign at about -75 mV[37,38]

but performed on frog atrial tissue. A controlled potential was maintained at various levels following the first of a series of repetitive action potentials. For potentials positive to -73 mV, as in Vassalle's result, the current changes slowly in an inward (downward) direction. Figure 3B shows the result of an experiment on the frog sinus venosus in which a voltage step (from -50 to -30 mV for 2 s) was used in place of an action potential. Both of these sets of records illustrates another important feature of the slow current changes involved: they reverse direction at a fairly negative level of membrane potential. Moreover, this level of potential varies with the extracellular potassium concentration in the manner expected of a potassium current (Purkinje fibres: Noble and Tsien[18], Peper and Trautwein[19], SA node: Noma and Irisawa[20, 21]). We may therefore conclude that the decay of a potassium current underlies at least part of the pacemaker depolarization.

But what process activates this current? Hall, Hutter and Noble[10] first described slow conductance changes that they attributed to activation of a potassium current by membrane depolarization in Purkinje fibres. This result was confirmed by McAllister and Noble[22] using the voltage clamp technique, and a full kinetic analysis was performed by Noble and Tsien[18]. This work has shown that the potassium conductance mechanism involved resembles that described by Hodgkin and Huxley[23] in nerve fibres, except that the speed of activation and the absolute magnitude of membrane current are much smaller.

Figure 4 summarizes the kinetics of the potassium current, i_{K2}, involved in controlling Purkinje fibre pacemaker activity. A threshold potential for activating the current exists at about -90 mV and the system is fully activated by about -60 mV. It was originally thought that this current was the only potassium current in the Purkinje fibre with voltage and time-dependence of the Hodgkin–Huxley type. It is now known that the overall picture is more complex (see discussion in Noble and Tsien[24], and, for a mathematical summary of the currents in Purkinje fibres, see McAllister et al.[25]). Other potassium currents (usually called i_x) are activated at a more positive range of potentials in Purkinje fibres. Moreover, it is now clear that the time-dependent potassium currents observed in atrial muscle[13, 26–30]; and in ventricular muscle[31, 32]; bear a closer resemblance to i_x in Purkinje fibres than to i_{K2}. This fact is of some importance in studying the actions of autonomic transmitters, as we shall see later in this chapter.

INWARD CURRENTS INVOLVED IN PACEMAKER ACTIVITY

The decay of potassium conductance simply reduces the rate at which positive charge leaves the cell. In order to depolarize, positive charge must actually enter the cell (or negative charge leave it). Pacemaker activity can be modulated by changes in anions in the bathing fluid[33] but it continues even in the presence of impermeable anions. We may therefore be sure that some cations enter the cell during the pacemaker depolarization. The obvious candidates are sodium and calcium, the free concentrations of which are much larger outside the cell than inside it. Three inward current mechanisms have been described as being involved in pacemaker depolarization.

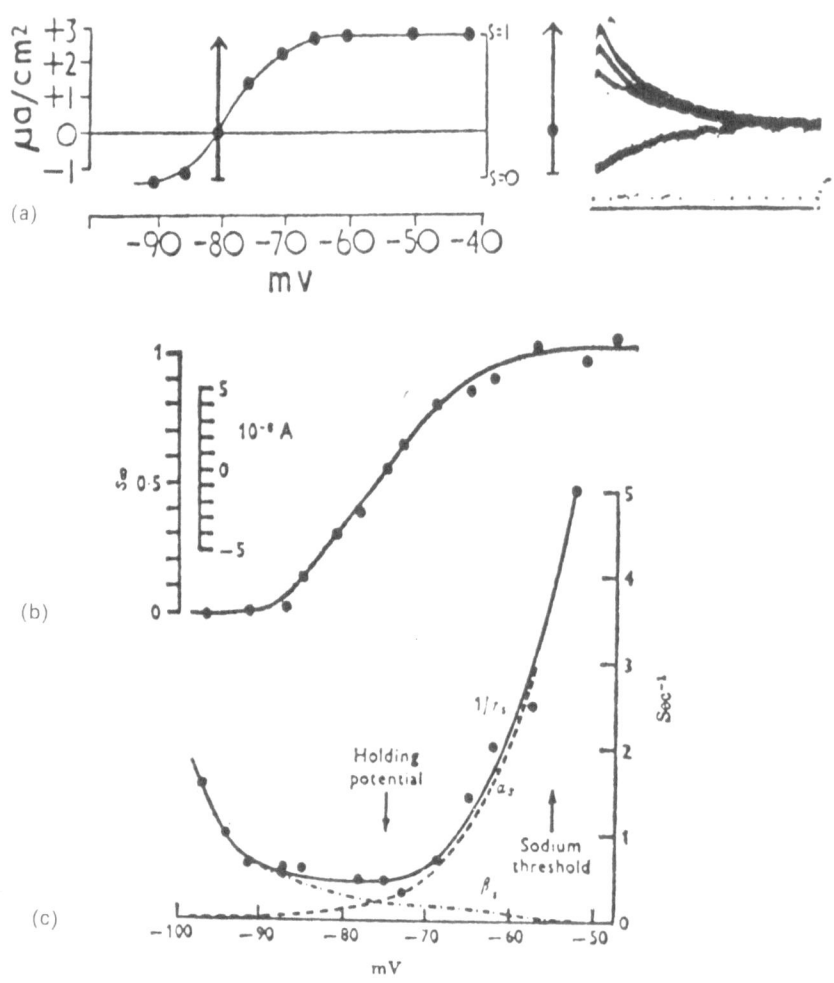

Figure 4 Kinetics of pacemaker potassium current i_{K2} in sheep Purkinje fibres. (*a*) Illustration of the way in which the steady state activation curve, s_∞, is obtained from the amplitudes of recovery tails (points 1–4). (*b*) Activation curve obtained by same technique in another preparation. (*c*) Rate coefficients of activation, a_s, and deactivation, β_s, as functions of membrane potential obtained from same fibre as (*b*)[18]

First, it is known that even at very negative potentials (at which we may suppose that conductances of the Hodgkin–Huxley type are not activated) some leak of charge into the cell occurs. This is called the inward background current since it is always present. This current is presumed to be carried by the resting flux of sodium ions. Replacement of sodium by choline does not usually cause substantial hyperpolarization, but it is known that the cardiac cell membrane is permeable to choline[34]. The inward background current may therefore be fairly non-selective. It is even conceivable that it may represent a 'leak' of other cations through the channels carrying the potassium background current, i_{K1} (see Noble[35], chap. 9 for a further discussion of the nomenclature and functions of background currents). In Noble and Tsien's original analysis of the Purkinje fibre pacemaker potential[18] it was proposed that the inward background current, assisted by the time- and voltage-dependent falls in potassium permeability, was sufficient to account for pacemaker activity.

It is now clear that the analysis was too simple. To account for some of the properties of the pacemaker potential in this tissue it is necessary to suppose that some small degree of activation of the Hodgkin–Huxley sodium conductance occurs during the last third or so of the depolarization[25]. The transition to the fast upstroke of the action potential is then a matter of degree, and the pacemaker depolarization can be viewed as composed of two not very distinct phases: an early phase primarily controlled by the time-dependent decay of i_{K2} and by the inward background current, and a later phase involving activation of g_{Na} and the voltage-dependent fall in i_{K2}. At very low frequencies it is even possible for the phases to become more distinct. The pacemaker depolarization then shows an inflection characteristic of Purkinje pacemaker activity.

When all these factors are taken into account it is possible to reproduce the properties of the Purkinje pacemaker quite accurately. Figure 5 shows

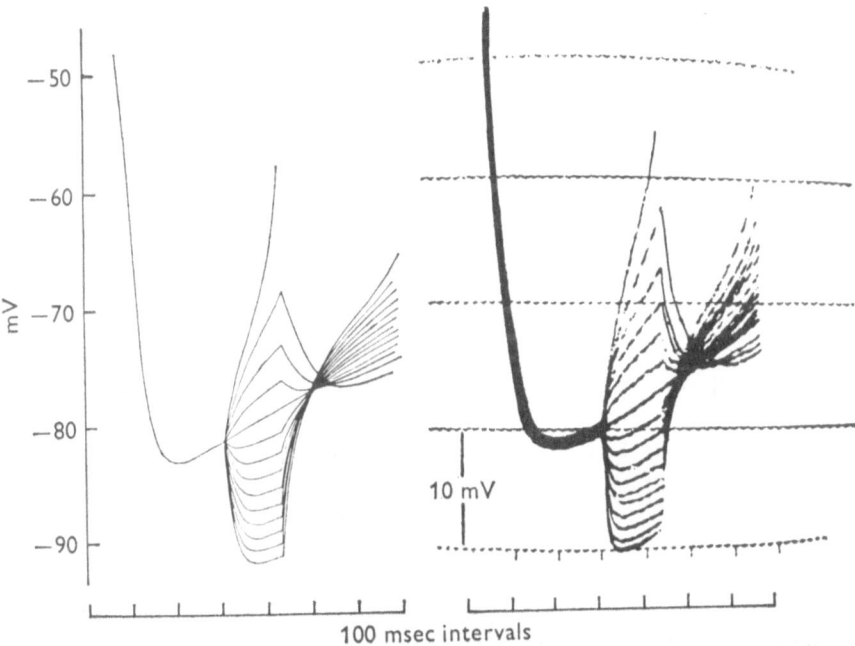

Figure 5 Comparison between the behaviour of a model of pacemaker activity[25] and the influence of small depolarizing and hyperpolarizing current pulses on the Purkinje fibre pacemaker potential[8]. *Left:* computed responses. *Right:* experimental responses. In each case depolarizing pulses are followed by a slowing of pacemaker depolarization due to reactivation of i_{K2} whereas hyperpolarizing pulses are followed by an acceleration due to faster deactivation of i_{K2}. The computations were done by O. Hauswirth

how successfully the model described by McAllister, Noble and Tsien[25] reproduces the responses to short current pulses obtained by Weidmann[8]. One of the important aspects of recent work on pacemaker activity is that the Purkinje fibre has been found to have some important limitations as a model for pacemaker activity in atrial and sinus tissue. We shall discuss the comparison in relation to control by the sympathetic nervous system later. First it is important to note a very important difference in the role played by voltage- and time-dependent inward current. It is well known that sinus pacemaker activity is insensitive to the sodium current blocker, tetrodo-toxin[36-38]. The rapidly activated sodium conductance cannot, therefore, be involved in the way it is in Purkinje fibres. This is not an unexpected result. The pacemaker potential in Purkinje fibres takes place at a very negative

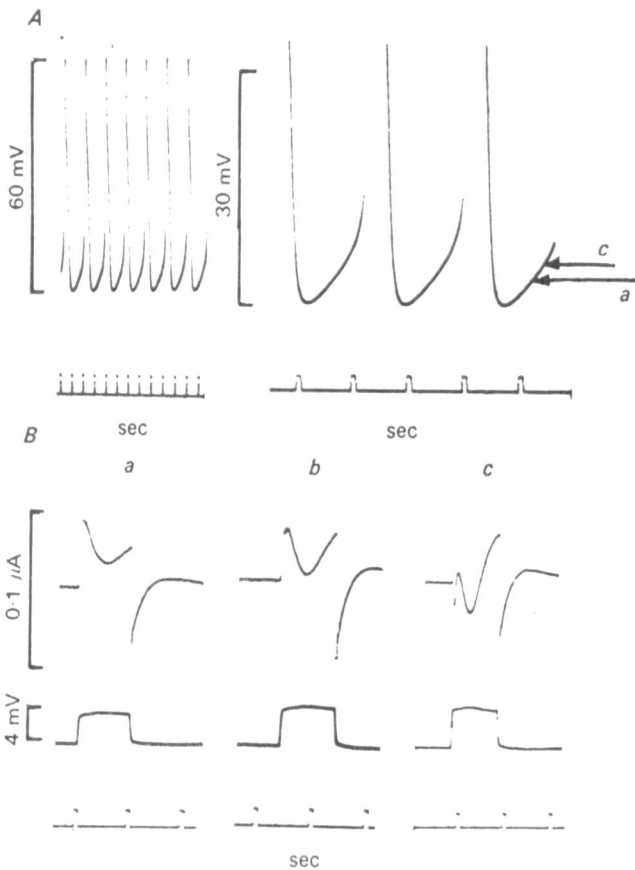

Figure 6 *A*, spontaneous activity of a frog sinus preparation in TTX-Ringer solution. *Left:* lower gain record. *Right:* higher gain record to show the pacemaker depolarization in more detail. Levels to which voltage clamp pulses *a* and *c below* depolarized the membrane are marked against the pacemaker potential. *B*, the preparation was then clamped at the maximum diastolic potential and depolarizing pulses of +4, +5 and +6 mV applied (*a*, *b* and *c*). The corresponding current records are shown above each voltage pulse and show the onset of slow inward current[37,38]

range of potentials (−90 to −60 mV) at which the TTX-sensitive sodium conductance is available for activation. By contrast, the pacemaker potential in sinoatrial tissue often occurs at a much less negative range (usually positive to −50 mV) at which it would be expected that the TTX-sensitive current would be largely inactivated. The inward current activated towards the end of the pacemaker depolarization in this case has been shown to be the second inward current, which is thought to be carried at least partly by calcium ions[20, 21, 37–39].

Figure 6 shows the result of an experiment on frog sinus in which the currents in response to very small depolarizations in the pacemaker range were recorded. It is clear that a potential and time-dependent inward current is activated by pulses that displace the potential into the second half of the pacemaker range. This current is the second inward current. Notice that in this range of potentials its activation is very slow. In the case of pulse C it requires 200–300 ms for the inward current to reach its peak. This is *very* much slower than the activation of the TTX-sensitive sodium current (which typically activates in about 1 ms).

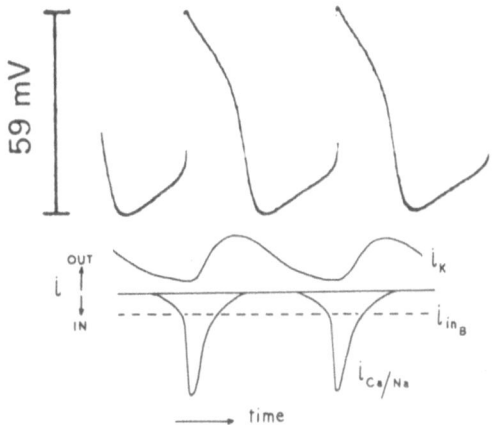

Figure 7 Diagram showing changes in inward and outward ionic currents thought to occur during sinus pacemaker activity. The inward background current is represented here as a constant, though it probably does vary with time through being voltage-dependent, but this voltage-dependence is as yet unknown. The potassium current activates slowly during each action potential and then decays during the pacemaker potential. The slow inward (calcium/sodium) current activates towards the second half of the pacemaker depolarization[62]

Figure 7 summarizes the role of outward and inward currents in the genesis of pacemaker activity in frog sinus. The dotted line indicates the zero current level. The time-independent inward current (the background current) is shown as a constant (this may not be strictly correct but the voltage-dependence of this current is as yet unknown: it is not possible to separate it from the background outward current i_{K1}). The line labelled i_K shows the activation and decay of the voltage and time-dependent potassium current (also called i_x) and the line labelled $i_{Ca/Na}$ shows the activation and inactivation of the second inward current.

INHIBITION OF PACEMAKER ACTIVITY BY ACETYLCHOLINE

In addition to his work on the myogenic origin of the heartbeat, Gaskell investigated its control by the nervous system. He was the first to show that stimulation of the vagus nerve produces an increased resting potential in auricular tissue. This finding was amply confirmed by microelectrode techniques[40, 41]. The use of these techniques, together with radioactive tracer

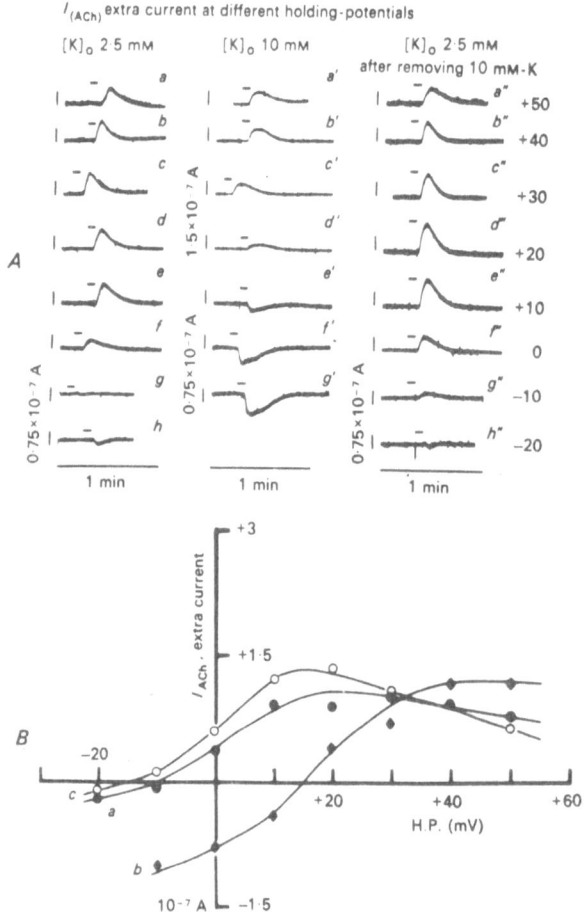

Figure 8 *A.* records of membrane current in frog atrium at various potentials (expressed as mV positive or negative to the holding potential) during application of acetylcholine. Positive to a certain potential (initially −10 mV) the current is outward. Negative to this potential the current is inward. Increasing the K concentration from 2.5 to 10 mM shifts this reversal potential by about 25 mV. The shift is reversible. *B.* current–voltage relations for the maximum value of acetylcholine-induced current[43]

studies, led to the view that the hyperpolarization is produced by a specific increase in potassium permeability (see review by Hutter[42]).

The recent use of voltage clamp techniques has confirmed this view[43], but has also shown that it is incomplete. Changes in calcium conductance are also involved in the inhibitory action of acetylcholine[44-47] in both atrial and sinus tissue.

Figure 8 shows records of membrane current obtained under voltage clamp conditions in frog atrial muscle by Garnier et al.[43]. On applying acetylcholine there is an increase in outward current at potentials positive to the reversal potential. The latter varies with the extracellular potassium concentration in the way expected for a potassium selective current.

That this is not the complete story is in fact clear from some of the earlier microelectrode records. Thus, Hutter and Trautwein[41] (in a figure reproduced here as Figure 9) found that the action potential is still greatly reduced in

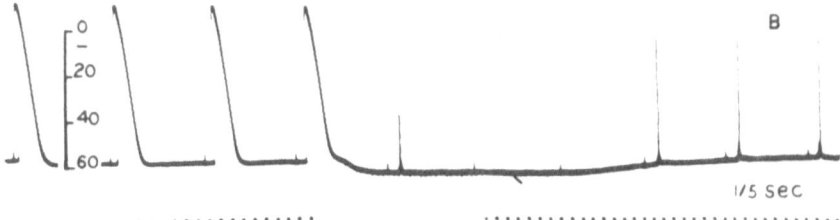

Figure 9 Action and resting potentials in tortoise sinus venosus during and following stimulation of the vagus nerve, indicated by interruption in dotted line. During stimulation the membrane hyperpolarizes and action potentials are either very short (1st response) or entirely suppressed (2nd and 3rd responses). After stimulation has ceased, the resting potential returns to its original level but the action potentials remain very short (4th, 5th and 6th responses)[41]

duration even when the hyperpolarization has completely subsided. If the hyperpolarization is used as an index of the increased potassium permeability then the action potential can be greatly affected at a time when the potassium permeability has returned to normal levels. The ionic basis of this effect is shown in Figure 10, which shows current records and current-voltage diagrams obtained in frog atrial muscle before and after the application of acetylcholine at a concentration of 3×10^{-8} M and at 1.2×10^{-7} M. At 3×10^{-8} M there is a large decrease in the inward current activated at potentials between -30 mV and $+40$ mV, whereas no change in current is recorded negative to -40 mV. Since the fast sodium current is blocked by tetrodotoxin, the current involved is the second inward current. Thus, the second inward current may be greatly reduced at a level of acetylcholine that is insufficient to increase the potassium permeability. Moreover, the reduction in strength of contraction produced by acetylcholine is strongly correlated with the effect on the calcium current. This is shown in Figure 11 which shows the dose-response curves for second inward current, contraction and potassium current obtained by Garnier et al.[48].

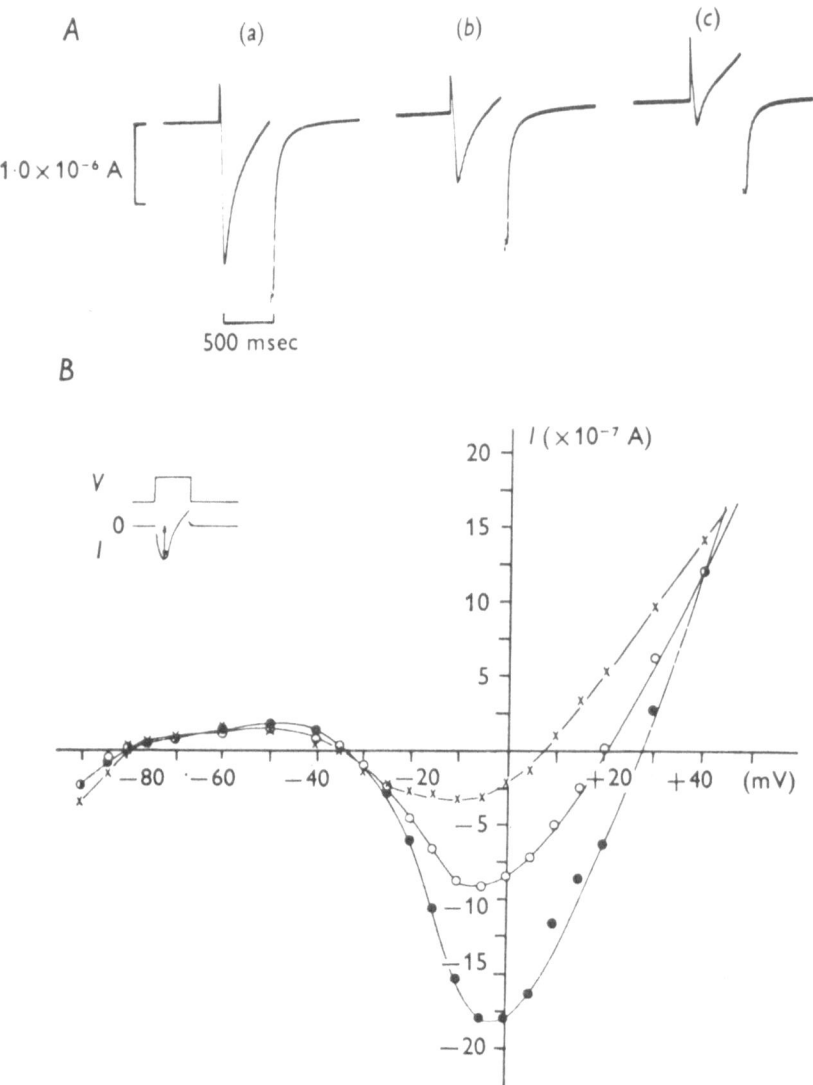

Figure 10 Ionic basis of action potential shortening in the absence of increased potassium permeability and membrane hyperpolarization. *A*. Pen recorder tracings of slow inward current in response to 500 ms, 80 mV depolarization from the resting potential (-80 mV) in frog atrium. (*a*) is the control record, and (*b*) and (*c*) were recorded after application of 3×10^{-8} M and 1.2×10^{-7} M acetylcholine respectively. *B*. The peak inward or minimum outward current is plotted against membrane potential. Control (Ringer solution +TTX 2×10^{-6} g/ml), 3×10^{-8} M ACh (O) and 1.2×10^{-7} M ACh ($\times$)[46]

These results raise the question how far each of the two actions of acetylcholine are involved physiologically in mediating the inhibition produced by the parasympathetic nervous system. It is difficult to answer this question

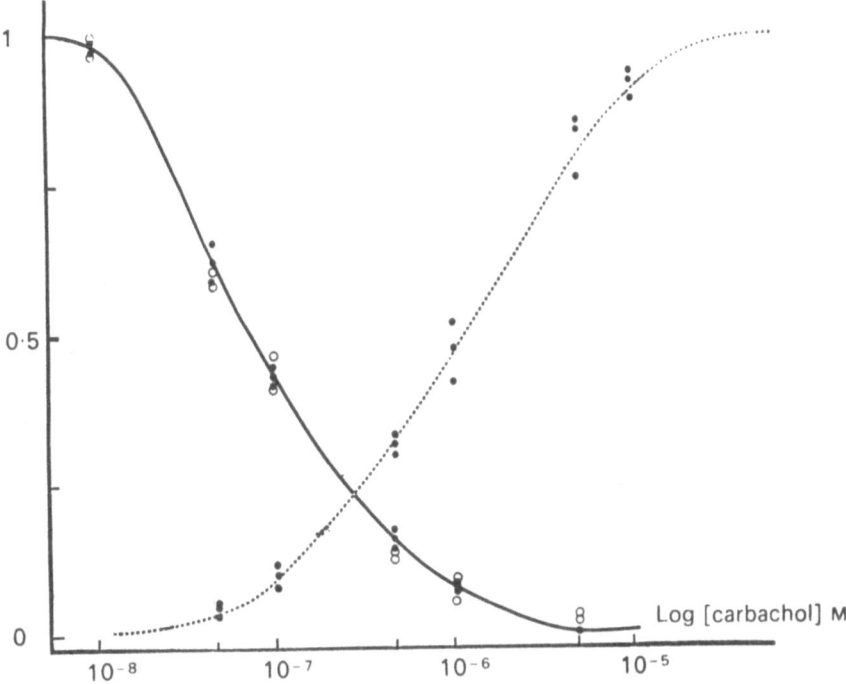

Figure 11 Reduction of calcium/sodium current (●) and of contraction (○) in frog atrium by carbachol. These effects are proportional to each other. They begin at 10^{-8} M and the apparent K_m is $<10^{-7}$ M. The interrupted line (---- ----) shows the increase in potassium current. This effect starts at a higher concentration (5×10^{-8}) and has an apparent K_m of 10^{-6} M[48]

with certainty, since it is not known precisely what level of acetylcholine surrounds the pacemaker tissue during stimulation of the vagus nerve. Complete arrest *is* accompanied by hyperpolarization[41]. On the other hand, slowing of pacemaker activity in the frog sinus may occur without any hyperpolarization[37, 38]. There may also be a difference between the frog and the mammal. In the mammalian atrium relatively high doses of acetylcholine were required by Ten Eick *et al.*[42] to reduce the second inward current.

ACCELERATION OF PACEMAKER ACTIVITY BY ADRENALINE

Attention was drawn earlier to the significant differences that exist between the pacemaker mechanisms in Purkinje fibres and in sinoatrial tissue. These differences become of fundamental importance in analysing the mechanism by which the sympathetic nervous system produces acceleration.

Since adrenaline has no effect on the rapidly activated sodium conductance, it seemed likely that the mechanism by which it accelerates pacemaker activity in Purkinje fibres would lie in an action on the potassium current involved. Hauswirth *et al.*[49] found that the threshold for activating i_{K2} is displaced to less negative potentials under the influence of adrenaline. This enables a larger and faster decay of potassium current to occur during diastole and so increases the rate of depolarization. This action of adrenaline has been investigated in further detail by Tsien[50,51] and by Hauswirth *et al.*[52]. Tsien *et al.*[53] have shown that, like other actions of adrenaline, it may be mimicked by, and is probably mediated by, an increase in the intracellular concentration of cyclic AMP.

Quite small displacements of the i_{K2} activation curve produce substantial increases in pacemaker frequency[25]. This action therefore seemed sufficient to account for the dramatic increase in frequency produced by the sympathetic nervous system. More recently, however, it has been found that adrenaline has an additional action on the potassium system, which is to increase the potassium gradient across the i_{K2} channels and so displace the i_{K2} reversal potential in a negative direction[54].

Figure 12 shows the current records obtained during voltage displacements to -80 mV which in this preparation was the potential at which the time-dependent current change reverses direction. The record is therefore initially flat. On application of adrenaline, two effects are observed: first the holding current (the current required to maintain the holding potential of -70 mV) shifts in an inward direction. This effect is attributable to the decrease in i_{K2} produced by the positive shift of the i_{K2} activation curve[49]. Second, the current during the pulse to -80 mV is no longer flat. An outward tail

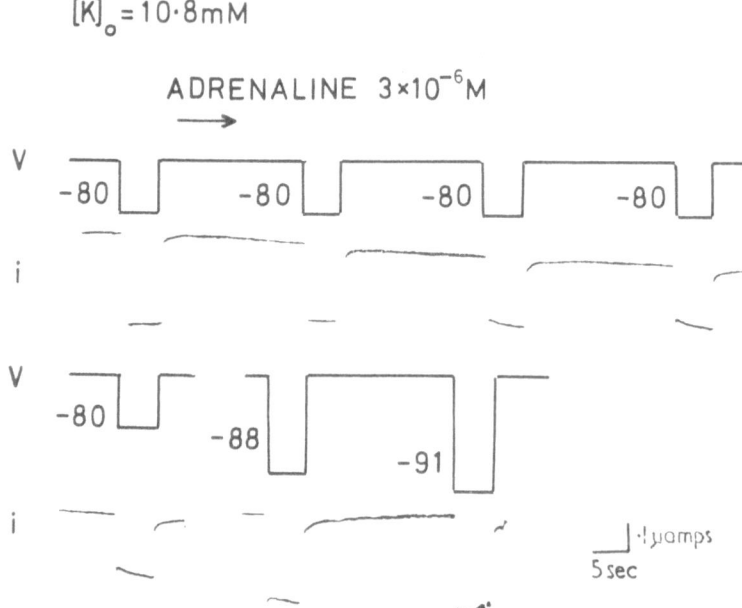

Figure 12 Displacement of i_{K2} reversal potential in a sheep Purkinje fibre under influence of adrenaline (3×10^{-6} M). Before application of adrenaline a voltage clamp pulse to -80 mV is close to the reversal potential. After adrenaline the current at this potential is no longer flat and a pulse to -91 mV is required to reach the reversal potential[54]

appears and it is now necessary to clamp to −91 mV to reach the reversal potential.

One possible explanation for this effect is that adrenaline has disturbed the balance of factors determining the potassium concentration in the extra-cellular cleft spaces, perhaps by stimulating the sodium–potassium exchange pump, and has decreased the extracellular K^+ concentration. It is well known that this leads to a decrease in outward K^+ current[55] and this may also contribute to the acceleration of pacemaker activity. Figure 13 shows the results of computations that demonstrate this effect using the mathematical model described by McAllister et al.[25].

We turn now to the action of adrenaline on sinoatrial tissue. It has proved difficult to investigate the mechanism in frog sinus and mammalian SA nodal tissue. Most of the experimental information therefore comes from work on pacemaker activity in frog atrial muscle[56,57]. The action of adrena-line on the potassium current i_x involved in pacemaker activity in this tissue has been found to be strikingly different from that on i_{K2} in Purkinje fibres. First, there is no change in the threshold potential for activating i_x and, instead of decreasing the steady state K current at some potentials, adrenaline

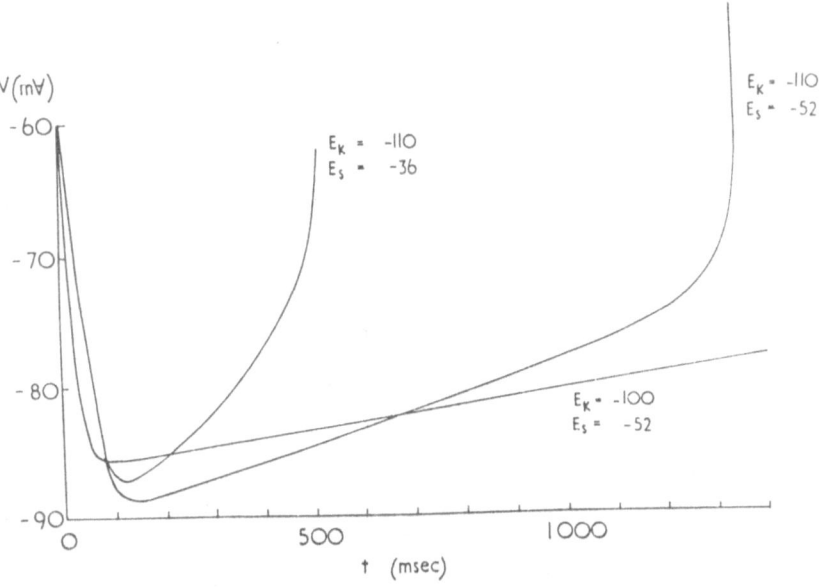

Figure 13 Influence of negative shift in i_{K2} reversal potential and of positive shift in s activation curve on pacemaker activity in Purkinje fibres. E_{rev} for i_{K2} is − 100 mV in the control computation. Shift by 10 mV to − 110 mV produces a steeper pacemaker potential and an increased maximum diastolic potential. Also shifting S by 10 mV in positive direction produces a further acceleration and reduces the maximum diastolic potential (although this is still more negative than in the control case). Calculations were made using the model of McAllister et al.[25] as extended by Cohen et al.[54]

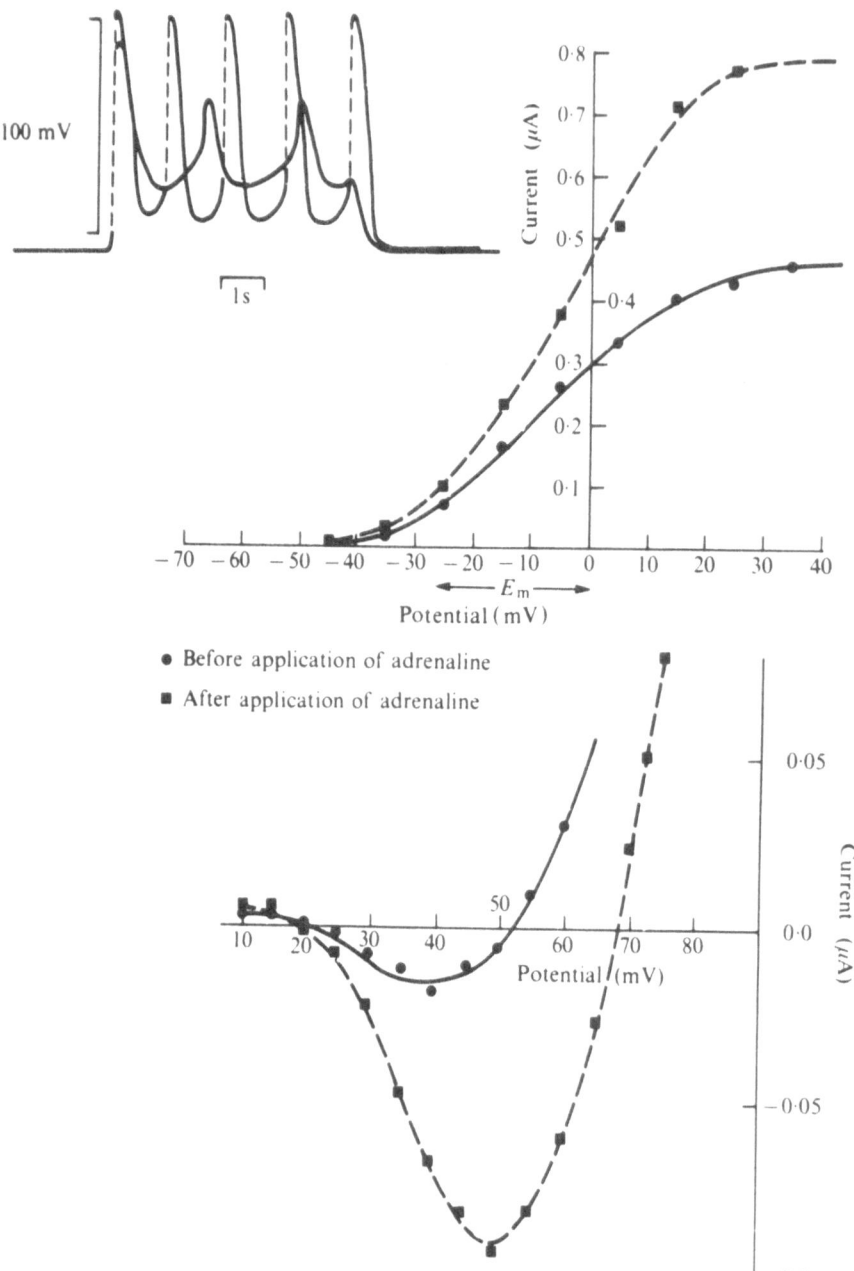

Figure 14 *Top:* influence of adrenaline (10^{-8} M) on potassium activation curve in frog atrium. The amplitude of the current is increased by 50% but there is no shift in the threshold potential (about -40 mV). *Bottom:* influence of adrenaline (5×10^{-9} M) on second inward current[56]

increases it over the whole activation range, as shown in Figure 14. The result is consistent with the hypothesis that, instead of acting largely on the gating mechanism, as in the case of i_{K2}, adrenaline acts by increasing either the conductivity or the number of channels carrying the current i_x. The activation curves shown in Figure 14 are obtained by measuring the total time-dependent outward current activated. This current includes some current change due to K^+ accumulation in addition to i_x[29,30,35,58]. This makes it difficult to be certain that there is no change in the shape of the activation curve[59]. We can, however, be certain that the net outward current is increased rather than decreased, and that this is in the *opposite* direction to the change required to accelerate pacemaker activity. Acceleration must therefore be the result of an action of adrenaline on another ionic current.

It was noted earlier that in sinoatrial tissue, unlike Purkinje fibres, the activation of the second inward current is involved in reinforcing the pacemaker depolarization. Moreover this current is increased in amplitude by adrenaline[12,60]. As shown in Figure 14 this effect can be proportionately much larger than the effect on the potassium current. It seems likely therefore that the acceleration of the pacemaker depolarization is primarily attributable to an increase in the calcium current and that the increased potassium current is involved in preventing the prolongation of the action potential duration that might otherwise occur.

The results of Figure 14 were obtained on frog atrium. A full analysis of the action of adrenaline on ionic currents in the sinus or SA node has not yet been achieved. However, preliminary results suggest that the picture may be very similar in the natural pacemaker. Figure 15 shows voltage clamp currents in response to step depolarizations from -30 to -15 mV in the

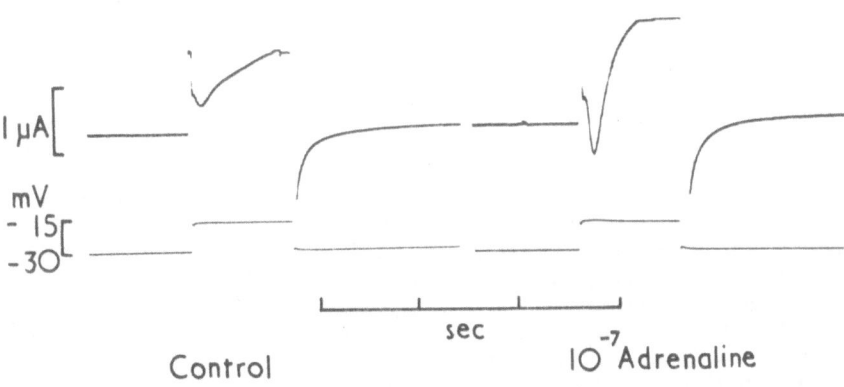

Figure 15 Action of adrenaline (10^{-7} M) on ionic currents in tortoise sinus venosus. *Left:* response to depolarization from -30 to -15 mV in the control solution. The second inward current is relatively small. *Right:* response to same voltage pulse after adding adrenaline. Both the second inward and the delayed outward currents are increased (the full increase in the latter is not recorded). (Brown, H. F., DiFrancesco, D. and Noble, S. J., unpublished)

tortoise sinus venosus before and after applying adrenaline (10^{-7} M). Before adrenaline the inward current activated by this pulse is insufficient to produce a net inward ionic current. After adrenaline, the current is greatly increased and a net inward current is then recorded. It is also clear that the time-dependent outward current is increased. After applying adrenaline the outward current rapidly exceeds the maximum value recorded by the apparatus.

Thus the action of adrenaline on the sinus pacemaker resembles that on the atrium rather than on the normal Purkinje fibre pacemaker mechanism.

References

1. Bottazzi, F. (1964). Leonardo as physiologist. In *Leonardo da Vinci*, pp. 373–387. (London: Leisure Arts)
2. Gaskell, W. H. (1883). On the innervation of the heart, with especial reference to the heart of the tortoise. *J. Physiol.*, **4,** 43
3. Hill, C. (1964). William Harvey and the idea of monarchy. *Past and Present*, 27. Reprinted in Webster, C. (ed.) (1974). *The Intellectual Revolution of the Seventeenth Century*, pp. 160–181. (London and Boston: Routledge & Kegan Paul)
4. Whitteridge, G. (1965). William Harvey: a royalist and no parliamentarian. *Past and Present*, 30. Reprinted in Webster, C. (ed.) (1974). *The Intellectual Revolution of the Seventeenth Century*, pp. 182–188. (London and Boston: Routledge & Kegan Paul)
5. Hill, C. (1965). William Harvey (no parliamentarian, no heretic) and the idea of monarchy. *Past and Present*, 31. Reprinted in Webster, C. (ed.) (1974). *The Intellectual Revolution of the Seventeenth Century*, pp. 189–196. (London and Boston: Routledge & Kegan Paul)
6. Arvanitaki, A. (1938). *Propriétés rythmiques de la matière vivante. II. Etude expérimentale sur le myocarde d'Helix*. (Paris: Hermann)
7. Bozler, E. (1943). The initiation of impulses in cardiac muscle. *Am. J. Physiol.*, **138,** 273
8. Weidmann, S. (1951). Effect of current flow on the membrane potential of cardiac muscle. *J. Physiol.*, **115,** 227
9. Noble, D. and Tsien, R. W. (1972). The repolarization process of heart cells. In: *Electrical phenomena in the heart* (ed. de Mello), pp. 133–161. (New York: Academic Press)
10. Hall, A. E., Hutter, O. F. and Noble, D. (1963). Current–voltage relations of Purkinje fibres in sodium-deficient solutions. *J. Physiol.*, **166,** 225
11. Deck, K. A., Kern, R. and Trautwein, W. (1964). Voltage clamp technique in mammalian cardiac fibres. *Pfluegers Arch. Gesamte Physiol.*, **280,** 50
12. Rougier, O., Vassort, G., Garnier, D., Gargouil, Y.-M. and Coraboeuf, E. (1969). Existence and role of a slow inward current during the frog atrial action potential. *Pfluegers Arch. Gesamte Physiol.*, **308,** 91
13. Brown, H. F. and Noble, S. J. (1969). Membrane currents underlying delayed rectification and pacemaker activity in frog atrial muscle. *J. Physiol.*, **204,** 717
14. Morad, M. and Trautwein, W. (1968). The effect of the duration of the action potential on contraction in the mammalian heart tissue. *Pfluegers Arch. Gesamte Physiol.*, **299,** 66
15. Beeler, G. W. and Reuter, H. (1970). Voltage clamp experiments on ventricular myocardial fibres. *J. Physiol.*, **207,** 165

16. Vassalle, M. (1966). Analysis of cardiac pacemaker potential using a 'voltage clamp' technique. *Am. J. Physiol.*, **210**, 1335
17. Lederer, W. J. and Tsien, R. W. (1976). Transient inward current underlying arrhythmogenic effects of cardiotonic steroids in Purkinje fibres. *J. Physiol.*, **263**, 73
18. Noble, D. and Tsien, R. W. (1968). The kinetics and rectifier properties of the slow potassium current in cardiac Purkinje fibres. *J. Physiol.*, **195**, 185
19. Peper, K. and Trautwein, W. (1969). A note on the pacemaker current in Purkinje fibres. *Pfluegers Arch. Gesamte Physiol.*, **309**, 356
20. Noma, A. and Irisawa, H. (1976a). Membrane currents in rabbit sinoatrial node cells studied by the double microelectrode method. *Pfluegers Arch. Gesamte Physiol.*, **364**, 45
21. Noma, A. and Irisawa, H. (1976b). The time- and voltage-dependent potassium current in the rabbit sino-atrial node cell. *Pfluegers Arch. Gesamte Physiol.*, **366**, 251
22. McAllister, R. E. and Noble, D. (1966). The time and voltage dependence of the slow outward current in cardiac Purkinje fibres. *J. Physiol.*, **186**, 632
23. Hodgkin, A. L. and Huxley, A. F. (1952). A quantitative description of membrane current and its application to conduction and excitation in nerve. *J. Physiol.*, **117**, 500
24. Noble, D. and Tsien, R. W. (1969). Outward membrane currents activated in the plateau range of potentials in cardiac Purkinje fibres. *J. Physiol.*, **200**, 205
25. McAllister, R. E., Noble, D. and Tsien, R. W. (1975). Reconstruction of the electrical activity of cardiac Purkinje fibres. *J. Physiol.*, **251**, 1
26. deHemptinne, A. (1971a). Properties of the outward current in frog atrial muscle. *Pfluegers Arch. Gesamte Physiol.*, **329**, 321
27. deHemptinne, A. (1971b). The frequency dependence of outward current in frog auricular fibres. *Pfluegers Arch. Gesamte Physiol.*, **329**, 332
28. Ojeda, C. and Rougier, O. (1974). Kinetic analysis of delayed outward currents in frog atrium. Existence of two kinds of preparation. *J. Physiol.*, **239**, 51
29. Brown, H. F., Clark, A. and Noble, S. J. (1976a). Identification of the pacemaker current in frog atrium. *J. Physiol.*, **258**, 521
30. Brown, H. F., Clark, A. and Noble, S. J. (1976b). Analysis of pacemaker and repolarization currents in frog atrial muscle. *J. Physiol.*, **258**, 547
31. Katzung, B. G. and Morgenstern, J. A. (1977). Effects of extracellular potassium on ventricular automaticity and evidence for a pacemaker current in mammalian ventricular myocardium. *Circ. Res.* **40**, 105
32. McDonald, T. F. and Trautwein, W. (1978). The potassium current underlying delayed rectification in cat ventricular muscle. *J. Physiol.*, **274**, 217
33. Hutter, O. F. and Noble, D. (1961). The anion conductance of cardiac muscle. *J. Physiol.*, **157**, 335
34. Bosteels, S., Vleugels, A. and Carmeliet, E. E. (1970). Choline permeability in cardiac muscle cells of the cat. *J. Gen. Physiol.*, **55**, 602
35. Noble, D. (1975). *The Initiation of the Heartbeat.* (Oxford: Clarendon Press)
36. Brooks, C. McC. and Lu, M. M. (1972). *The Sinoatrial Pacemaker of the Heart.* (Illinois: Charles C. Thomas)
37. Brown, H. F., Giles, W. R. and Noble, S. J. (1977a). Cholinergic inhibition of frog sinus venosus. *J. Physiol.*, **267**, 38
38. Brown, H. F., Giles, W. R. and Noble, S. J. (1977b). Membrane currents underlying activity in frog sinus venosus. *J. Physiol.*, **271**, 783

39. Brown, H. F., Giles, W. R. and Noble, S. J. (1976). Voltage clamp of frog sinus venosus. *J. Physiol.*, **258**, 78

40. Burgen, A. S. V. and Terroux, K. G. (1953). On the negative inotropic effect in the cat's auricle. *J. Physiol.*, **120**, 449

41. Hutter, O. F. and Trautwein, W. (1956). Vagal and sympathetic effects on the pacemaker fibres in the sinus venosus of the heart. *J. Gen. Physiol.*, **39**, 715

42. Hutter, O. F. (1957). Mode of action of autonomic transmitters on the heart. *Br. Med. Bull.*, **13**, 176

43. Garnier, D., Nargeot, J., Ojeda, C. and Rougier, O. (1978a). The action of acetylcholine on background conductance in frog atrial trabeculae. *J. Physiol.*, **274**, 381

44. Giles, W. and Tsien, R. W. (1975). Effects of acetylcholine on the membrane currents in frog atrial muscle. *J. Physiol.*, **246**, 64

45. Ikemoto, Y. and Goto, M. (1975). Nature of the negative inotropic effect of acetylcholine on the myocardium. An elucidation on the bullfrog atrium. *Proc. Japan Acad.*, **51**, 501

46. Giles, W. and Noble, S. J. (1976). Changes in membrane currents in bullfrog atrium produced by acetylcholine. *J. Physiol.*, **261**, 103

47. Ten Eick, R., Nawrath, H., McDonald, T. F. and Trautwein, W. (1976). On the mechanism of the negative inotropic effect of acetylcholine. *Pfluegers Arch. Gesamte Physiol.*, **361**, 207

48. Garnier, D., Nargeot, J., Ojeda, C. and Rougier, O. (1978b). Action of carbachol on atrial fibres: induced extra current and slow inward current inhibition. *J. Physiol.*, **273**, 27

49. Hauswirth, O., Noble, D. and Tsien, R. W. (1968). Adrenaline: mechanism of action on the pacemaker potential in cardiac Purkinje fibres. *Science*, **162**, 916

50. Tsien, R. W. (1974a). Effect of epinephrine on the pacemaker potassium current of cardiac Purkinje fibres. *J. Gen. Physiol.*, **64**, 293

51. Tsien, R. W. (1974b). The mode of action of chronotropic agents in cardiac Purkinje fibres. *J. Gen. Physiol.*, **64**, 320

52. Hauswirth, O., Wehner, H. D. and Ziskoven, R. (1976). α adrenergic receptors and pacemaker current in cardiac Purkinje fibres. *Nature (Lond.)*, **263**, 155

53. Tsien, R. W., Giles, W. R. and Greengard, P. (1972). Cyclic AMP mediates the action of adrenaline on the action potential plateau of cardiac Purkinje fibres. *Nature, New Biol.*, **240**, 181

54. Cohen, I., Eisner, D. A. and Noble, D. (1978). The action of adrenaline on pacemaker activity in cardiac Purkinje fibres. *J. Physiol.* (in press)

55. Noble, D. (1965). Electrical properties of cardiac muscle attributable to inward-going (anomalous) rectification. *J. Cell. Comp. Physiol.*, **66** (Suppl. 2), 127

56. Brown, H. F. and Noble, S. J. (1974). Effects of adrenaline on membrane currents underlying pacemaker activity in frog atrial muscle. *J. Physiol.*, **238**, 51

57. Brown, H. F., McNaughton, P. A., Noble, D. and Noble, S. J. (1975). Adrenergic control of cardiac pacemaker currents. *Phil. Trans. Roy. Soc.*, **B270**, 527

58. Brown, H. F., DiFrancesco, D., Noble, D. and Noble, S. J. (1978). The contribution of potassium accumulation to outward currents in frog atrium. *J. Physiol.* (submitted)

59. Eisner, D. A., Cohen, I. and Attwell, D. (1978). Voltage clamp and tracer flux data: effects of a restricted extracellular space. (In preparation)

60. Reuter, H. (1967). The dependence of slow inward current in Purkinje fibres on the extracellular calcium concentration. *J. Physiol.*, **192**, 479

61. Brown, H. F., Clark, A. and Noble, S. J. (1972). Pacemaker current in frog atrium. *Nature, New Biol.*, **235,** 30
62. Brown, H. F., Giles, W. R. and Noble, S. J. (1978). Membrane currents underlying rhythmic activity in frog sinus venosus. *Scientific American.* (In press)

5
Human cardiac electrophysiology

D. DURRER, M. J. JANSE, K. I. LIE AND F. J. L. VAN CAPELLE

'Shrimp' and its Dutch equivalent 'herneel' are two of the few non-Latin words of the *Exercitatio*[1]. Why did Harvey know this word 'herneel'? Probably because he was born in Folkestone, a small fishing town with a more or less romantic trade in smuggling, lying close to the Low Countries[1]. Both activities might have attracted Dutch and Flemish fishermen; their boats were often leaking structures which sometimes had to be kept afloat by liberal use of the pump. This was a relatively recent invention, for which therefore a Latin word did not exist. The construction is depicted in Figure 1, taken from a marine dictionary, published in 1793[2]. Now the striking thing is that the Dutch name for the essential element of this pump, whose function might be compared with a valve, links two words essential in the circulation: pump and heart, because it is called 'pomphartje', the diminutive of 'pomphart'.

Harvey, as a boy walking among these boats, may have seen this pump and heard the word 'pomphart'. One might speculate—I will accept the verdict that it is a hazardous undertaking—that reversing the sequence of these words, giving 'heartpump', might be one of the roots of Harvey's discovery!

THE BEGINNING AND THE FIRST CENTURY OF CARDIAC ELECTROPHYSIOLOGY

About two centuries later cardiac electrophysiology was born, when Matteucci in 1843 discovered that a pile of pigeon hearts, cut in half, generated electricity between the intact part of the first and the cut surface of the last[3]. This led to investigations on a massive scale, which however did not result in the formulation of fundamental concepts. Indeed, the history of cardiac electrophysiology is in many respects a comedy of errors, the fun of mistaken identities. It was nearly a century later that Craib and Wilson found about 1930 the correct approach to the physical problems involved[4-5].

PUMPENSCHUH.

Holl. Pump-hartje, zuiger.
Dän. Pompefkoe.
Schw. Pumpfko.
Engl. Upper box of a pump.

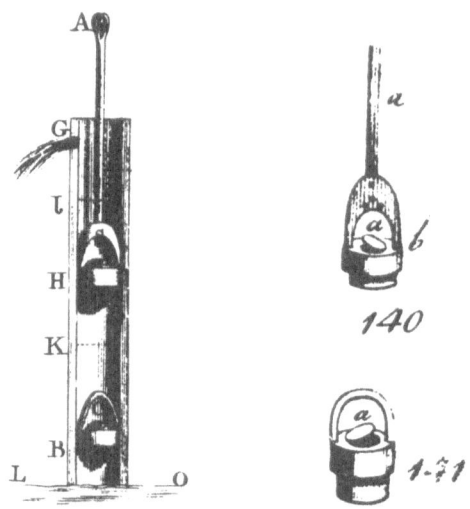

Figure 1 Reproduction of a pump from Röding: *Handbuch des Marine*. The 'pomphartje', —upper box of a pump—is shown in detail (140). The valve (a) is like a tilting disc of a Björck–Shiley type of valve prosthesis

HUMAN CARDIAC ELECTROPHYSIOLOGY

Human cardiac electrophysiology is the study of:

1. impulse formation and conduction in the normal and diseased heart, of its cells and structures;
2. the relation of the normal and diseased heart as an electric generator with the body surface potentials (forward problem)
3. the inverse relation, which is the 'decoding' of the body surface potentials into electrophysiological mechanisms (inverse problem). The latter two will not be discussed in this article.

Human cardiac electrophysiology, the basis of electrocardiography, asks for close cooperation between cellular electrophysiologists, physicists, biochemists, computer experts, pathologists and cardiologists. They represent the disciplines which have greatly contributed to our knowledge in this field. The role of the clinician is an important one, because it is his problems which have to be solved.

EXPERIMENTAL TECHNIQUES AND MODELS AND THEIR LIMITATIONS

The data and concepts presented here are obtained from experimental models which are, where possible, of human origin; however, if important gaps in our knowledge exist, data from experimental animals are given. The experimental techniques used must be critically examined. Only the outer layer of 150 μm thickness of superfused preparations survives after some hours for the inner core has become necrotic. Moreover when intramural electrodes are introduced into the heart, the heart muscle is damaged. This might influence some of the results, despite the sealing-off process. The same process also occurs with micro-electrodes at a microscopic level.

SOME ELECTROPHYSIOLOGICAL FIRST PRINCIPLES

Relation of depolarization and contraction

The almost complete synchronicity between depolarization and the beginning of contraction found in contracting cells from foetal myocardial tissue cultures also applies for the intact heart: the pathway of depolarization is the pathway of the beginning of contraction. This relation, which has been demonstrated recently in the intact human heart[6], explains why the pre-excited region in the Wolff–Parkinson–White (WPW) syndrome contracts before the normally activated part of the ventricles. New evidence suggests that the reverse relation must also be considered. A changed contraction pattern in paced dog hearts with total block may cause a myofibrillar disarray after 3 months[7]. Post-pacing T-wave changes might be related to this phenomenon.

Transmembrane action potential and extracellular currents

Two factors are responsible for the extracardiac electrical manifestations:

(a) the transmembrane action potential which represents the electrical activity of each of the 10^{10} cells constituting the heart;
(b) the differences in time of occurrence of this electrical activity in the heart, a consequence of the fact that it is a propagated phenomenon (Figure 2). If all cells were activated synchronously, no QRS would be present. Synchronous repolarization results in an absent T-wave.

There is a close relationship between the form of the transmembrane action potential, the propagation velocity through the cardiac tissues and the strength and direction of the extracellular currents which generate the potential fluctuations inside and outside the heart[8]. The strength of the intramural equivalent dipole layer is about 40 mV[9].

Intrinsic deflection and transmembrane action potential

The upstroke of the transmembrane action potentials recorded from sites

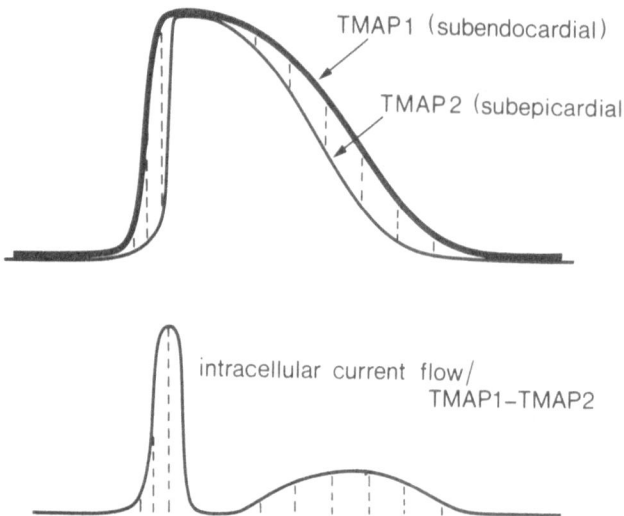

Figure 2 Recordings from epicardial and endocardial cells, from the same part of the ventricular wall, give information about strength and direction of intracellular and extra-cellular currents during depolarization and repolarization in this region

at the epicardial surface of the heart is synchronous with the rapid part of the intrinsic deflection in unipolar electrograms from this site, and is therefore caused by the synchronous firing of the many myocardial cells directly under the exploring electrode. Thus it is truly a local phenomenon. It disappears in acute ischaemia and information about the time of firing of the ischaemic cells can only be obtained by intracellular recordings from these cells.

Desynchronized depolarization

It can be demonstrated in the same way that desynchronized, late depolarization is responsible for the multiple, small deflections in the electrogram recorded from the border zone of infarcted regions[10,11]. They are caused by organized depolarization of a complex network of conducting cells, separated by strands of fibrous tissue, which is constant in successive beats. They have nothing to do with 'local fibrillation'[12]. Desynchronized conduction is also found in strips of atrial tissue obtained from patients with mitral stenosis.

Conduction velocity

The following values for conduction velocity in the cardiac structures have been found in *some* isolated human hearts, during surgery in a few patients, and some strips of atrial muscle:

Atria	normal	75 cm/s
	strips of muscle of patients with mitral stenosis and atrial fibrillation	10–20 cm/s[9]
Ventricles	normal muscle	
	transmural	30 cm/s
	parallel with fibres	50–60 cm/s
	acute ischaemia	some centimetres/second or less (millimetres?)
Specific conduction system	normal large branches	$2\frac{1}{2}$ m/s
Subendocardial Purkinje system	normal	50–75 cm/s
	diseased	20–25 cm/s

Repolarization

The transmembrane action potentials we recorded in one isolated human heart clearly demonstrated that with increasing frequency the duration of phase 2 shortens, while the time-course of phase 3 remains constant. If this occurs in all myocardial cells, the form of the T-wave will change little with increased rate.

SOME ELECTROPHYSIOLOGICAL CONCEPTS IN ARRHYTHMIAS

Important unifying concepts, if properly applied, explain greatly different types of arrhythmias[9,13-21].

Re-entry

Single or repetitive, 'reciprocation', can cause a multitude of arrhythmias, from innocent to potentially dangerous. The echo pathway may be preformed as in the WPW syndrome or caused by the cardiac disease process (e.g. infarction). The necessary conditions for the occurrence of re-entry are illustrated in Figure 3. Re-entry circuits have been demonstrated in many cardiac structures. They may be large, as in the WPW syndrome, or small, as in reciprocating sinus- or atrioventricular nodal tachycardia.

Focal activity (automaticity)

Caused by synchronized phase 4 depolarization of a group of cells, or of the subendocardial Purkinje fibres[22]. A triggered focus may be elicited by electric stimulation of human atrial muscle. There is some evidence that the injury current caused by ischaemia causes ventricular muscle automaticity[23,24].

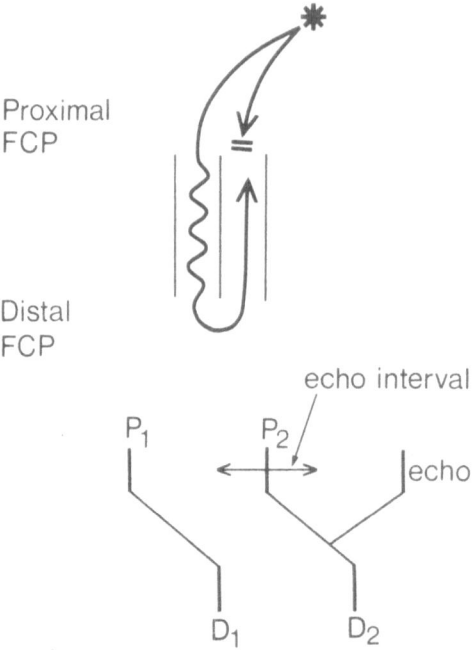

Figure 3 Schematic representation of pathways involved in re-entry. Both pathways connect a proximal final common pathway (FCP) with a distal final common pathway (FCP). During regular driving of P, causing P_1, premature beats P_2 elicited in P are blocked in the pathway on the right with a slightly longer refractory period, but (slowly) conducted in the other one on the left. If sufficiently slowed, activation of the faster pathway may occur in a retrograde (D–P) direction and cause an echo. These echoes only follow ventricular premature beats elicited in a well-defined coupling interval (echo interval). The size of the echo pathway may differ from 10 cm or more (Wolff–Parkinson–White) to some millimetres

Synchronization

Synchronization of a parasystolic focus located in the ischaemic subendo-cardial Purkinje system with atrial activity, may cause WPW-like complexes.

Concealed conduction

This indicates the influence of a non-conducted beat on subsequent impulse conduction and formation, and occurs frequently in the atrioventricular junction, less in the ventricles and atria. In the isolated rat heart it was possible to measure the degree of 'concealment' by using an appropriate stimulation pattern[25]. Very early atrial premature beats have no appreciable effect on conduction of subsequent impulses. For non-conducted atrial premature beats occurring later, the degree of 'concealment' rapidly increases and is greatest when the atrial premature beat is just not conducted. This is caused by progressively deeper penetration of A2 in the atrioventricular functional tissue. This can be demonstrated by the effect of pre-excitation of the ventricles, which 'peel off' a part of the peripheral refractory barrier.

CLINICAL CARDIAC ELECTROPHYSIOLOGY

Programmed stimulation

The clinical stimulation technique and His bundle recording have opened new perspectives in the study of arrhythmias[26-30]. However, the application of current to the cardiac tissues causes a complex electrophysiological situation in the stimulated region. The area involved is related to the size of the stimulating electrode and the strength of the applied current. Depolarizing and hyperpolarizing potentials in different cells in the vicinity of an extracellular electrode have been registered. Local re-entry mechanisms near the site of stimulation may cause spontaneous ventricular premature beats of similar form to the stimulated beat[31]. Ventricular tachycardias are often initiated during right ventricular driving (which is an artificial ventricular rhythm), or there may be an induction of two or three ventricular premature beats. Very complex electrophysiological situations can easily occur in diseased human hearts. Therefore, the ventricular tachycardias elicited may have different mechanisms from those that occur spontaneously.

His bundle recording

The recording of electrical activity of the His bundle has resulted in a breakthrough. A method suitable for the similar exploration of the activity of the deeper branches of the specific conduction system would be of great importance, but this system is probably very sensitive to pressure. Programmed stimulation clearly cannot solve the problem of the mechanism responsible for the spontaneous beat which initiates tachycardia and fibrillation.

Suction electrode

We do not use this method because we doubt the value of the records obtained.

SPECIAL HUMAN CARDIAC ELECTROPHYSIOLOGY

In this section the electrophysiological properties of the structures of the human heart involved in impulse formation and conduction, and in the initiation and perpetuation of arrhythmias, will be described briefly.

Sinus node

The recording of sinus nodal electrical activity with intracardiac electrodes would allow the accurate diagnosis of abnormalities in the sinus node function[32,33]. However, no intrinsic sinus node deflections have been identified convincingly in intracavitary electrograms. Close contiguous electrodes applied on the epicardial surface of this region of a dog heart sometimes showed two or three small oscillations, beginning 10 ms before a series of small and rapid atrial deflections caused by activation of perinodal muscle[34] (Figure 4). The slow deflections may indicate the presence of a process related to synchronization of pacemaking nodal cells. A slow and low-voltage pre-auricular deflection in unipolar electrograms from the nodal regions was recently described by Théry et al., following functional isolation of the sinus node with tetrodotoxin (TTX) injected into the sinus nodal artery[35].

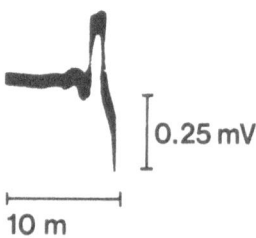

0.25 mV

10 m

Figure 4   Sinus nodal potentials preceding activity of perinodal atrial cells in the exposed dog heart, recorded with a pair of contiguous electrodes placed upon the pacemaking region

These results indicate that sinus nodal function in man can only be studied with programmed stimulation of the atria. However, rapid atrial stimulation or early premature atrial beats may depress its pacemaking function[22]. Very early atrial premature beats may cause echo beats from the sinus node.

This process may become repetitive and a circulating excitation wave of small dimensions, involving a part of the sinus node and perinodal tissue, may manifest itself as a reciprocating sinus tachycardia[36]. Patients with sinus node disease frequently have attacks of supraventricular arrhythmias. The details of the pathways involved in the isolated preparations are not well known, but recently Alessie and Bonke have demonstrated in one sinus-nodal preparation of the rabbit heart that the circus movement was completely intranodal[37].

Atrium

Studies of atrial excitation in the isolated revived human heart and in the superfused preparation of a 3-month-old foetal heart give no electrophysio-logical evidence for the presence of an atrial specialized conduction system[38]. In the atrial muscle of patients with rheumatic heart disease conduction velocity is greatly slowed, which contributes to the occurrence of atrial arrhythmias[39,40]. Fibrous tissue dispersed through the atrial muscle causes desynchronized activation, which during premature stimulation of super-fused human atrial strips increased greatly. With unidirectional block at certain sites, all conditions are present for the occurrence of single or repetitive atrial echo beats. Diffuse changes of this nature set the scene for atrial fibrillation.

Weldo *et al.* suggested that circulating activation waves may involve various parts of the atria, particularly around one or more of the vessels which enter the atria inferiorly[41]. They obtained evidence about their presence in lower parts of the left or right atria, even when other parts of the atria followed driving stimuli applied from a site in the high right atrium. We studied atrial epicardial activation of a patient with atypical flutter and had to conclude that every depolarization was initiated in a small region, located posteriorly in the atria, either with focal activity or harbouring a small circulating wave[42].

Atrioventricular node

Cellular characteristics and structural design are responsible for its delaying function[40,43,44]. Decreased atrioventricular nodal function may result in a more rapid transit of the impulse. A very short conduction time of less than 0.12 s, as present in the Lown–Ganong–Levine syndrome, does not necessarily indicate therefore the existence of a nodal bypass tract. Autonomic influences greatly change its function[45,46]; vagal impulses during sleep are probably responsible for type II atrioventricular conduction disturbances recorded during sleep in normal persons[47] (Figure 5). The response pattern of the atrioventricular node to induced atrial stimuli in a conscious unrestrained trained dog was unpredictable. This is in sharp contrast with the deterministic response pattern of the isolated rabbit heart[25].

Specific conduction system in the left ventricle of the human heart; left anterior hemiblock

Our present results indicate that, in the left ventricle, three subendocardial areas are activated in the first 10 s of depolarization, which merge after 20 s; only one is present in the right ventricle, near its anterior papillary muscle[48]. We assume therefore, that the left bundle divides into three fasciculi: anterior, posterior and a small septal one. The anterior region is larger than the posterior one, and the regions are not located symmetrically in respect to the large axis of the left ventricle for the upper part of the anterior region extends in a basal direction. Block in the anterior or posterior fasciculi—hemiblock —causes changes in time-course of depolarization in that part activated by the blocked fasciculi, which result in changes in QRS form and electrical axis[49]. These are well known in dog and monkey heart[50,51], but not in the human heart.

Wolf–Parkinson–White syndrome

The recent developments in the WPW syndrome make it a successful chapter of human cardiac electrophysiology. The syndrome is caused by one, sometimes two, anomalous conducting pathways, located at any part of the atrio-

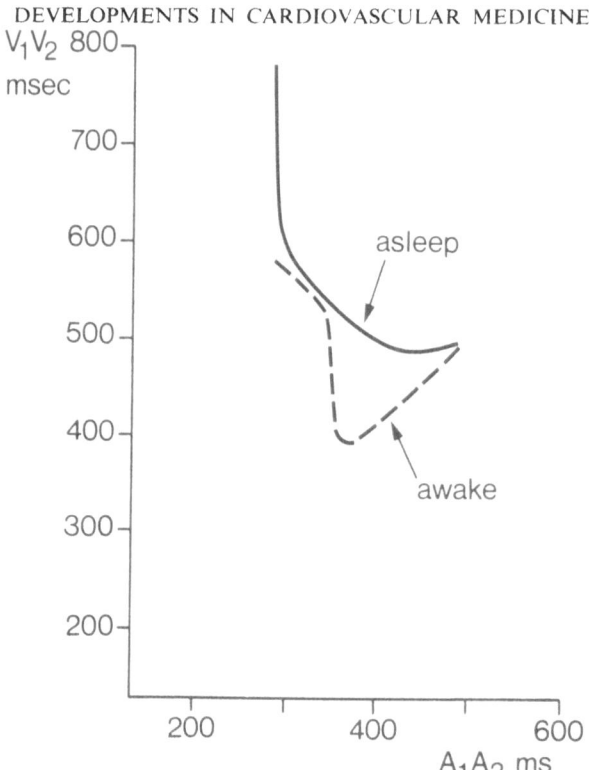

Figure 5 Atrioventricular response pattern following atrial premature beats. A_1A_2 is the interval between the last beat of the regular basic rhythm A_1 and the induced atrial premature beat A_2; V_1-V_2 is the interval between their ventricular responses. When the patient fell asleep immediate changes in the response pattern, compatible with increased vagal tone, were found

ventricular boundary, connecting adjacent parts of the atria and ventricles[30,52,53]. Conduction through the anomalous pathway may be possible in both atrioventricular and ventriculoatrial direction and the conduction time is usually approximately 40–50 ms. However, prolongation of conduction in one or both directions has been found. Of great clinical importance is the presence of unidirectional block which is often in the AV direction with an intact VA conduction. These patients have attacks of supraventricular tachycardia due to a circus movement tachycardia of the usual type. However, they never show WPW complexes during sinus rhythm: there is a concealed bypass. The absence of retrograde conduction can be suspected in those patients which have a constant WPW pattern, without attacks of tachycardia which can be related to a bypass. Block in both directions explains those instances in which an anomalous pathway was found in a heart without any indication that during life an arrhythmia was present.

The relatively simple diagrams given in 1967 for the several types of tachycardia which one might expect and the necessary electrophysiological conditions for their occurrence are still valid[52]. Supraventricular tachycardia is dependent on the conditions for retrograde conduction. The refractory period of the AV node must be longer than that of the anomalous pathway. The AV node must provide a sufficiently long delay for antegrade conduction to reach the anomalous pathway after its refractory period has ended. If the atrial refractory period is long, the circus movement stops and this also occurs if the AV node does not conduct the early atrial echo, for example due to vagal influences.

The occurrence of ventricular fibrillation in this syndrome has been amply documented[54]. The causative mechanism is as yet incompletely known. Atrial fibrillation and an anomalous pathway with short refractory period might be responsible, but other initiating mechanisms may be possible.

Surgical intervention in a 16-year-old boy with intractable attacks of ventricular tachycardia and ventricular fibrillation made it possible to explore the earliest activated region. An intramural electrode with ten terminals was introduced into the earliest activated region. It is evident that a very unusual intramural depolarization pattern is present, which can be explained by intramural branching of the anomalous pathway, causing multiple, small and closed depolarization fronts. The electrical activity of the anomalous pathway has not been recorded convincingly as yet. However, the well-developed very early deflection, recorded in the outer layer of the early activated region, which precedes the irregularly formed intramural, bipolar complexes, could be caused by depolarization of the anomalous pathway. The form of the intramural complexes recorded in this patient indicate an epicardial insertion of the anomalous pathway (Figure 6).

Many problems remain to be solved[55-57]. Why does the anomalous pathway function intermittently? Why can the bundle be dormant for many years and suddenly become responsive and cause a catastrophe? What is the relation between anatomical and histological features and its electrophysiological properties? The diameter of the bundle at origin and insertion, the form and length must be important factors. The nature of the constituting cells is a matter of dispute. What is the role of the branching pattern of the bundle in the myocardium in the occurrence of these arrhythmias, which suggest that pacemaking properties exist in the anomalous pathway?

ACUTE LOCAL ISCHAEMIA AND INFARCTION OF THE MYOCARDIUM

The ΣST concept is used clinically as an index for the degree of ischaemic injury and for the detection of 'directional changes of injury' following certain interventions. The concept has attracted great attention from clinicians. The genesis of the characteristic ischaemic QRST changes is not understood in detail[58,59]. We approached this problem along the lines outlined above in the isolated pig heart, where the ischaemic changes occur nearly uniformly in the affected region[23,60]. Transmembrane action potentials of ischaemic and normal cells were recorded, together with the usual epicardial and intramural complexes using DC coupled amplifiers, non-polarizable electrodes and a zero potential.

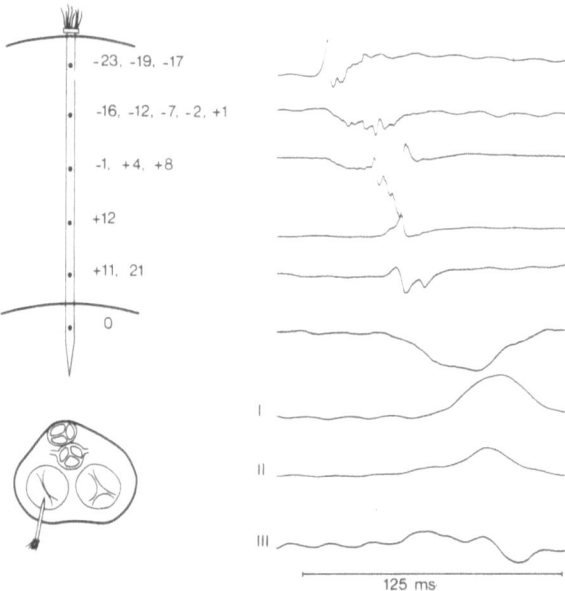

Figure 6 Intramural bipolar complexes from the left ventricular region activated earliest by an anomalous pathway in Wolff–Parkinson–White syndrome. The upper tracing reflects electrical activity of the subepicardial layer, activated directly by the anomalous pathway. Intramural activation is recorded in the close bipolar leads from the adjacent deeper layers of the wall and is highly irregular, indicating possible intramural penetration of the anomalous pathway for about 4 mm. The well-developed initial deflection in the upper record, occurring after the P-wave, may be caused by activation of the anomalous pathway. At the left side the position of the intramural electrode in the ventricular wall is depicted schematically. The upper border is the epicardial surface. The figures indicate time of activation in ms, with the beginning of the left ventricular cavity complex as zero-reference

Ischaemic changes of transmembrane action potential

The changes in the transmembrane action potential in the ischaemic region of the intact heart follow a rather uniform pattern of development[23,60,61] (Figure 7). The first change is a decrease in the resting membrane potential from 90 mV to about 75 mV, without appreciable changes in its form and duration. In the following minutes the velocity of the upstroke decreases, the duration of the transmembrane action potential shortens, the peak voltage (overshoot) decreases, phase 2 of the transmembrane action potential does not reach the zero potential line. The resting potential diminishes to about −65 mV, when the cells become inexcitable.

Ischaemic changes in epicardial and intramural electrograms

These are a direct consequence of the cellular changes. The time of activation of ischaemic cells is gradually delayed and the decreasing strength of the extracellular currents during depolarization is reflected in its decrease in size,

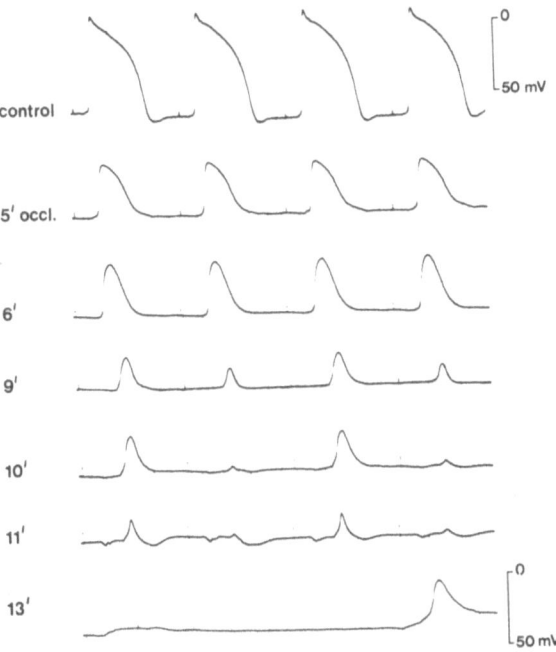

Figure 7 Intracellular potentials following coronary artery occlusion in the isolated pig heart. They are similar to those occurring in the isolated human heart. Alternation is present after 9 min of occlusion, with block after 13 min

rapidity of downstroke and time of occurrence of the intrinsic deflection. The remnant of this deflection eventually disappears completely in the mono-phasic QRST complexes.

Mechanism of ST elevation

ST elevation in epicardial electrograms is caused by a diastolic and a systolic phenomenon (Figure 8). The diastolic phenomenon is a TQ depression caused by the decreased resting membrane potential of the ischaemic cells. Intracellular current flows from the less negative (−75 mV) injured cells to the adjacent normal cells (−90 mV), leaks to the extracellular space and there causes a current in the reverse direction. The ischaemic region will appear negative in respect to the surrounding normal muscle. This TQ shift causes a relative ST elevation, because the depressed T–Q portion is used as the baseline in the clinical evaluation of ST shift. The systolic phenomenon, which begins a few minutes later, is caused by the shortening of transmem-brane action potential duration and the decrease in overshoot. During systole the intra- and extracellular current flow changes direction. The ischaemic region will now be positive in respect to the normal myocardium (true ST elevation).

The ST segment shift is therefore a consequence of the electrical inter-action between ischaemic and normal cells. ST elevation can be influenced

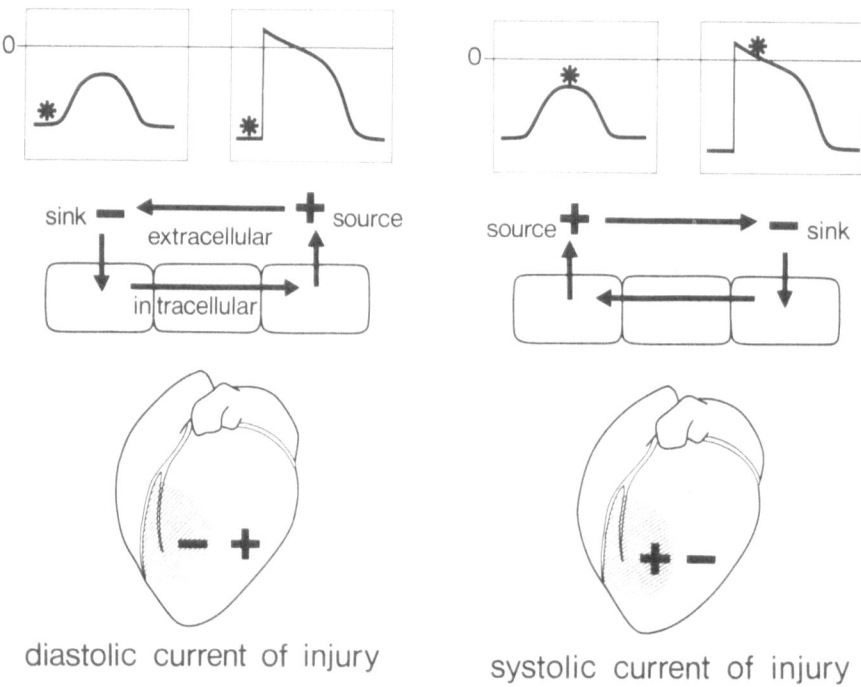

diastolic current of injury   systolic current of injury

Figure 8 The diastolic injury current is caused by a decrease in the diastolic resting membrane potential (left side). This results in negativity of the injured region in the extracellular space. During systole the situation is reversed due to shortening of the ischaemic transmembrane action potential and decrease of its overshoot which does not reach the zero line

by changes in transmembrane action potentials of normal or ischaemic cells or both. The oldest method used to influence the degree of ischaemia is a glucose–insulin–potassium solution, introduced in 1963 by Sodi-Pallaris et al.[62]. The electrophysiological analysis of ST shift, as given above, makes it possible to give an alternative explanation. The increased extracellular K^+ concentration will reduce the resting potential of the normal cells, with little or no damage to the potential of the completely or partially ischaemic cells. These effects will reduce the diastolic intracellular current between ischaemic and normal cells with a resultant decrease in TQ depression which, if recorded with the usual AC amplifier ECG apparatus, would be interpreted as a decreased ST elevation.

Strength of the injury current in border zone

Recently we have measured the strength of the currents flowing between ischaemic and normal myocardium[23]. The maximal current density was $1 \mu A/mm^2$ during late systole, the current flowing towards the normal myocardium. It is of sufficient strength to consider the possibility that it may initiate automaticity of ventricular muscle[24,63].

Border zone

Electrophysiological and histological investigations demonstrated that in the pig heart the boundary between ischaemic (infarcted) and normal regions is very sharp. There appears to be no twilight zone which can be 'saved'[64]. For the human heart with multi-vessel coronary heart disease and a complex intramyocardial perfusion pattern, this conclusion may not apply.

Ventricular arrhythmias and delayed activity in ischaemic myocardium

Delayed depolarization of smaller or larger clusters of ischaemic cells also causes delayed repolarization of these cells[23]. Delayed repolarization is

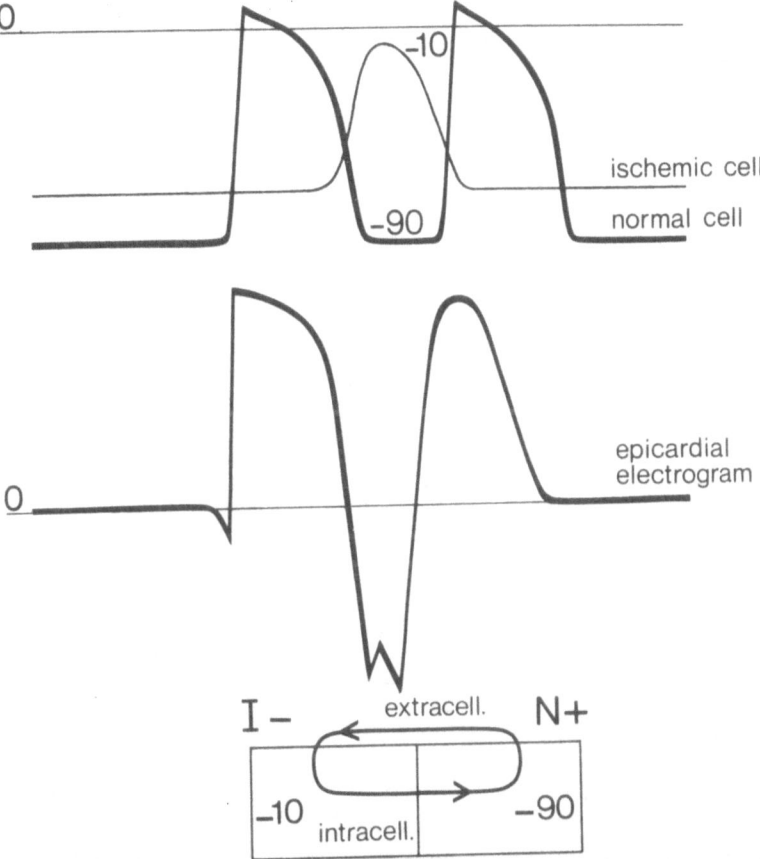

Figure 9 The upper two tracings were recorded in a patient with variant form of angina pectoris. During pain, monophasic deflections are recorded which have a pronounced negative T-wave, followed by a monophasic ventricular premature beat. In the lower panel from a dog heart, the electrogram of the ischaemic region is recorded synchronously with a transmembrane action potential of an ischaemic cell. Its upstroke coincides with the beginning of a deep negative deflection, notched near its apex. Therefore, the 'T-wave' is caused by delayed electrical activity of a cluster of ischaemic cells

indicated by a deep and broad negative 'T-wave' in the electrogram from this region. If this cluster is situated relatively close to the normal myocardium, current flow in the intracellular and extracellular spaces will be as depicted in Figure 9. At a time when the normal cells are repolarized, intracellular current will flow from relatively positive ischaemic cells towards the normal cells, act as a depolarizing current, and a ventricular premature beat may follow.

ECG changes in variant form of angina pectoris

Multichannel recordings of patients with variant angina pectoris show sequences of complexes which suggest that this mechanism is responsible for some of the ventricular premature depolarizations occurring during the attacks. In Figure 10 the lower tracing was obtained in a dog heart; the epicardial complex from the ischaemic region was recorded synchronous

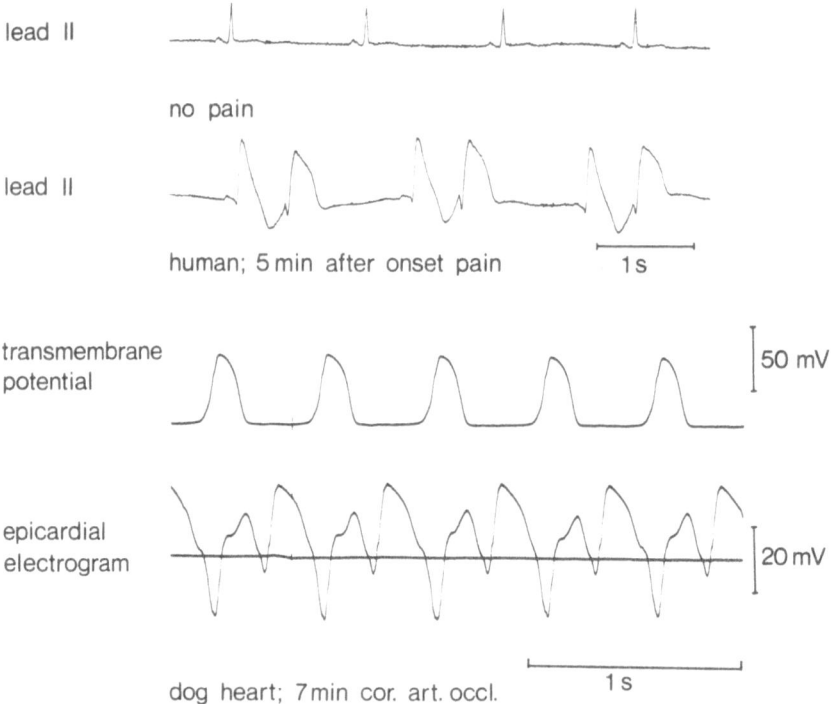

Figure 10 *Upper panel:* the transmembrane action potential of an ischaemic cell is situated between two transmembrane action potentials of an adjacent normal cell. *Lower panel:* epicardial electrogram of ischaemic region. Intracellular current during deep negative deflection in the electrogram is determined by the difference between the intracellular potentials of the ischaemic (-10 mV) and the normal cells (-90 mV). This current is directed from ischaemic cells towards normal cells; the extracellular current will be in the reverse direction and cause negativity of the ischaemic surface. During the latter part of this deflection the non-ischaemic part of the ventricles is activated

with a transmembrane action potential of an ischaemic cell. The upper tracing is the precordial ECG of a patient with variant form of angina pectoris during an attack. The correspondence between the tracings is striking.

Ventricular arrhythmias in acute myocardial infarction

In the early stages of myocardial infarction ventricular arrhythmias may be caused by excitation waves, initiated by delayed activated epicardial regions[65-67]. In the dog ischaemic heart an inward spread of depolarization is favoured by several factors. The ischaemic changes in the outer layers decrease because collateral circulation gradually improves. In some sites of the considerably changed ischaemic inner layers, where a network of surviving ischaemic cells may be present, normal outward depolarization is blocked, but conduction in the opposite direction is possible (Figure 11). In this

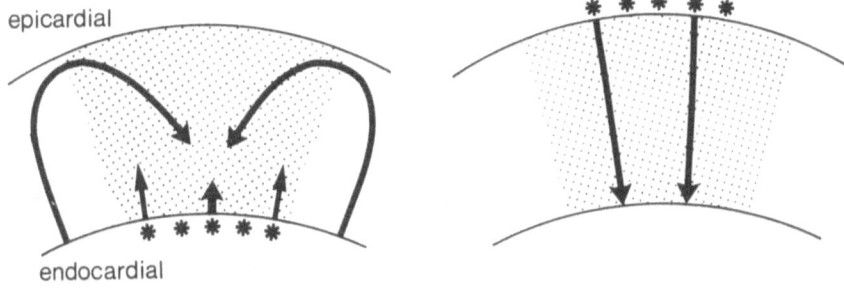

endocardial stimulation   epicardial stimulation

Figure 11 During acute ischaemia and infarction normal outward-moving depolarization may be blocked at some subendocardial layers. This remains so after stimulation of five subendocardial terminals. During these beats inward-moving depolarization waves can be found in the outer layers of the ischaemic region, which may also be present during normal beats. Following subepicardial stimulation of five terminals the inward-moving depolarization wave may cross the endocardial layers, which therefore have a unidirectional block

respect it is interesting that Ashman demonstrated that conduction from normal into damaged muscle may be possible, while conduction in the other direction is blocked[68]. This inward-moving excitation wave has been recorded in some instances of ventricular premature beats and ventricular tachycardia in dog hearts (Figure 12). The mechanism of arrhythmias in the later stages of experimental myocardial infarction was studied extensively by Scherlag, El Sherif and Lazzara et al.[67-69].

Ventricular tachycardia in coronary heart disease

The electrophysiology of the mechanisms responsible for the ventricular arrhythmias such as ventricular premature depolarization, ventricular

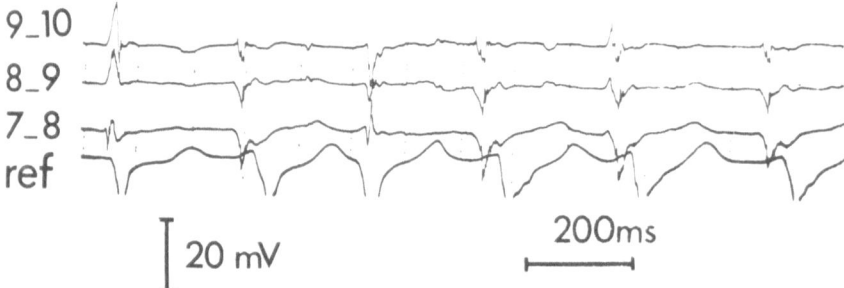

Figure 12 Bipolar complexes between consecutive terminals of an intramural electrode. Number 10 is located in the subepicardium, number 7 closer to the subendocardium. Positivity of bipolar complexes indicates outward spread of depolarization, while negativity is caused by inward spread. The reference complex is from the left ventricular cavity. Ischaemia and infarction were present following occlusion of the coronary artery, several hours previously. The electrode was therefore situated at the border of the region. The first complex is a normally conducted sinus beat with outward-spreading depolarization through the wall and is followed by ventricular premature beats which all show inward-moving intramural depolarization. The tachycardia is therefore caused by re-entry

tachycardia and ventricular fibrillation in patients with old myocardial infarction often associated with disease of many vessels is now studied when surgical intervention is contemplated because of intractable attacks[12,70,76].

The results of isolated human heart studies suggest the presence of abundant opportunities for re-entering mechanisms, occurring in regions dispersed throughout the ventricular walls[10]. Many small or larger regions with a highly irregular activation pattern can be found. If located in the subepicardial region of a transmural scar, a series of small rapid deflections following the QS complex can be found in the epicardial electrograms[10,11,71]. Here too a network of surviving slowly conducting myocardial fibres is present in which re-entering wavelets might occur easily (Figure 13). In some dog hearts with old myocardial infarction we have elicited ventricular premature beats from points located at the circumference of the infarction. Many of them penetrated the intra-infarction network without eliciting return beats. However, at some sites re-entry beats could be elicited. Geometric–electric conditions—as yet unknown—may be responsible for this re-entry phenomenon. In some instances repetitive activity did occur, causing ventricular tachycardia, which sometimes deteriorates to ventricular fibrillation.

Intramural circulating waves in human heart and re-entry

Different mechanisms may be expected in hearts with extensive coronary heart disease. In a revived heart of a patient with an old apical and a recent large postero-inferior myocardial infarction, excitation started in the left

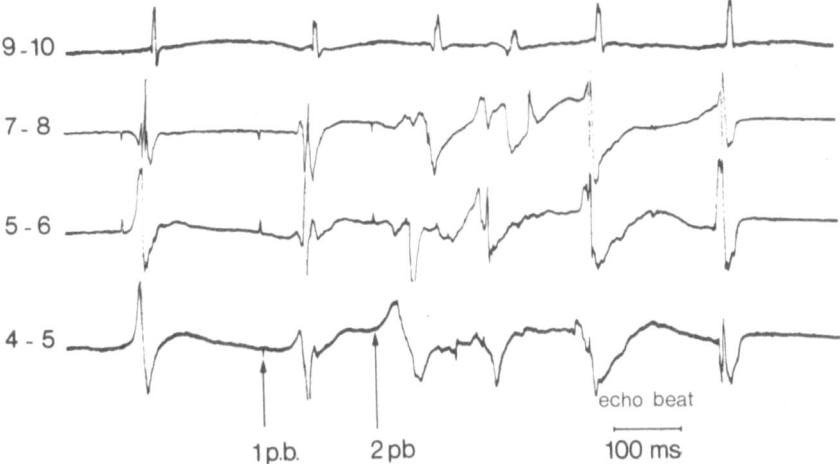

Figure 13 An intramural electrode was situated in the middle of an old myocardial infarction in the dog heart. During driving from the right ventricle two ventricular premature beats (1pb, 2pb) were induced. The intramural complexes following the second ventricular premature beat indicate that a highly irregular excitation pattern was present in all layers except 9–10. About 300 ms after the second ventricular premature beat an echo beat occurs. There is no appreciable intra-infarction electrical activity after this complex

side of the anterior ventricular septum[10]. Intramural excitation in the anteroseptal region was very unusual because the successive layers were activated nearly synchronously. This was caused by an intramural depolarizing front oriented almost perpendicularly to the normal inward–outward spreading depolarization front. It rotated slowly from the anterior insertion of the septum through anterior and lateral ventricular wall towards the postero-inferior infarction, where it stopped. Ventricular tachycardias occurred readily, but their mechanism could not be elucidated. Some relation with this rotating depolarizing front seems likely, because here only one pathway suffices to cause a circulating wave. The diffuse fibrotic changes found in the specific conduction system, Purkinje system and myocardium set the scene for this unusual excitation pattern.

Ventricular fibrillation and the initiating beat

The genesis of the first, spontaneously occurring depolarization wave initiating ventricular fibrillation is as yet unknown[72]. In ischaemia and infarction an early, depolarization wave re-entering through this region might initiate ventricular fibrillation, probably by setting up secondary excitation waves in this region[65,73,74]. There are indications that ventricular fibrillation starts in a relatively small region before it invades the ventricles, and that this usually occurs within seconds[74,75]. The fibrillating region acts as a focus, and might be responsible for the tachysystolic phase of ventricular fibrillation. In the Coronary Care Unit attacks of seconds' duration of irregular, rapid ventricular tachycardia may be recorded, which may occur repetitively and eventually cause ventricular fibrillation. One might speculate that these attacks are caused by local fibrillation[74].

This short survey is a presentation 'in a nutshell', with some characteristics of a desert-island approach, because the selection from the impressive body of information available necessarily had to be a subjective one.

References

1. Harvey, W. (1894). *An Anatomical Dissertation upon the Movement of the Heart.* Fascimile edition with a translation and memoir by G. Moreton (Canterbury)
2. Röding, J. H. (1793). *Allgemeines Wörterbuch der Marine* (Hamburg)
3. Matteucci, C. (1894). *Traité des Phénomènes Electrophysiologiques des Animaux,* pp. 59–60. (Paris)
4. Craib, W. H. (1930). The electrocardiogram. *Med. Res. Counc. Spec. Rep. Ser.* **147,** 1
5. Wilson, F. N., Macleod, A. G. and Barker, P. S. (1933). The distribution of the action currents produced by heart muscle and other excitable tissues immersed in extensive conducting media. *J. Gen. Physiol.,* **16,** 423
6. Clayton, P. D., Bulawa, W. F. and Urie, H. W. (1977). The characteristic pattern for the onset of contraction in the normal left ventricle. *Circulation,* **56,** II, 126
7. Adomian, G. E., Beazell, J. W. and Furmanski, M. (1977). The production of myofibrillar disarray in hearts of normal dogs produced by chronic electronic pacing. *Circulation,* **56,** II, 205
8. Noble, D. (1975). *The Initiation of the Heart Beat.* (Oxford: Clarendon Press)
9. Janse, M. J., Van Capelle, F. J. L. and Freud, G. E. (1971). Circus movement within the A–V node as a basis for supraventricular tachycardia as shown by multiple microelectrode recording in the isolated rabbit heart. *Circ. Res.,* **28,** 403.
10. Durrer, D. (1966). The human heart: some aspects of its excitation. *Trans. Coll. Phys. Philadelphia,* **33,** 159
11. Durrer, D., Van Lier, A. A. W. and Büller, J. (1964). Epicardial and intramural excitation in chronic myocardial infarction. *Am. Heart J.,* **68,** 765
12. Josephson, M. E., Horowitz, L. N. and Farshidi, A. (1978). Recurrent sustained ventricular tachycardia: *Circulation,* **57,** 431, 440
13. Langendorf, R. (1953). Ventricular premature beats with postponed compensatory pause. *Am. Heart J.,* **46,** 401
14. Pick, A. (1953). Parasystole. *Circulation,* **8,** 251
15. Langendorf, R. (1976). Newer aspects of concealed conduction of cardiac muscle. In H. J. J. Wellens, K. I. Lie and M. J. Janse (eds.). *The Conduction System of the Heart,* pp. 410–423. (Leiden)
16. Pick, A. (1972). The electrophysiologic basis of parasystole and its variants. In H. J. J. Wellens, K. I. Lie and M. J. Janse (eds.). *The Conduction System of the Heart,* pp. 143–162 (Leiden)
17. Pick, A. (1973). Mechanism of cardiac arrhythmias: from hypothesis to physiologic fact. *Am. Heart J.,* **86,** 249
18. Spurrell, R. A. J. (1976). Reciprocation. *Am. Heart J.,* **91,** 409

19. Krikler, D. M. and Goodwin, J. F. (1975). *Cardiac Arrhythmias*. (London: W. B. Saunders Co. Ltd.)

20. Moe, G. K. and Mendez, C. (1965). The physiological basis of reciprocal rhythm. *Prog. Card. Dis.*, **8**, 460

21. Mendez, C. and Moe, G. K. (1966). Demonstration of a dual A–V nodal conduction system in the isolated rabbit heart. *Circ. Res.*, **19**, 378

22. Lange, G. (1965). Action of driving stimuli from intrinsic and extrinsic sources on in situ cardiac pacemaker tissues. *Circ. Res.*, **17**, 449

23. Kleber, A. G., Janse, M. J. and Van Capelle, F. J. L. (1978). Mechanism and time course of ST and TQ segment changes during acute regional myocardial ischemia in the pig's heart determined by extracellular and intracellular recordings. *Circ. Res.*, **42**, 603

24. Katzung, B., Hondeghem, L. M. and Grant, A. O. (1975). Cardiac ventricular automaticity induced by current of injury. *Pfluegers Arch. Gesamte Physiol.*, **360**, 193

25. Van Capelle, F. J. L., du Perron, J. C. and Durrer, D. (1971). Atrioventricular conduction in isolated rat heart. *Am. J. Physiol.*, **221**, 284

26. Scherlag, B. J., Lau, S. H. and Helfant, R. H. (1969). Catheter technique for recording His bundle activity in man. *Circulation*, **39**, 13

27. Latour, H. and Puech, P. (1957). *Electrocardiographie Endo-cavitaire*. (Paris: Masson et Cie)

28. Puech, P. and Grolleau, R. (1972). *l'Activité du Faisceau de His Normale et Pathologique*. (Paris: Edition Sandoz)

29. Wellens, H. J. J. (1978). Value and limitation of programmed electrical stimulation of the heart in the study and treatment of tachycardias. *Circulation*, **57**, 845

30. Durrer, D. (1968). Electrical aspects of human cardiac activity: a clinical-physiological approach to excitation and stimulation. *Cardiovasc. Res.*, **2**, 1

31. Fleischmann, D. W., Pop, T. and de Bakker, J. M. T. (1977). Evidence for re-entry within the His–Purkinje system in man. In Kulbertus (ed.). *Re-entrant Arrhythmias*, p. 256. (Lancaster: MTP Press) 256

32. Hecht, H. H. and Woodbury, L. A. (1950). Excitation of human auricular muscle and the significance of the intrinsicord deflection of the auricular electrogram. *Circulation*, **2**, 37

33. Hombach, V., Behrenbeck, N. and Hilger, H. H. (1978). Die Ableitung von Sinusknotenpotentialen beim Menschen. *Z. Kreislaufforsch.*, **67**, 155

34. Van der Kooi, M. W., Durrer, D. and Van Dam, R. Th. (1956). Electrical activity in sinus node and atrioventricular node. *Am. Heart J.*, **51**, 684

35. Théry, Cl., Asseman, Ph. and Adamantidis, M. (1978). Enregistrement de l'echocardiogramme du noeud sinusal. *Arch. Mal. Coeur*, **71**, 121

36. Curry, P. V. L., Gallowhill, E. A. and Krikler, D. M. (1976). Paroxysmal reciprocating sinus tachycardia. *Br. Heart J.*, **38**, 311

37. Alessie, M. A. and Bonke, F. I. M. Direct demonstration of sinus node re-entry in the rabbit heart. (Submitted for publication)

38. Janse, M. J., Anderson, R. H. and van Capelle, F. J. L. (1976). A combined electrophysiological and anatomical study of the human fetal heart. *Am. Heart J.*, **91**, 556

39. Van Dam, R. Th. and Durrer, D. (1961). Excitability and electrical activity of human myocardial strips from the left atrial appendage in cases of rheumatic mitral stenosis. *Circ. Res.*, **9**, 509

40. Van Capelle, F. J. L., Janse, M. J. and Varghese, G. E. (1972). Spread of excitation in the atrioventricular node of isolated rabbit heart studied by multiple microelectrode recordings, *Circ. Res.*, **31**, 602

41. Waldo, A., MacLean, W. A. H. and Karp, R. B. (1977). Entrainment and interruption of atrial flutter with atrial pacing. *Circulation*, **56**, 737, 1977

42. Wellens, H. J. J., Janse, M. J., van Dam, R. Th., (1971). Epicardial excitation of the atria in a patient with artrial flutter. *Br. Heart J.* **33**, 233

43. Hoffman, B. F. and Cranefield, P. F. (1960). *Electrophysiology of the Heart.* (New York: McGraw-Hill)

44. Mendez, C. and Moe, G. K. (1966). Some characteristics of transmembrane potentials of AV nodal cells during propagation of premature beats. *Circ. Res.*, **19**, 993

45. Schuilenburg, R. M. and Durrer, D. (1968). Atrial echobeats in the human heart elicited by induced atrial premature beats. *Circulation*, **37**, 680

46. Moore, E. N. and Spear, J. F. (1976). Effect of autonomic activity on pacemaker function and conduction. In H. J. J. Wellens, K. I. Lie and M. J. Janse (eds.). *The Conduction System of the Heart*, pp. 100–110

47. Clarks, J. M., Shelton, J. R. and Hamer, J. (1976). The rhythm of the normal human heart. *Lancet*, **2**, 508

48. Durrer, D., Van Dam, R. Th. and Freud, G. E. (1970). Total excitation of the isolated human heart. *Circulation*, **41**, 899

49. Rosenbaum, M. B., Elizari, M. V. and Lazzari, J. O. (1970). *The hemiblocks.* (Oldsman, Florida: Tampa Tracings)

50. Watt, T. B., Freud, G. E. and Durrer, D. (1968). Left anterior arborization block combined with right bundle branch block in canine and primate hearts: an electrocardiographic study. *Circ. Res.*, **22**, 57

51. Pruitt, R. D. and Watt, T. B. (1971). On block of something less than a bundle branch, or of something more. *Circulation*, **43**, 775

52. Durrer, D., Schoo, L. and Schuilenburg, R. M. (1967). The role of premature beats in the initiation and the termination of supraventricular tachycardias in in the WPW syndrome. *Circulation*, **36**, 644

53. Gallagher, J. J., Gilbert, M. and Svenson, R. H. (1975). Wolff–Parkinson–White syndrome: the problem, evaluation and surgical correction. *Circulation*, **51**, 767

54. Laham, J. (1969). Le syndrome de Wolff–Parkinson–White. *Actualités Electro-cardiographiques* (Paris: Librairie Maloine, S.A.)

55. Becker, A. E., Anderson, R. H. and Durrer, D. (1978). The anatomical substrates of the Wolff–Parkinson–White syndrome: a clinico-pathologic correlation in 7 patients. *Circulation*, **57**, 870

56. Durrer, D. and Wellens, H. J. J. (1974). The Wolff–Parkinson–White syndrome anno 1973. *Eur. J. Cardiol.*, **1**, 347

57. Gallagher, J. J., Pritchett, E. L. C. and Sealy, W. C. (1978). The pre-excitation syndromes. *Prog. Cardiovasc. Dis.*, **20**, 285.

58. Fozzard, H. A. and Das Gupta, D. S. (1976). ST-segment potentials and mapping. *Circulation*, **54**, 533

59. Holland, R. P. and Brooks, H. (1975). Precordial and epicardial surface potentials during myocardial ischemia in the pig heart. A theoretical and experimental analysis of the TQ and ST segment. *Clin. Res.*, **37**, 471

60. Downar, E., Janse, M. J. and Durrer, D. (1977). The effect of acute coronary occlusion on subepicardial transmembrane potentials in the intact porcine heart. *Circulation*, **56**, 217

61. Samson, W. E. and Scher, A. M. (1960). Mechanism of ST–T segment alteration during acute myocardial injury. *Circ. Res.*, **8**, 780

62. Sodi-Pallares, D., Bisteni, A. and Mediano, G. A. (1963). The polarizing treatment of acute myocardial infarction – possibility of its use in other cardiovascular conditions. *Dis. Chest*, **43**, 424

63. Dekker, E. (1970). Direct current make and break threshold for pacemaker in the canine ventricle. *Circ. Res.*, **27**, 811

64. Janse, M. J., Cinca, J. and Moréna, H. The 'borderzone' in myocardial ischemia, an electrophysiological, metabolic and histochemical correlation in the pig heart. (Submitted for publication)

65. Durrer, D., Van Dam, R. Th. and Freud, G. E. (1971). Re-entry and ventricular arrhythmias in local ischemia and infarction in the intact dog heart. *Kon. Ned. Academie v. Wetenschappen* (Proceedings Series C), **74**, 321

66. Scherlag, B. J., El Sherif, N. and Hope, R. R. (1974). Characterization and localization of ventricular arrhythmias resulting from myocardial ischemia and infarction. *Circ. Res.*, **35**, 372

67. Scherlag, B. J., Hope, R. R. and Williams, D. O. (1976). Mechanisms of ectopic rhythm formation due to myocardial ischemia: effects of heart rate and ventricular premature beats. In H. J. J. Wellens, K. I. Lie and M. J. Janse (eds.). *The Conduction System of the Heart*, pp. 633–649 (Leiden)

68. Ashman, R. and Hull, E. (1945). *Essentials of Electrocardiography* (New York: MacMillan)

69. El-Sherif, N., Lazzara, R. and Hope, R. R. (1977). Re-entrant ventricular arrhythmias in the late myocardial infarction period. *Circulation*, **55**, 686; **55**, 702; **56**, 225; **56**, 395

70. Wellens, H. J. J., Düren, D. R. and Lie, K. I. (1976). Observations on mechanisms of ventricular tachycardia in man. *Circulation*, **54**, 237

71. Fontaine, G., Guiraudon, G. and Fraule, R. (1975). La cartographie epicardique et le traitement chirurgicale par simple ventriculotomie de certaines tachycardies rebelles par réentrée. *Arch. Mal. Coeur*, **68**, 113

72. Wiggers, C. J. (1940). The mechanism and nature of ventricular fibrillation. *Am. Heart J.*, **20**, 399

73. Durrer, D. (1977). Les mécanismes de certaines arythmies au cours de l'insuffisance coronaire aiguë et chronique. *Bull. Mém. l'Acad. Roy. Méd. de Belgique*, **132**, 551

74. Garrey, W. E. (1924). Auricular fibrillation. *Physiol. Rev.*, **4**, 215

75. Moe, G. K., Harris, A. S. and Wiggers, C. J. (1941). Analysis of the initiation of fibrillation by electrocardiographic studies. *Am. J. Physiol.*, **134**, 473

76. Wellens, H. J. J., Schuilenburg, R. M. and Durrer, D. (1972). Electrical stimulation of the heart in patients with ventricular tachycardia. *Circulation*, **46**, 216

6
Human intracardiac electrocardiography

P. PUECH

DEVELOPMENT OF INTRACARDIAC ELECTROCARDIOGRAPHY

Intracardiac electrocardiography was first carried out in man 33 years ago, when Lenègre and Maurice, using a conductive filament introduced within a Cournand catheter, recorded electrical potentials from the right atrium and ventricle[1]. The field of intracardiac exploration of the right side of the heart developed rapidly both in Europe and North America[2-12], to be followed by indirect recording of the activity of the left atrium via the coronary sinus[13-15] and of left ventricular potentials by retrograde arterial catheterization[16-19]. The Montpelier School has used this method, in particular, in the study of cardiac arrhythmias[20,21]. The first intracardiac recordings of electrical activity in the bundle of His in man was made by us in 1957, while studying a patient with a congenital heart disorder (pulmonary stenosis with intact interventricular septum). The tracing, recorded with a unipolar electrode introduced through the brachial vein, is shown in Figure 1. Similar recordings were obtained by our group and published in 1960[22]. Ten years later Watson et al.[23] reported a case of Ebstein's anomaly in whom a His bundle electrogram was recorded; they concluded that the abnormal insertion of septal leaflet of the tricuspid valve had rendered this feasible. The decisive step in the history of intracardiac recording of electrical activity from the bundle of His was the demonstration by Scherlag and Damato[24] that this could be accomplished via a catheter electrode passed through a leg vein and that this could be done percutaneously through the femoral space. Activity from the bundle of His was recorded when the tip of the catheter was placed near the superior margin of the tricuspid valve. The activity of the proximal portion of the right bundle branch is quite often detected in the same way. An electrogram from the bundle of His may also be obtained during retrograde arterial catheterization when the tip of the catheter is placed in the region of the posterior aortic cusp. Figure 2 shows the different positions from which His bundle electrograms can be recorded. Activity from the left bundle branch can be demonstrated when the tip of the electrode is placed about 1.5 cm below the aortic valve, towards the interventricular septum[25-27].

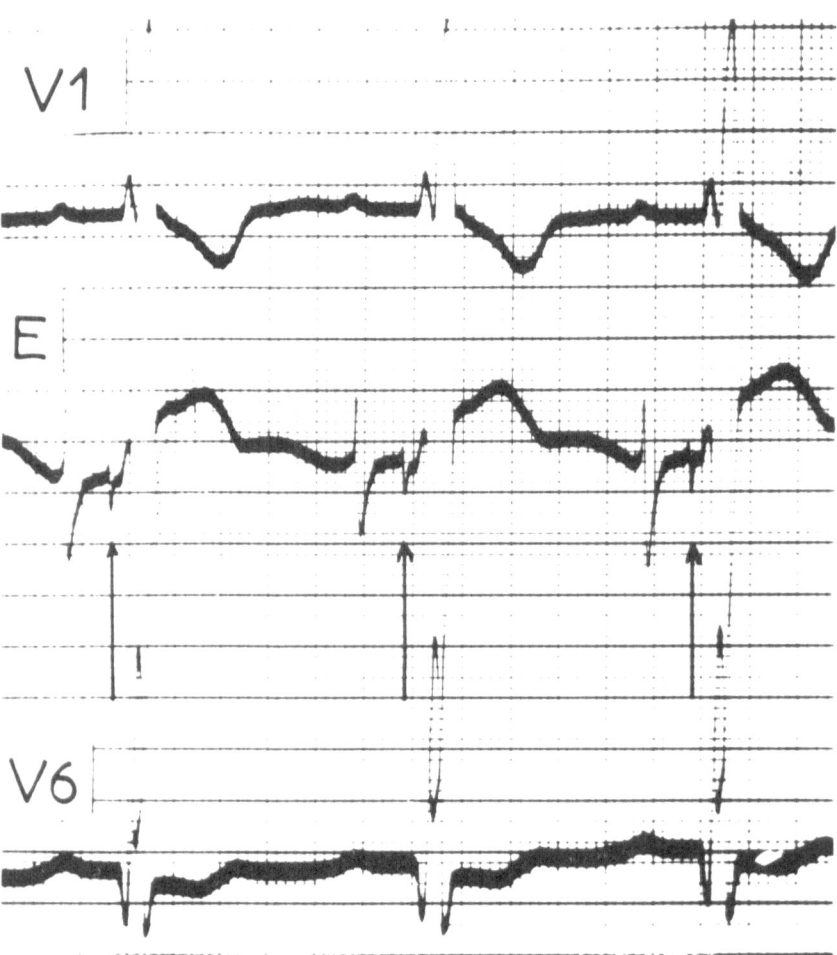

Figure 1 First recording of the activity of the bundle of His (indicated by the arrows) obtained in 1957 by an intracardiac unipolar electrode introduced through the brachial vein

TECHNICAL ASPECTS OF INTRACARDIAC ELECTROCARDIOGRAPHY

Catheter electrodes

Various models of catheter electrodes are available, the choice of type depending upon the purpose for which it is to be used.

The simplest catheter has a floating or semi-floating electrode (with balloon tip) which can be introduced without fluoroscopic observation. This technique is adequate to study atrial activity and one can occasionally record activity from the bundle of His[28], but is not appropriate for detailed intraventricular study.

Intracardiac electrocardiography may also be undertaken with a catheter size 5 or 6 F and bipolar electrodes with an interelectrode distance of up to 10 mm. Tripolar and quadripolar electrodes are also used frequently, in order to obtain simultaneous recordings of activity from the right atrium and bundle of His, or in the technique when one pair of electrodes is used for recording and one pair for intracardiac electrical stimulation.

More elaborate intracardiac recordings may be made with multipolar electrodes with varying distances between the electrodes[29,30]. In order to assist positioning in different areas, a special bipolar electrode can be modified with a Brockenbrough guide wire[31].

Recordings by the unipolar and bipolar techniques

UNIPOLAR RECORDINGS

The electrodes are influenced by local phenomena (activation of the endo-cardial portion of the wall close to the electrode) and those at a distance (activation of the whole heart), in relation to the distance which separates the electrode from the wall. The differences of potential recorded in the unipolar electrodes are usually larger than those with bipolar methods. The shape and polarity indicate the general direction of cardiac activation, thus a negative electrogram represents an activation process travelling away from the electrode while a positive complex represents activation towards the electrode. A rapid deflection in a unipolar electrogram represents change in electrical activity in the neighbouring portion of the endocardium. It is only possible to utilise unipolar recordings to measure the exact time of local activation if the electrode is very close to the part to be studied (large deflection, rapid change and a small contribution from more distant changes). Unipolar recordings are particularly useful for studying slowly changing events, for example atrial repolarisation and in particular that of the auricles, which are not seen on surface recordings[20]. Recently unipolar epicardiac recordings have made it possible to study the slow activation of the sino-atrial node which precedes the rapid potential due to atrial depolarization[32-36]. Demonstration of activity in the atrioventricular node[22] needs to be confirmed.

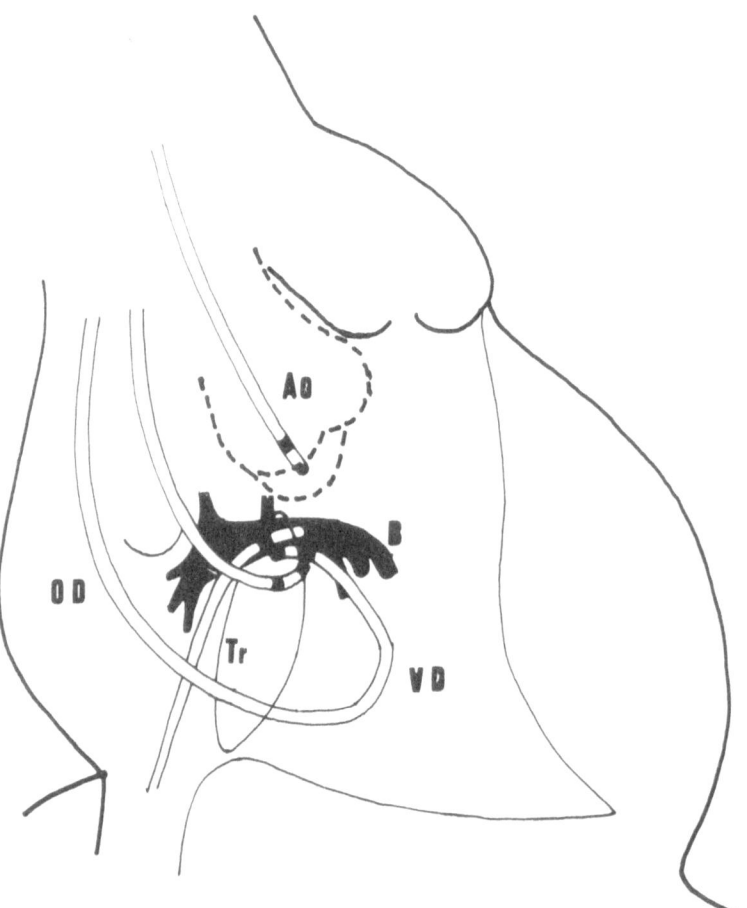

Figure 2 Position of catheter electrodes for recording of activity from the bundle of His. OD = right atrium; VD = right ventricle; H = bundle of His; B = bundle branch.

Bipolar electrograms reflect the differences in potential between the two electrodes; depending on the type, these are between 1 and 10 mm apart. They reflect local activity, with only negligible contribution from distant electrical events. Thus maximal deflections in the bipolar electrogram provide accurate representations of activation in neighbouring structures (atrium, bundle of His, ventricle). Maximum precision is achieved with minimum separation of the electrodes. Bipolar electrograms can only be used for analysis of the local potential, for the filters are usually set at between 40 and 500 Hz, which improves the stability of the baseline without interfering with the high frequency changes which predominate during depolarization of the atrium, the ventricle and the bundle of His and its branches.

Recordings within the right side of the heart

Numerous transvenous approaches to the right atrial and ventricular cavities are possible and may be used simultaneously for the introduction of several electrodes for detailed intracardiac study. They include, currently, unilateral and bilateral percutaneous femoral approaches and approach through the brachial vein at the elbow, with or without exposure of the vein. The jugular and subclavian vein are only rarely justified.

The object of right-sided intracardiac study is essentially the mapping of the cavities and the recording of activity from the conducting tissues. Mapping of the right atrium may be undertaken directly, but while occasionally that of the left may be achieved at the same time, when there is a patent foramen ovale, it is usually achieved indirectly. Recording from the orifice of the coronary sinus reflects the activity of the posterio-inferior part of the left atrium, those in the pulmonary artery trunk reflect the left atrium while those from the beginning of the right pulmonary artery represent those at the top of the left atrium[20,37,38]. Recording the activity in the bundle of His and in the proximal portion of the right bundle branch are usually easy via the femoral route, but may be impossible (e.g. in inferior vena cava thrombosis, amputation), difficult (in obesity) or dangerous (e.g. local infection, phlebitis, heart failure with oedema). The alternative approach via the brachial vein is possible and the positioning of the electrode in the region of the bundle of His is facilitated by certain special techniques[39,40]. Epicardial maps obtained in the dog[41,43] and in man during surgery[42] have demonstrated that the great veins show electrical activity. After starting from the right atrium the activation spreads in the wall of the superior vena cava in man for a distance of 4 to 5 cm and after leaving the left atrium, depolarization penetrates the walls of the pulmonary veins as far as the line of reflection of the pericardium. In the dog spread along the veins is even further. The double deflections which may be recorded frequently in intracardiac electro-cardiography in the superior vena cava and the pulmonary veins are perhaps due to the interaction of electrical changes in the vein and in adjacent areas of the atrium. The fact that the region of the coronary sinus shows a high automatic potential[15] is confirmed by studies on isolated portions of coronary veins[44].

Recordings within the left side of the heart

In addition to the opportunity to study the left atrium and ventricle afforded by septal defects, they can also be explored by retrograde catheterization via the brachial or femoral artery.

Exploration of the left side makes it possible to record the activity of the bundle of His and the left bundle branch and to map the left ventricular cavity. It is currently restricted to a group of patients for whom coronary arteriography and/or left ventricular investigation is justified, in particular when surgical intervention is contemplated for recurrent ventricular tachycardia[45].

APPLICATIONS OF INTRACARDIAC ELECTROCARDIOGRAPHY

Atrial conduction in sinus rhythm

Internodal conduction corresponds to the interval separating the initial atrial depolarization in the region of the sinus node and the activation of the

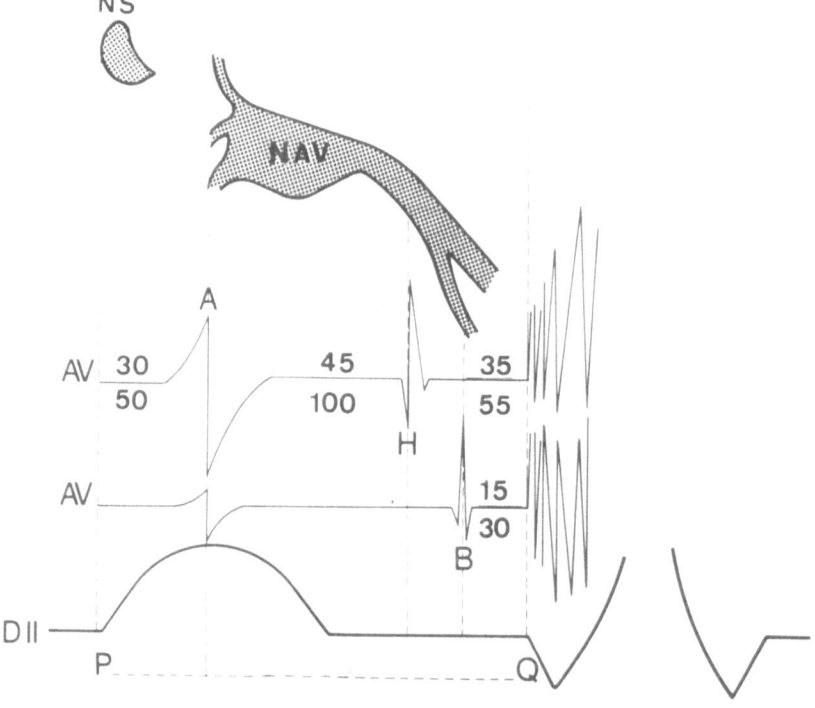

Figure 3 Schematic representation of study of atrioventricular conduction in intracardiac studies. NS = sinus node; NAV = atrioventricular node; AV (above) recording of electrogram from the bundle of His (H); AV (below) recording of activity of the right branch (B). The figures expressed in milliseconds, represent the minimum and maximum physiological conduction intervals. PA = Inter-nodal conduction time; AH = Conduction time through the AV node; HV = Conduction time in the His–Purkinje tissue

interatrial septum in the region of the atrioventricular node (PA interval). This interval is measured from the beginning of the P-wave on a surface lead (or the earliest deflection in the upper portion of the right atrium) and the deflection in the electrogram which corresponds with the start of activity in the bundle of His (Figure 3). The normal time for this interval is, in our experience, between 30 and 50 ms in the adult. It only represents a fraction of the intra-atrial conduction time[46].

Detailed atrial study enables one to measure the inter-atrial conduction time between the superior parts of the right and left atria; this is shown by the difference between the atrial defections in the high right atrial electrogram and that recorded from the proximal portion of the right pulmonary artery[20,38]. The interval between the onset of right atrial activity and the end of left atrial depolarization recorded in the great coronary vein determines

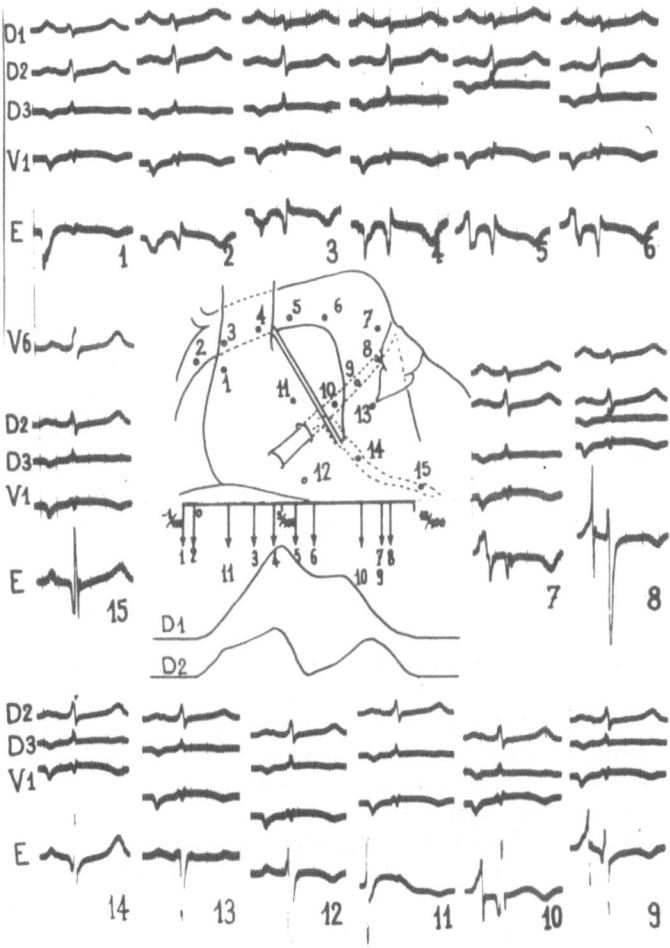

Figure 4 Atrial map in a case of left atrial dilatation with slowing of inter-atrial conduction

the *maximal intra-atrial conduction time*. Physiologically left atrial depolarisation recorded via the pulmonary trunk precedes that in the lowest portion of the left atrium.

Atrial mapping thus enables one to obtain evidence of conduction abnormalities within and between the atria. Figure 4 is an example of a detailed atrial map, recorded 25 years ago with a unipolar electrode catheter, showing slowing and prolongation of left atrial depolarization in a patient with mitral valve disease.

Retrograde atrial conduction

Retrograde atrial conduction may be seen during episodes of paroxysmal reciprocating supraventricular tachycardia or when ventricular stimuli are propagated to the atria. The value of atrial mapping in these subjects with paroxysmal tachycardia, with or without over ventricular pre-excitation in sinus rhythm has been reinforced during the past few years by the need for better definition of the mechanism should the possibility of surgical intervention need consideration[47-50].

Initial depolarization of the lower part of the septum, followed by ascending and symmetrical activation of the right and left atria shows that the retrograde excitation of the atria may orginate from the AV node (intra-nodal re-entry, ectopic AV rhythm, ectopic ventricular rhythm with retrograde propagation through the normal pathways), or from a region of the septum close to the AV junction (accessory atrio-nodal bypass, atrio-His bypass, bundle of Kent lying within the septum).

Asymmetric retrograde depolarization of the atria with the depolarization of one atrium preceding that of the septum and other atrium is very characteristic of the presence of a lateral accessory atrio-ventricular bypass (parietal bundle of Kent). Atrial mapping during tachycardia with reciprocal rhythm permits the recognition of concealed accessory bypasses, in the absence of Wolff–Parkinson–White syndrome in sinus rhythm. With overt pre-excitation during sinus rhythm, atrial mapping shows whether the accessory pathway is utilized in the reciprocal rhythm (distinguishing a reciprocal intranodal rhythm: providing evidence of dual accessory bypasses).

Figure 5 is an example of paroxysmal tachycardia with reciprocal rhythm using a left parietal bundle of Kent, inapparent during sinus rhythm. In tachycardia atrial depolarization is recorded first in the distal portion of the coronary sinus then activation is seen at the base of the atrial septum (site of the bundle of His) and the atrial free wall activated last. The appearance of functional left bundle branch block in the course of tachycardia does not modify the order of retrograde atrial depolarization but prolongs the VA interval and slows the tachycardia, a further argument in favour of the presence of an accessory bypass between the left atrium and ventricle[51-58].

The retrograde depolarisation of the left atrium in the presence of a left parietal bundle of Kent gives rise to a negative P-wave following the QRS complex in surface lead I as shown in Figure 6. This sign, which we have previously described[55,58] and which has been confirmed[59], is useful for recognizing concealed left accessory bypasses.

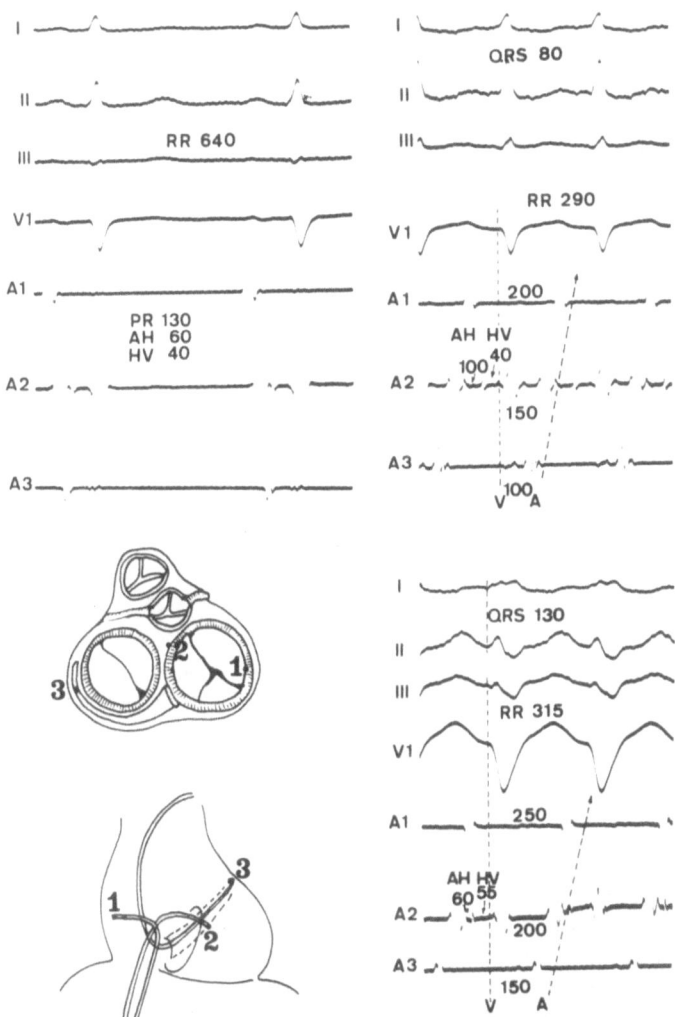

Figure 5 Latent left accessory parietal atrioventricular conduction pathway. *Left upper portion*: in sinus rhythm depolarization of the right atrium (1) preceeds that of the base of the atrial septum (recording from the bundle of His – 2) and that of the left atrium (recording from distal coronary sinus – 3). *Right upper portion*: in reciprocating paroxysmal tachycardia, retrograde depolarization of the left atrium precedes that of the base of the atrial septum and of the right atrium. *Right lower portion*: functional left branch block slows the tachycardia by lengthening the VA interval to retrograde conduction, but the left atrium remains the first area to be depolarized.

85

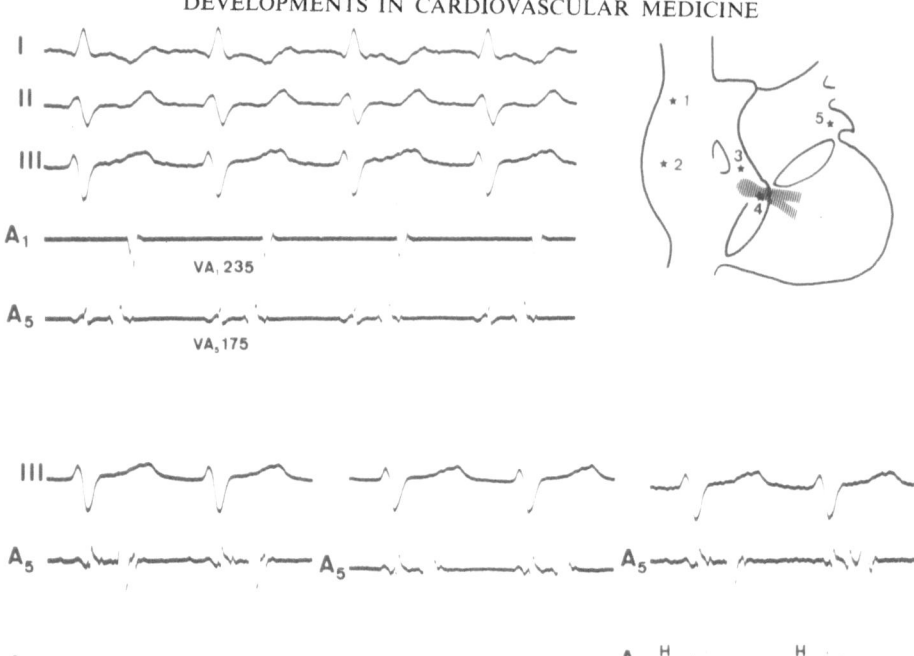

Figure 6 Tachycardia with reciprocal rhythm using a left parietal bundle of Kent. The first atrial depolarisation (shortest VA interval) is recorded in the left atrium. Note negative P-wave in lead I

Atrial fusion beats

Here simultaneous depolarization of both atria occurs from two waves of excitation through different regions. It implies synchronous activation of the high right atrium from the sinus node and of the distal atria by impulses derived from the AV junction[20] or by a simultaneous double retrograde atrial depolarization in the course of ventricular stimulation, the excitation being derived at the same time along the normal passage from the AV node-bundle of His axis as well via an accessory atrio-ventricular pathway (personal unpublished observations).

Activity in atrial arrhythmias

Atrial mapping in the *common form of atrial flutter* shows a specific pattern of atrial depolarization, ascending the atrial septum and left atrium and descending the right atrial free wall, associated, in our experience, with considerable prolongation of right intra-atrial conduction[60], as seen in some experimentally produced flutters[61]. Atrial depolarization is different in atypical (the uncommon form of) flutter and in atrial tachycardias[60].

During *atrial fibrillation* intracardiac recording shows diffuse desynchronization of the atria and the presence of some areas where the electrical activity is less rapid and more organized, in particular the region between the superior vena cava and the right atrium[20].

The coexistence of different ectopic rhythms in the atria has been documented[62,63]. Figure 7 is an example of the association of the common form of atrial flutter and of atrial fibrillation localized, to a limited area of the base

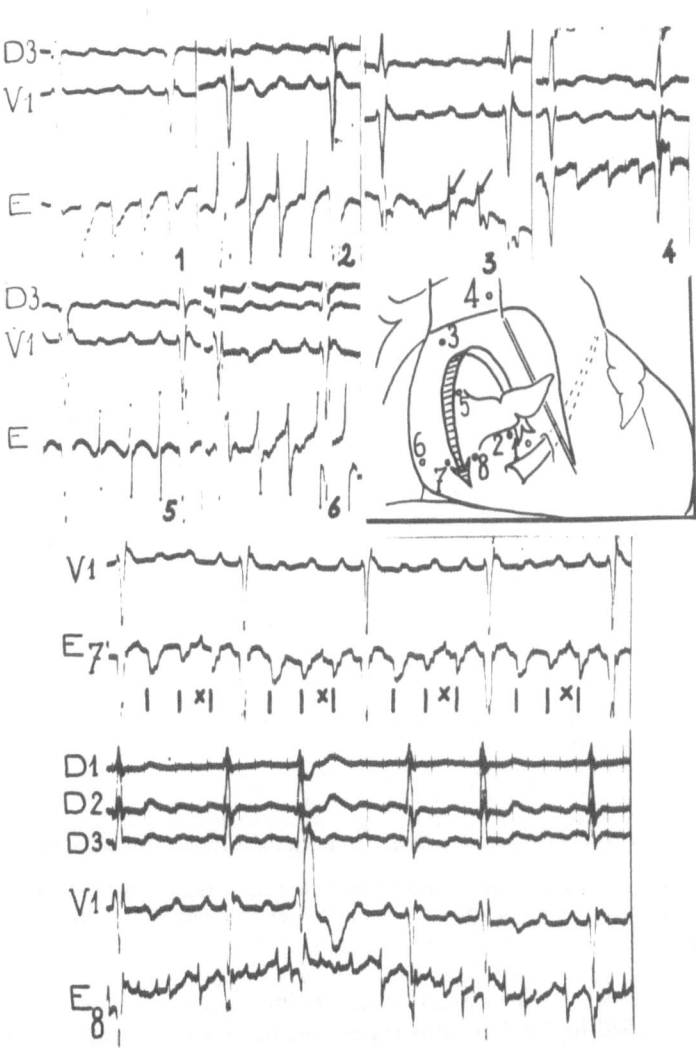

Figure 7 Association of typical atrial flutter (as recorded with surface electrodes) and localized atrial fibrillation in the lower part of the right atrium (position E8). In the border zone (position E7) there is additional regular electrical activity after four flutter waves (indicated by **X**)

of the right auricle, at the same time that atrial activity appears normally organized in the surface leads and in the other intracardiac recordings.

Figure 8 illustrates a case of typical (common) atrial flutter with localised intra-atrial Wenckebach phenomenon in the region at the junction of the superior vena cava and the right auricle. The Wenckebach phenomenon or 2:1 intra-atrial block can be demonstrated by incremental atrial pacing in patients who frequently show the 'sick sinus syndrome'[64-68]. Complete intra-atrial dissociation is very rare and in the majority of reported cases the signs represent artefacts of respiratory origin.

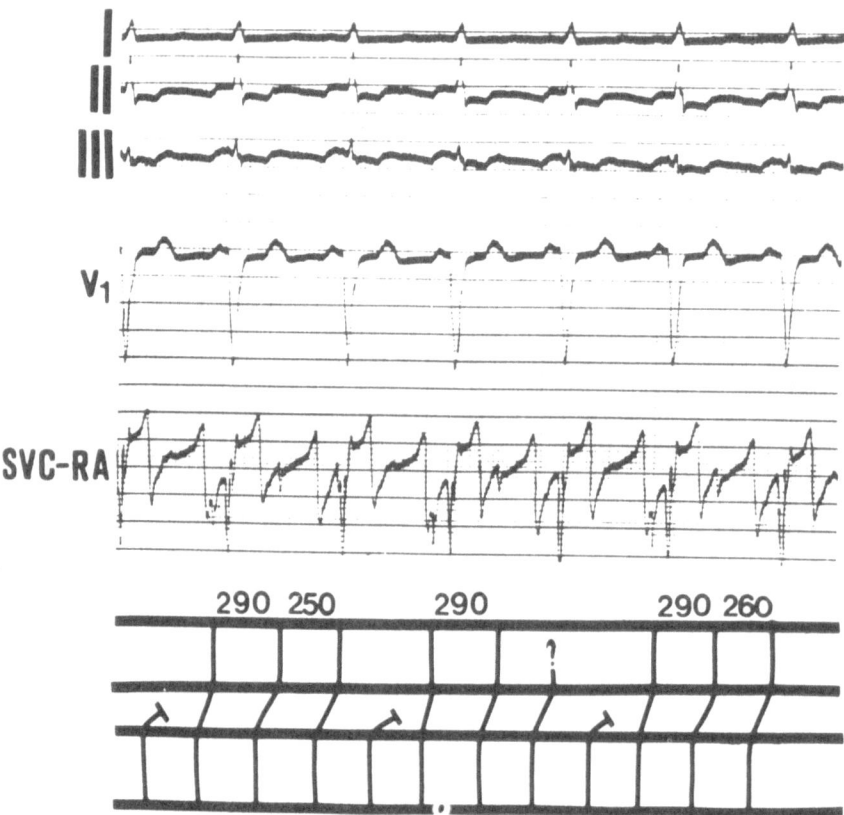

Figure 8 Intra-atrial Wenckebach phenomenon recorded from the right atrium and the superior vena cava during an episode of common atrial flutter in the rest of the right atrium

Figure 9 shows a slow parasystolic activity, at a rate of less than 35 a minute, recorded in the peri-sinus region during atrial tachycardia and after DC conversion of the tachycardia.

Atrial paralysis, either transient or persistent is shown by the absence of activity in intracardiac electrograms and inability to stimulate the quiescent areas[68-71].

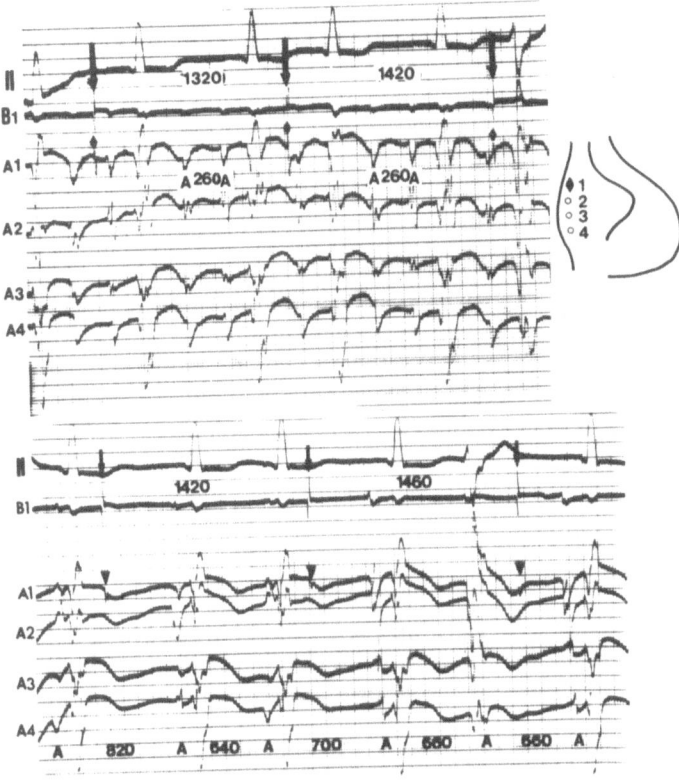

Figure 9 *Upper portion:* regular atrial tachycardia (cycle length 260 ms). A1 to A4 = unipolar recording from right atrium; B1 = bipolar recording (inter-electrode distance 1 mm) from the upper part of the right right auricle, the unipolar (A1) and the bipolar (B1) recordings show not only the rapid activity associated with the atrial tachycardia but also slow atrial activity (cycle 1320–1420 ms—and parasystolic in origin) totally dissociated from the other (indicated by the arrows). *Lower portion:* after cardioversion, the rapid atrial tachycardia has been abolished. Atrial rhythm at the base shows a cycle of 640–820 ms and atrial activity is polymorphic. Parasystolic atrial activity (indicated by the arrow) persists and is localized to the upper part of the right atrium.

Atrioventricular conduction

Normal atrial conduction consists of two components that can be subdivided on the His bundle electrogram, within the totality of excitation from the sinus node to the first depolarization recorded from the interventricular septum (Figure 3). The PA interval represents inter-nodal conduction (see above) and is followed by the AH interval, which is measured from the rapid atrial deflection and the onset of the His bundle deflection. It represents conduction through the AV node and reflects rapid conduction to the bundle of His, the normal value of 50–100 ms corresponds to an average conduction speed of 1.5 m/s[72]. The HV interval represents conduction in the specific intraventricular conducting system (His–Purkinje system) and measures

30–50 ms. It is shorter below the age of 15 years[72]. The conduction time in the bundle branches, measured between either the left or the right branch and the first ventricular depolarization is less than 30 ms. Direct measurement of the rate of conduction during open heart surgery suggests that the intervals between depolarization in the bundle branches and in the ventricles are longer: right bundle branch to ventricle 18–35 ms and left bundle branch to ventricle 20–39 ms[72]. Thus there is some variability in the conduction time, which means that identification of specific areas by measurement of the conduction interval has only limited value.

Studies of abnormal atrioventricular conduction have greatly benefited from recording from the bundle of His[73,74]. It has shown that surface recordings are inadequate to make accurate topographical diagnosis in conduction abnormalities, that it is possible to find evidence of slow conduction when the PR interval on the surface is within normal limits, and has defined the frequency of abnormalities in AV conduction. Blocks above the bundle of His (between A and H) can be interpreted as an abnormality in the region of the atroventricular node, block within the bundle (splitting of the His potential) corresponds to a focal lesion in the trunk of the bundle of His, and blocks below the bundle of His (between H and V) reflect bilateral lesions in the intraventricular conduction pathways.

Figure 10 shows an example of complete AV block with a subsidiary ventricular rhythm with wide QRS complexes. The absence of the H-potential after the P-waves and the presence of the electrogram of the bundle of His before each ventricular complex indicates that the block is proximal to

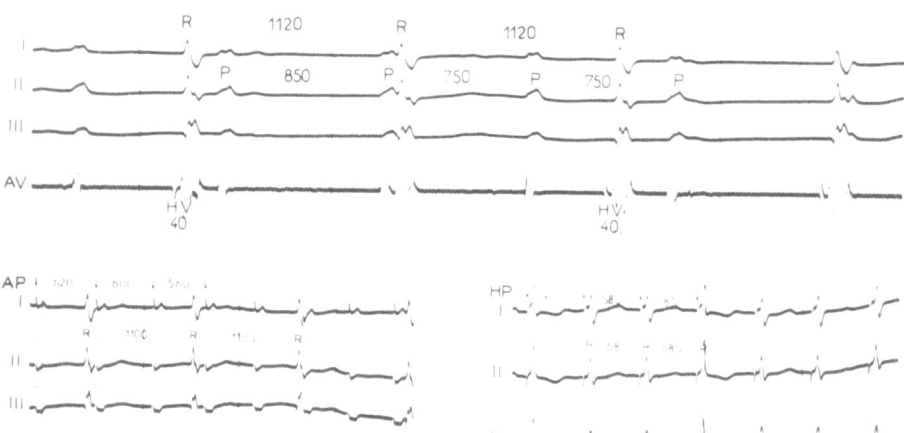

Figure 10 Complete AV block proximal to the bundle of His with right branch block. *Upper portion* (speed 100 mm/s): recording from the bundle of His (AV) shows that the block is proximal to the bundle of His: the A wave is not followed by an H-potential, while there are normal HV intervals (40 ms) with each ventricular escape. *Lower left portion* (speed 50mm/s): atrial stimulation (AP) with persistence of complete AV block. *Right lower portion* (speed 50 mm/s): stimulation of the bundle of His with 1:1 ventricular response.

the bundle of His and that the widening of the QRS complex is due to right bundle branch block. Stimulation of the bundle of His was followed by 1:1 transmission to the ventricles without a change in QRS morphology, confirming the proximal site of the AV block.

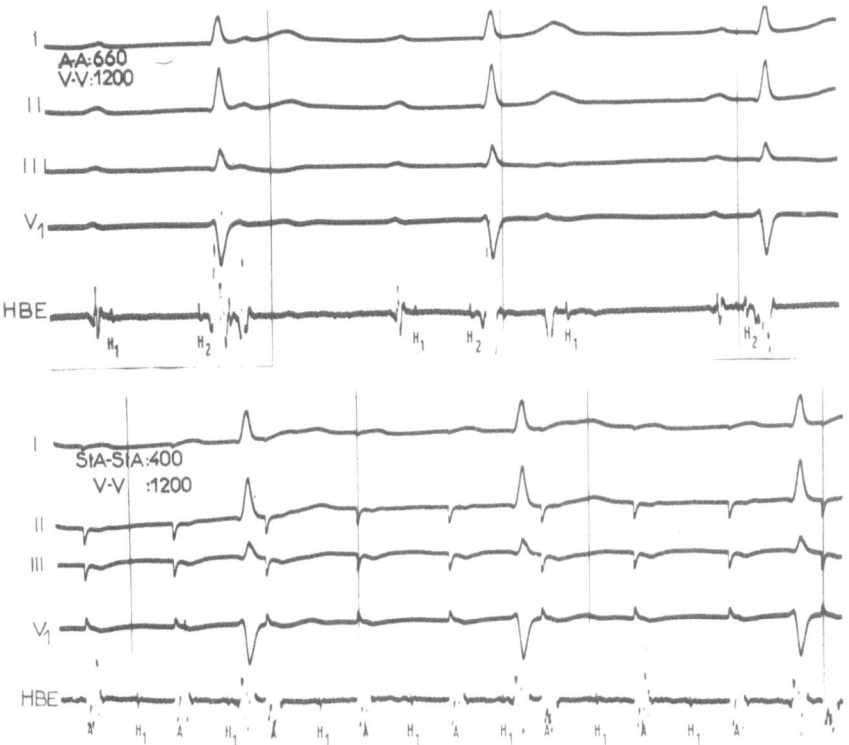

Figure 11 Complete AV block within the bundle of His. *Upper portion:* recording from the bundle of His (HBE) showing the presence of a split H. H1 is linked to the atrial activity while H2 precedes ventricular depolarization. The complexes AH1 and H2V are totally dissociated. The normal ventricular complexes indicate that the lesion is an isolated one of the bundle of His. *Lower portion:* atrial stimulation at a rate of 150/min (StA = 400 ms) detaches the H1 potential from A (the intra-nodal conduction is prolonged) and shows that H1 represents the activity in the proximal portion of the bundle of His not the end of atrial depolarization.

Figure 11 is an example of a congenital complete AV block, with a ventricular escape rhythm showing narrow QRS complexes. The recording of two separate dissociated His tracings, one related to the atrial tracings and corresponding to the proximal part of the bundle of His and the other preceding each QRS and corresponding to the distal part of the bundle demonstrates that the block is in the bundle of His itself.

Figure 12 illustrates a case of third degree block below the bundle of His, unidirectional in nature. The spontaneous sinus P waves are followed by evidence of depolarisation in the bundle of His, while the separate widened QRS complexes are not preceded by H potentials (showing that the abnormal focus is situated beyond the bifurcation of the bundle of His). Stimulation of the ventricle is followed by retrograde 1:1 atrial conduction with H-potentials between the ventricular and atrial deflections, showing that retrograde conduction is possible although there is anterograde block.

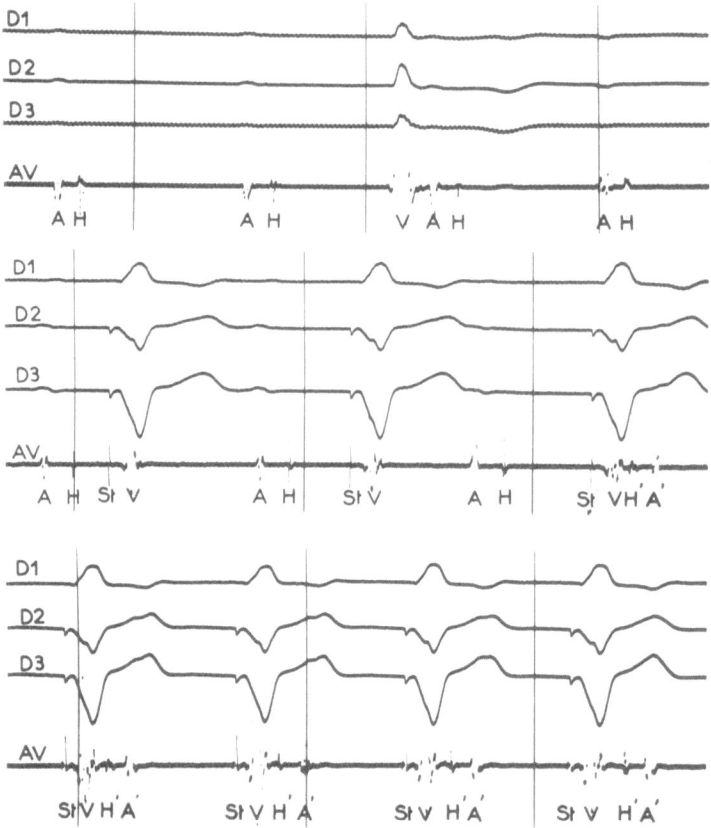

Figure 12 Unidirectional AV block below the bundle of His. *Upper portion:* complete AV block below the bundle of His: the atrial tracing is followed by an H potential but no ventricular response. The ventricular escape rhythm is not preceded by H complexes. *Middle and lower portion:* ventricular stimulation at increasing rates. From the last complex of the middle tracing there is a 1:1 retrograde conduction from ventricular stimulation. There is an H-potential after each QRS complex and before the retrograde atrial activity, showing that VA conduction follows the normal route.

Recording the His bundle electrogram in the *Wolff–Parkinson–White syndrome* shows the respective parts played by the normal and the accessory pathways in ventricular depolarization and that the H-potential migrates into the delta wave when the degree of pre-excitation is increased[75–77].

Intraventricular conduction

In the course of *normal ventricular depolarization* the activation of the septum from left to right is responsible for the initial positive deflections seen with unipolar electrodes in the right ventricle (morphology rs) and of the negative deflection within the left ventricle (morphology QS). In corrected transposition of the great vessels the ventricular inversion is accompanied by inversion of the bundle branches, producing mirror-image appearances in intracavitary electrograms from the right and left ventricles, in comparison with the normal pattern (Figure 13).

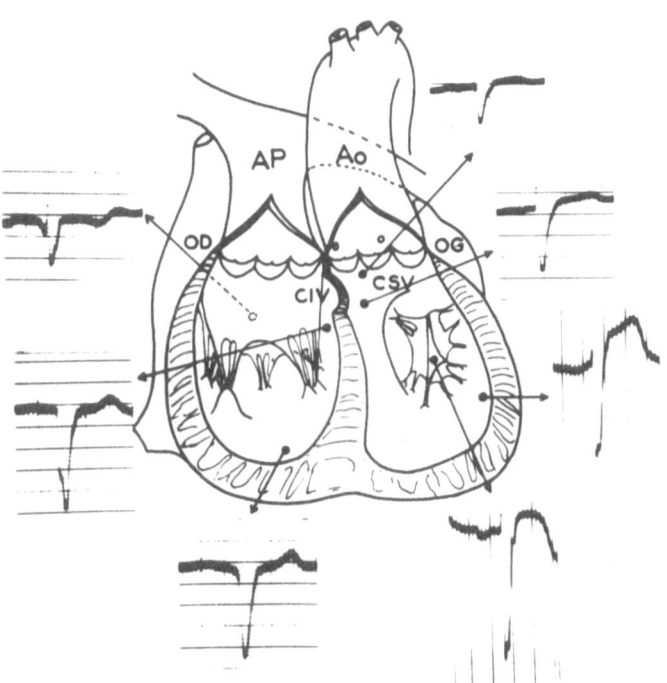

Figure 13 Transposition of the great vessels. The inversion of the ventricular cavities and of the atrioventricular valves is accompanied by reversal of septal activity: negative QRS complexes recorded from the right (morphologically the left ventricle) and positive pattern from the left (morphologically the right ventricle).

Intraventricular mapping has contributed to our understanding of the sequence of ventricular depolarization in *branch block* and in the *Wolff–Parkinson–White syndrome*[21,78–80]. Recordings from the bundle of His enable us to diagnose ventricular aberration when a widened QRS complex is preceded by an H potential with either a normal or a prolonged HV interval and thus differentiate the disorder from ectopic ventricular rhythms[81,82].

Stimulation of the bundle of His in cases of bundle branch block, particularly affecting the left bundle branch sometimes causes the QRS to become normal (Figure 14). This was thought to represent functional longitudinal dissociation of the bundle of His[83,84], but it may be due to a lesion localized to at the origin of the left bundle branch[85] as was seen in one of our cases studied both clinically and anatomically.

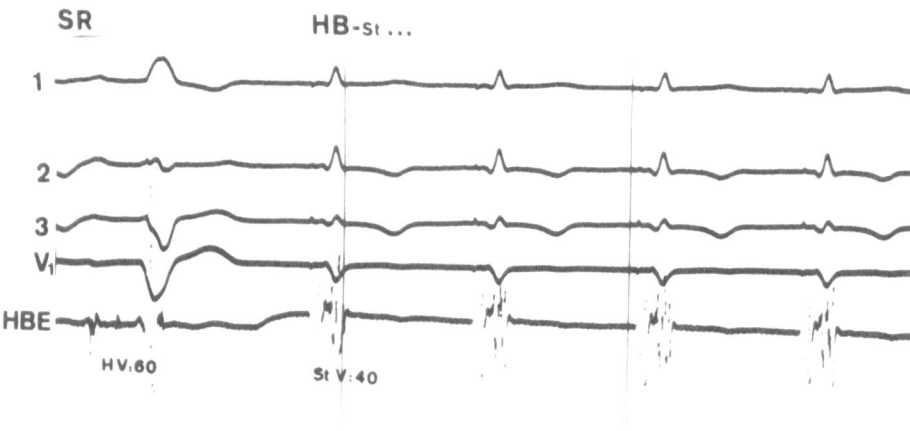

Figure 14 Left bundle branch block. Normalization of QRS by stimulation of the bundle of His. The first sinus complex (SR) shows complete left bundle branch block. The interval HV is prolonged to 60 ms. Stimulation of the bundle of His following the second complex (HB.St) produces normalisation of QRS with disappearance of left axis deviation. The interval between the stimulus and the normalized ventricular complex is 40 ms

Left-sided intracardiac exploration in patients with recurrent paroxysmal tachycardia after a myocardial infarct has shown the presence of slow after-potentials following depolarization of the ventricles, asynchronous activation at the margins of ventricular aneurysms, and the presence of localised areas of ventricular fibrillation during the episodes of tachycardia[86].

RECORDING OF MONOPHASIC ACTION POTENTIALS

The recording of monophasic action potentials (MAP) with an electrode attached by suction to the endocardium is another possibility offered by intracardiac study. The method was utilized very extensively in experimental studies before the introduction of microelectrodes for cellular electrophysio-logical studies and was introduced for human use about 10 years ago[87,88], being popularized by Olsson et al.[89].

The recordings are made by a unipolar or bipolar electrode introduced by the percutaneous femoral route[90,91]. The electrode is situated within the lumen of the catheter and is held in contact with the endocardium by suction with an aspiration system that can produce a pressure of —350 mmHg.

The MAPs have a shape and duration similar to the action potentials of the cells in the immediate neighbourhood[92]. The atrial MAP has a triangular shape and the ventricular MAP shows a well defined plateau (Figure 15).

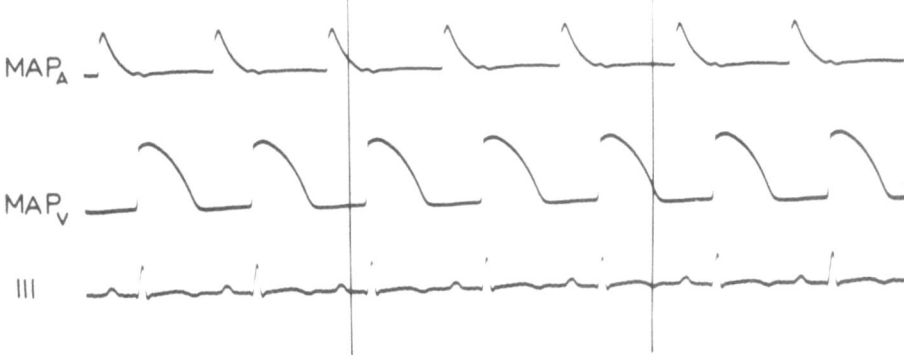

Figure 15 Monophasic potentials (MAP) recorded simultaneously in the atrium (upper portion) and in the right ventricle (lower portion)

The value of MAP tracings lies in the stability of the recordings, the precision of estimating the time of local depolarization, on the basis of the rapid rise of the potential, and the opportunity to measure the duration of repolarization. However there is a problem in recording the MAP in man. Suction exceeding 2 min may produce endocardial damage, which means that the duration of recording in any one zone must be briefer than the suction time. Furthermore, topographical exploration is more limited than with the conventional electrodes.

INTRACARDIAC STIMULATION

In addition to its therapeutic importance, not considered here, intracardiac stimulation is an indispensable complement to all electrophysiological studies. Coumel in France[93], Durrer and Wellens in Holland[94,95] and Damato *et al.* in the USA[96] were the first to demonstrate its applications.

There are two methods of stimulation: incremental increase in the rate of pacing, and the 'extrastimulus method', pacing during diastole with a stimulus that is coupled to the heart cycle (spontaneous or paced) with a coupling interval which is progressively shortened until the refractory period of the tissue under study is reached.

Sinus function is studied indirectly[97–99] by determining the sinus node recovery time and the sino-atrial conduction time which only give approximations.

The *atrioventricular conduction capacity* is defined by the 1:1 AV transmission under the effect of atrial stimulation at progressively increasing rates; the development of second-degree AV block corresponds to the 'Wenckebach point.'

The *refractory periods* are studied at different levels in the heart by extrastimuli to the atria (anterograde conduction refractory period) and to the ventricles (retrograde refractory period). The absolute refractory period of the atrium, the node and the ventricle and the relative refractory period, both effective and functional of the atrium, of the specialized conduction tissue and the ventricle are defined as in Table 1. The refractory period varies in relation to age and to the heart rate. In the same subject the refractory periods differ in the anterograde and retrograde directions[103]. The same principles apply in the study of accessory conduction pathways[104].

Table 1   Conduction refractory periods

Area	Refractory period	Definition
Atrium	Effective	Longest S1–S2 (A) not followed by A2
	Functional	Shortest A1–A2 from S1–S2
AV Node	Effective	Longest A1–A2 not followed by H2
	Functional	Shortest H1–H2 from A1–A2
His–Purkinje	Effective	Longest H1–H2 not followed by V2
	Relative	Longest H1–H2 followed by lengthening of H2–V2 and/or ventricular aberration
Ventricle	Effective	Longest S1–S2 (V) not followed by V2

S1–S2: interval between the basic stimulus (S1) auricular (A) or ventricular (V) and the extrastimulus (S2).
A1–A2, H1–H2, V1–V2: response intervals of atrium, bundle of His and ventricule which follow at intervals between the basic stimulus and the extrastimulus (S1–S2).

Cardiac stimulation may reproduce certain tachycardias and thereby suggest their mechanisms. Re-entrant tachycardias may be induced by stimulation of the sinus node or its neighbourhood[105,106] or the AV node, or by involving latent or overt accessory pathway[107–110], or may be localized to the ventricles[111,112]. Deliberate induction of atrial fibrillation in patients with the Wolff–Parkinson–White syndrome makes it possible to recognize patients at high risk from this arrhythmia because they respond with a very rapid ventricular response[113,114].

Anti-arrhythmic drugs may be classified on the basis of their effects on conduction and the refractory periods of the atrium, the AV node, the His–Purkinje system, the ventricle and the accessory pathways[115–118]. With this we start a new chapter in pharmaco-electrophysiology.

References

1. Lenegre, J. and Maurice, P. (1945). La dérivation directe, intracavitaire des courants électriques de l'oreillette et du ventricule droits. *Arch. Mal. Coeur*, **38**, 298

2. Hecht, H. H. (1946). Potentials variations of the right auricular and ventricular cavities in man. *Am. Heart J.*, **32,** 39

3. Battro, A. and Bidoggia, H. (1947). Endocardiac electrocardiogram obtained by heart catheterization in man. *Am. Heart J.*, **33,** 604

4. Sodi Pallares, D., Vizcaino, M., Soberon, J. and Cabrera, D. (1947). Comparative study of the intracavitary potential in man and in dog. *Am. Heart J.*, **33,** 819

5. Coelho, E., Da Fonseca, J. M., Paiva, E. and Nunes, A. (1948). Les dérivations intracardiaques (cavités droites) dans les hypertrophies ventriculaires et dans les blocs de branches. *Arch. Mal. Coeur*, **41,** 577

6. Duchosal, P. W., Ferrero, L., Doret, J. P., Andereggen, P. and Rilliet, B. (1948). Les potentiels intracardiaques recueillis par cathétérisme chez l'homme. *Cardiologia*, **13,** 113

7. Kert, M. and Hoobler, W. (1949). Observations on the potential variations of the cavities of the right side of the human heart. *Am. Heart J.*, **38,** 97

8. Gibert Queralto, J., Forner, M., Paravisini Parra, J. and Morato Portell, J. M. (1949). El electrograma intraauricular e intraventricular derecho. *Med. Clinica*, **12,** 299

9. Levine, H. D., Hellems, H. K., Winttenborg, M. H. and Dexter, L. (1949). Studies in intracardiac electrocardiography in man. I. The potential variations in the right atrium. *Am. Heart J.*, **37,** 46

10. Levine, H. D., Hellems, H. K., Dexter, L. and Tucker, A. S. (1949). Studies in intracardiac electrocardiography in man. II. The potential variations in the right ventricle. *Am. Heart J.*, **37,** 64

11. Schlesinger, P., Benchimol, A. M. and Cotrim, M. R. (1949). Intracavity and oesophaegeal potentials in right ventricular hypertrophy. *Am. Heart J.*, **37,** 1110

12 Kossmann, C. E., Berger, A. R., Bader, R., Brumlik, J., Briller, J. A. and Donnely, J. H. (1950). Intracardiac and intravascular potentials resulting from electrical activity of the normal human heart. *Circulation*, **2,** 10

13. Levine, H. D. and Goodale, W. I. (1950). Studies in intracardiac electrocardiography in man. IV. The potential variations in the coronary venous system. *Circulation*, **2,** 48

14. Giraud, G., Latour, H. and Puech, P. (1954). L'électrocardiographie du sinus coronaire. Première partie: etude générale et pathologie de base. *Arch. Mal. Coeur*, **47,** 900

15. Giraud, G., Latour, H. and Puech, P. (1954). L'électrocardiographie du sinus coronaire. Deuxième partie: etude électrocardiographique endocavitaire des dysrythmies du sinus coronaire chez l'homme. *Arch. Mal. Coeur*, **47,** 1008

16. Sodi Pallares, D., Estandia, A., Soberon, J. and Rodriguez, M. I. (1950). The left ventricular potential of the human heart. II. Criteria for diagnosis of incomplete left bundle branch block. *Am. Heart J.*, **40,** 655

17. Steinberg, M. F., Seligmann, A., Kroop, I. G. and Grishman, A. (1951). Catheterization of the left ventricle in man. Study of right bundle branch block by simultaneous intracardiac electrocardiography of both ventricles. *Circulation*, **3,** 198

18. Gibert Queralto, J., Torner Soler, M., Paravisini Parra, J. and Morato Portell, J. M. (1950). El electrocardiograma intraventricular izquierdo. *Med. Clinica*, **14,** 400

19. Zimmerman, H. A. and Hellerstein, H. K. (1951). Cavity potentials of the human ventricles. *Circulation*, **3,** 95

20. Puech, P. (1956). *L'activité électrique auriculaire normale et pathologique.* 1 vol., (Paris: Masson)

21. Latour, H. and Puech, P. (1957). *Electrocardiographie endocavitaire.* 1 vol. (Paris: Masson)

22. Giraud, G., Puech, P., Latour, H. and Hertault, J. (1960). Variations de potentiel liées à l'activité du système de conduction auriculo-ventriculaire chez l'homme. Enregistrement électrocardiographique endocavitaire. *Arch. Mal. Coeur*, **53**, 757

23. Watson, H., Emslie Smith, D. and Lowe, K. G. (1967). The intracardiac electrocardiogram of human atrioventricular conducting tissue. *Am. Heart J.*, **74**, 66

24. Scherlag, B. J., Lau, S. H., Helfant, R. H., Berkowitz, W. D., Stein, E. and Damato, A. N. (1969). Catheter technique for recording His bundle activity in man. *Circulation*, **39**, 13

25. Lau, S. H., Bobb, G. A. and Damato, A. N. (1970). Catheter recording and validation of left bundle branch potentials in intact dogs. *Circulation*, **42**, 375

26. Narula, O. S., Javier, R. P., Samet, P. and Maramba, L. C. (1970). Significance of His and left bundle recordings from the left heart in man. *Circulation*, **42**, 385

27. Puech, P., Grolleau, R., Latour, H., Dufoix, R., Cabasson, J. and Robin, J. (1971). Enregistrement de l'activité de la branche gauche du faiceau de His par voie endocavitaire. *Arch. Mal. Coeur*, **64**, 10

28. Meister, S. G., Banka, V. S., Chadda, K. D. and Helfant, R. H. (1974). A balloon tipped catheter for obtaining His bundle electrograms without fluoroscopy. *Circulation*, **49**, 42

29. Puech, P. (1974). The P wave: correlation of surface and intra-atrial electrograms, in complex electrocardiography. *Cardiovasc. Clin.*, **6**, 43

30. Torresani, J., Amichot, J. L., Picard, J. P. and Jouve, A. (1969). Acquisitions récentes dans les techniques d'exploration électrocardiographique des cavités cardiaques. *Arch. Mal. Coeur*, **62**, 193

31. Gallagher, J. J., Pritchett, E. L. C., Benditt, D. G., Tonkin, A. M., Campbell, R. W. F., Dugan, F. A., Bashore, T. M., Tower, A. and Wallace, A. G. (1977). New catheter techniques for analysis of the sequence of retrograde activation in man. *Eur. J. Cardiol.*, **6**, 1

32. Thery, Cl., Asseman, Ph., Adamanditis, M., Vincent, A., Dupuis, B. and Lekieffre, J. (1978). Enregistrement de l'électrogramme du noeud sinusal. Effets de l'injection de tétrodotoxine dans l'artère du sinus. *Arch. Mal. Coeur*, **71**, 121

33. Castillo-Fenoy, A., Valere, P. E. and Tricot, R. (1978). Identification du potentiel sinusal chez le chien par électrocardiographie épicardique. *Arch. Mal. Coeur*, **71**, 334

34. Ramlau, R. (1974). Electrograms of the sino-atrial node in dogs following surgical implantation of electrodes on the epicardium. *J. Electrocardiol.*, **7**, 137

35. Cramer, M., Hariman, R. J., Boxer, R. A., Krongrad, E. and Hoffman, B. F. (1978). Catheter recordings of sinoatrial node potentials in the in situ canine heart. *Am. J. Cardiol.*, **41**, 374 (Abst.)

36. Hariman, R. J., Krongrad, E., Boxer, R. A., Cramer, M., Bowman, F. O., Malm, J. R. and Hoffman, B. F. (1978). A method for recording of extracellular sinoatrial electrograms during cardiac surgery in man. *Am. J. Cardiol.*, **41**, 375 (Abst.)

37. Amat-y-Leon, F., Deedwania, P., Miller, R. H., Dhingra, R. C. and Rosen, K. M. (1977). A new approach for indirect recording of anterior left atrial activation in man. *Am. Heart J.*, **93**, 408

38. Ogawa, S., Dreifus, L. S., Kitchen, J. G., Shenoy, P. N. and Osmick, M. J.

(1978). Catheter recording of Bachmann's bundle activation from the right pulmonary artery. *Am. J. Cardiol.*, **41**, 1089

39. Gallagher, J. J., Damato, A. N., Lau, S. H., Tower, A. T., Caracta, A. R., Varghese, P. J. and Josephson, M. E. (1973). Antecubital vein approach for recording His bundle activity in man. *Am. Heart J.*, **85**, 199

40. Narula, O. S., Runge, M. and Samet, P. (1973). A new catheter technique for His bundle recordings via the arm veins. *Br. Heart J.*, **35**, 1226

41. Spach, M. S., Barr, R. C. and Jewett, P. H. (1972). Spread of excitation from the atrium into thoracic veins in human beings and dogs. *Am. J. Cardiol.*, **30**, 844

42. Zipes, D. P. and Knope, R. F. (1972). Electrical properties of the thoracic veins. *Am. J. Cardiol.*, **29**, 372

43. Castillo, A., Valere, P. and Guerot, Cl. (1974). Etude de l'excitabilité et de la conduction auriculaire normale chez le chien par stimulations auriculaires prématurées. *Coeur*, **6**, 745

44. Wit, A. L. and Cranefield, P. F. (1977). Triggered and automatic activity in the canine coronary sinus. *Circ. Res.*, **41**, 435

45. Josephson, M. E., Horowitz, L. N., Farshidi, A., Spear, J. F., Kastor, J. A. and Moore, E. N. (1978). Recurrent sustained ventricular tachycardia. 2. Endocardial mapping. *Circulation*, **57**, 440

46. Josephson, M. E., Scharf, D. L., Kastor, J. A. and Kitchen, J. G. (1977). Atrial endocardial activation in man. Electrode catheter technique for endocardial mapping. *Am. J. Cardiol.*, **39**, 972

47. Agha, A. S., Befeler, B., Castellanos, A. M., Sung, R. J., Castillo, A., Myerburg, R. J. and Castellanos, A. (1976). Bipolar catheter electrograms for study of retrograde activation pattern in patients without pre-excitation syndrome. *Br. Heart J.*, **38**, 641

48. Amat-y-Leon, F., Dhingra, R. C., Wu, D., Denes, P., Wyndham, C. and Rosen, K. M. (1976). Catheter mapping of retrograde atrial activation. Observations during ventricular pacing and AV nodal re-entrant paroxysmal tachycardia. *Br. Heart J.*, **38**, 355

49. Gallagher, J. J., Gilbert, M., Svenson, R. H., Sealy, W. C., Kasell, J., and Wallace, A. G. (1975). Wolff-Parkinson-White syndrome. The problem, evaluation and surgical correction. *Circulation*, **51**, 767

50. Coumel, P. and Attuel, P. (1974). Reciprocating tachycardia in overt and latent pre-excitation. *Eur. J. Cardiol.*, **1**, 423

51. Coumel, Ph., Waynberger, M., Fabiato, A., Slama, R., Aigueperse, J. and Bouvrain, Y. (1972). Problems in evaluation of multiple accessory pathways and surgical therapy. *Circulation*, **45**, 1216

52. Slama, R., Coumel, Ph. and Bouvrain, Y. (1973). Les syndromes de Wolff-Parkinson-White de type A inapparents ou latents en rythme sinusal. *Arch. Mal. Coeur*, **66**, 639

53. Spurrell, R. A., Krikler, D. M. and Sowton, E. (1974). Concealed bypasses of the AV node in patients with paroxysmal supraventricular tachycardias revealed by intracardiac stimulation and verapamil. *Am. J. Cardiol.*, **33**, 590

54. Zipes, D. P., De Joseph, R. L. and Rothbaum, D. A. (1974). Unusual properties of accessory pathways. *Circulation*, **49**, 1200

55. Neuss, H., Schlepper, M. and Thorman, J. (1975). Analysis of re-entry in three patients with concealed Wolff–Parkinson–White syndrome. *Circulation*, **51**, 75

56. Tonkin, A. M., Gallagher, J. J., Svenson, R. A., Wallace, A. G. and Sealy, W. C. (1975). Antegrade block in accessory pathways with retrograde conduction in reciprocating tachycardia. *Eur. J. Cardiol.*, **3**, 143

57. Puech, P. and Grolleau, R. (1977). L'onde P rétrograde négative en D1, signe de faisceau de Kent postero-lateral gauche. *Arch. Mal. Coeur*, **70**, 49

58. Puech, P., Grolleau, R. and Cinca, J. (1977). Reciprocating tachycardia using a latent left-sided accessory pathway. Diagnostic approach by conventional ECG. In H. E. Kulbertus (ed.). *Re-entrant Arrhythmias*, p. 117. (Lancaster: MTP Press)

59. Farshidi, A., Josephson, M. E. and Horowitz, L. N. (1978). Electrophysiologic characteristics of concealed bypass tracts: clinical and electrocardiographic correlates. *Am. J. Cardiol.*, **41**, 1052

60. Puech, P., Latour, H. and Grolleau, R. (1970). Le flutter auriculaire et ses limites. *Arch. Mal. Coeur*, **63**, 116

61. Boineau, J. P., Mooney, C. R., Hudson, R. D., Hughes, D. G., Erdin, R. A. Jr. and Wylds, A. C. (1977). Observations on re-entrant excitation pathways and refractory period distributions in spontaneous and experimental atrial flutter in the dog. In H. Kulbertus (ed.). *Re-entrant Arrhythmias*, p. 72. (Lancaster: MTP Press)

62. Zipes, D. and Dejoseph, R. L. (1973). Dissimilar atrial rhythms in man and dog. *Am. J. Cardiol.*, **32**, 618

63. Leier, C. V. and Schaal, S. F. (1977). Dissimilar atrial rhythm. A patient with interatrial block. *Br. Heart J.*, **39**, 680

64. Castellanos, A., Lyengar, R., Agha, A. and Castillo, C. A. (1972). Wenckebach phenomenon within the atria. *Br. Heart J.*, **34**, 1121

65. Narula, O. S., Runge, M. and Samet, Ph. (1972). Second-degree Wenckebach type AV block due to block within the atrium. *Br. Heart J.*, **34**, 1127

66. Puech, P., Grolleau, R., Cabasson, J., Baissus, C. and Latour, H. (1975). Blocs auriculo-ventriculaires du premier et du deuxième degré par trouble de conduction intra-auriculaire. *Arch. Mal. Coeur*, **68**, 19

67. Kerin, N. and Schwartz, H. (1975). Wenckebach phenomenon within the atria. *J. Electrocardiol.*, **8**, 61

68. Warin, J. F. and Fauchier, J. P. (1978). Les troubles de la conduction intra-auriculaire. In Roussel (ed.). *Les Troubles du Rythme Cardiaque*, (Paris)

69. Brechenmacher, C., Coumel, Ph. and Slama, R. (1975). Paralysie auriculaire apparente et trouble de la conduction auriculo-ventriculaire. Etude anatomoclinique. *Arch. Mal. Coeur*, **68**, 575

70. Rosen, K. M., Rahimtoola, S. H., Gunnar, R. M. and Lev, M. (1971). Transient and persistent atrial standstill with His bundle lesions. *Circulation*, **44**, 220

71. Donzeau, J. P., Constans, R., Fauchier, J. P., Levy, S., Vedel, J. and Bounhoure, J. P. (1978). Partial persistent right atrial standstill and atrial tachycardia. *Transactions of the European Society of Cardiology*, vol. I, no. 1, Brighton, June (Abst. 175).

72. Kupersmith, J. E., Krongrad, F. and Waldo, A. L. (1973). Conduction intervals and conduction velocity in the human cardiac conduction system: studies during open-heart surgery. *Circulation*, **47**, 776

73. Narula, O. S. (1975). Current concepts of atrioventricular block. In O. S. Narula (ed.). *His Bundle Electrocardiography and Clinical Electrophysiology*, p. 139. (Philadelphia: Davis Company)

74. Puech, P. (1975). Atrioventricular block: the value of intracardiac recordings. In D. M. Krikler and J. F. Goodwin (eds.). *Cardiac Arrhythmias*, p. 81. (London: Saunders Co.)

75. Castellanos, A., Chapunoff, E., Castillo, C., Maytin, O. and Lemburg, L. (1970). His bundle electrograms in two cases of Wolff–Parkinson–White (pre-excitation syndrome). *Circulation*, **41**, 399

76. Durrer, D. and Wellens, H. J. J. (1974). The Wolff–Parkinson–White syndrome: anno 1973. *Eur. J. Cardiol.*, **1**, 347
77. Puech, P. and Grolleau, R. (1972). L'activité du faiceau de His normale et pathologique. 1 vol. (Paris: Sandoz)
78. Castellanos, A. and Castillo, C. A. (1972). His bundle recordings in right bundle branch block coexisting with iatrogenic right ventricular pre-excitation. *Br. Heart J.*, **34**, 153
79. Kastor, J. A., Goldreyer, B. N., Moore, N., Shelburne, J. C. and Manchester, J. H. (1975). Intraventricular conduction in man studied with an endocardial electrode catheter mapping technique. Patients with normal QRS and right bundle branch block. *Circulation*, **51**, 786
80. Sung, R. J., Tamer, D. M., Garcia, O. L., Castellanos, A., Myerburg, R. J. and Gelband, H. (1976). Analysis of surgically-induced right bundle branch block pattern using intracardiac recording techniques. *Circulation*, **54**, 442
81. Puech, P. (1975). Ectopic ventricular rhythms: ventricular tachycardia and His bundle recordings. In O. S. Narula (ed.). *His Bundle Electrocardiography and Clinical Electrophysiology*, p. 243. (Philadelphia: Davis Co.)
82. Akhtar, M., Damato, A. N. and Caracta, A. R. (1976). Clinical use of His bundle electrocardiography. Part II. *Am. Heart J.*, **91**, 660
83. Narula, O. S. (1977). Longitudinal dissociation in the His bundle. *Circulation*, **56**, 996
84. El-Sherif, N., Amat-y-Leon, F., Schonfield, C., Scherlag, B. J., Rosen, K., Lazzara, R. and Wyndham, C. (1978). Normalization of bundle branch block patterns by distal His bundle pacing. *Circulation*, **57**, 473
85. Puech, P., Grolleau, R., Mellet, J. M. and Deceuninck, P. (1976). Affinement et normalisation de QRS par stimulation du faisceau de His dans les blocs complets de branche gauche. *71st European Congress of Cardiology*, Amsterdam, June (Abst. 656)
86. Josephson, M. E., Horowitz, L. N. and Farshidi, A. (1978). Continuous local activity: A mechanism of recurrent ventricular activity. *Circulation*, **57**, 659
87. Korsgren, M., Leskinen, E., Sjøstrand, U. and Varnauskas, E. (1966). Intracardiac recording of monophasic action potentials, in the human heart. *Scand. J. Clin. Lab. Invest.*, **18**, 561
88. Shabetai, R., Surawicz, B. and Hammil, W. (1968). Monophasic action potentials in man. *Circulation*, **38**, 341
89. Olsson, S. B. (1971). *Monophasic Action Potentials of Right Heart.* (Goteborg: Elanders Boktryckeri Aktiebolag ed.)
90. Gavrilescu, S., Cotoi, S. and Pop, T. (1972). The monophasic action potential of the right human atrium. A simple bedside suction technique and the first results in atrial arrhythmias. *Cardiology*, **57**, 200
91. Puech, P., Cabasson, J., Latour, H., Grolleau, R. and Baissus, C. (1974). Etude des potentiels d'action monophasique du myocarde par voie endocavitaire. Méthodologie. *Arch. Mal. Coeur*, **67**, 1117
92. Hoffman, B. F., Cranefield, P. F., Lepeschkin, E., Surawicz, B. and Herrlich, H. C. (1959). Comparison of cardiac monophasic action potentials recorded by intracellular and suction electrodes. *Am. J. Physiol.*, **196**, 1297
93. Coumel, Ph., Cabrol, C., Fabiato, A., Gourgon, R. and Slama, R. (1967). Tachycardie permanente par rythme réciproque. I. Preuves de diagnostic par stimulation auriculaire et ventriculaire. *Arch. Mal. Coeur*, **60**, 1830
94. Durrer, D. (1968). Electrical aspects of human cardiac activity. A clinical physiological approach to excitation and stimulation. *Cardiovasc. Res.*, **2**, 1
95. Wellens, H. J. J. (1971). *Programmed Electrical Stimulation of the Heart in the Study and Treatment of Tachyarrhythmias.* 1 vol., (Leiden: Stenfert Kroese ed.)

96. Damato, A. N., Lau, S. H., Patton, R. D., Stein, C. and Berkowitz, W. D. (1969). A study of atrioventricular conduction in man using premature atrial stimulation and His bundle recordings. *Circulation*, **39**, 297

97. Mandel, W. J., Hayakawa, H., Danzig, R. and Marcus, H. S. (1971). Evaluation of sino-atrial function in man by overdrive suppression. *Circulation*, **44**, 59

98. Narula, O. S., Samet, P. and Javier, R. P. (1972). Significance of the sinus node recovery time. *Circulation*, **45**, 140

99. Strauss, H. G., Saroff, A. L., Bigger, J. J. and Giardina, E. G. V. (1973). Premature atrial stimulation as a key to the understanding of sino-atrial conduction in man. *Circulation*, **47**, 86

100. Cagin, A. N., Kunstadt, D., Wolfish, P. and Levitt, B. (1973). The influence of heart rate on the refractory period of the atrium and AV conduction system. *Am. Heart J.*, **85**, 358

101. Denes, P., Wu, D., Dhingra, R., Pietras, R. J. and Rosen, K. M. (1974). The effect of cycle length on cardiac refractory period in man. *Circulation*, **49**, 32

102. Schuilenburg, R. (1976). Patterns of A-V conduction in the human heart in the presence of normal and abnormal A-V conduction. H. J. J. Wellens, K. I. Lie, and M. J. Janse (eds.). In *The conduction system of the Heart*, p. 485. (Leiden: Stenfert Kroese B.V.)

103. Akthar, M., Damato, A. N., Batsford, W. P., Ruskin, J. N. and Ogunkelu, J. B. (1975). A comparative analysis of antegrade and retrograde conduction patterns in man. *Circulation*, **52**, 766

104. Svenson, R. H., Miller, H. C., Gallagher, J. J. and Wallace, A. C. (1975). Electro-physiological evaluation of the W. P. W. syndrome. Problems in assessing antegrade and retrograde conduction over the accessory pathways. *Circulation*, **52**, 552

105. Narula, O. S. (1974). Sinus node re-entry: a mechanism for supraventricular tachycardia. *Circulation*, **50**, 1114

106. Curry, P. V. L. and Krikler, D. M. (1977). Paroxysmal reciprocating sinus tachycardia. In H. E. Kulbertus (ed.). *Re-entrant Arrhythmias*, p. 38. (Lancaster: MTP Press)

107. Coumel, Ph., Attuel, P. and Flammang, D. (1976). The role of the conduction system in supraventricular tachycardias. In H. J. J. Wellens, K. I. Lie and M. J. Janse (eds.). *The Conduction System of the Heart*, p. 424. (Leiden: Stenfert Kroese B.V.)

108. Coumel, Ph. (1975). Junctional reciprocating tachycardias. The permanent and paroxysmal forms of A-V nodal reciprocating tachycardias. *J. Electrocardiol.*, **8**, 79

109. Wellens, H. J. (1977). Modes of initiation of circus movement tachycardia in 139 patients with the Wolff–Parkinson–White syndrome. In H. E. Kulbertus (ed.), *Re-entrant Arrhythmias*, p. 153. (Lancaster: MTP Press)

110. Krikler, D. and Curry, P. (1977). Atypical initiation of reciprocating tachycardia in the Wolff–Parkinson–White syndrome. In H. E. Kulbertus (ed.). *Re-entrant Arrhythmias*, p. 144. (Lancaster: MTP Press)

111. Wellens, H. J. and Lie, K. I. (1975). Ventricular tachycardia: the value of programmed electrical stimulation. In D. M. Krikler and J. F. Goodwin (eds.). *Cardiac Arrhythmias*, p. 183. (London)

112. Fontaine, G., Guiraudon, G., Frank, R., Vedel, J., Grosgogeat, Y., Cabrol, C. and Facquet, J. (1977). Stimulation studies and epicardial mapping in ventricular tachycardia: study of mechanisms and selection for surgery. In H. E. Kulbertus (ed.). *Re-entrant Arrhythmias*, p. 350. (Lancaster: MTP Press)

113. Castellanos, A., Myerburg, R. J., Craparo, K., Befeler, B. and Agha, A. S.

(1973). Factors regulating ventricular rates during atrial flutter and fibrillation in pre-excitation (Wolff–Parkinson–White) syndrome. *Br. Heart J.*, **35**, 811

114. Wellens, H. J. J. (1976). The electrophysiologic properties of the accessory pathway in the Wolff–Parkinson–White syndrome. In H. J. J. Wellens, K. I. Lie and M. J. Janse (ed.). *The Cardiac Conduction System of the Heart*, p. 567. (Leiden: Stenfert Kroese B.V.)

115. Damato, A. N., Caracta, A. R., Akthar, M. and Lau, S. H. (1975). The effect of commonly used cardiovascular drugs on AV conduction and refractoriness. In O. S. Narula (ed.). *His Bundle Electrocardiography and Clinical Electrophysiology*, p. 105. (Philadelphia: Davis Company)

116. Neuss, H., Schaumann, H. J. and Stegaru, B. (1975). Drug effects on AV conduction. In B. Luderlitz (ed.). *Cardiac Pacing. Diagnostic and Therapeutic Tools*, p. 132. (Berlin: Springer-Verlag)

117. Puech, P. (1977). Etude électrophysiologique des anti-arrythmiques chez l'homme. *Ann. Cardiol. Angéiol.*, **26**, 41

118. Wellens, H. J. J. (1975). Effects of drugs on Wolff–Parkinson–White syndrome. In O. S. Narula (ed.). *His Bundle Electrocardiography and Clinical Electrophysiology*, p. 367. (Philadelphia: Davis Co.)

7

The application of electrocardiography to clinical medicine

D. KRIKLER

The introduction of indirect arterial and venous pulse recordings during the middle of the nineteenth century provided the clinician, for the first time, with a means of studying the activation of the heart, and of correlating the events observed with the stethoscope with cardiac rhythm changes. Great though this improvement was over the simple observation with eye and finger, it had only a limited value and did not render possible the diagnosis of the specific arrhythmias, except in a small number of cases. Thus, with the sphygmograph, MacKenzie was able to record total arrhythmia and explain it as 'nodal rhythm', parenthetically not too erroneous a description of ventricular activation, being entirely consistent with the fact that only some of the impulses from the fibrillating atria reached the ventricles, being filtered in the AV node.

One advantage that pulse tracings possessed was legibility. They were relatively easy to perform, and reproducible. Waller's application of the capillary electrometer to record the electrocardiogram[1] was a breakthrough, but an imperfect one. With it one could make recordings with great difficulty, and it was only when Einthoven used the string galvanometer for this purpose that electrocardiography became a feasible clinical tool. As Einthoven himself acknowledged[2], his development was brought into proper clinical perspective by Lewis[3], who systematically applied the instrument to the recording of a host of cardiac arrhythmias and conduction disturbances. It is a useful reminder of how shrewd an observer he was to go back to his early writings whenever one observes an apparently new phenomenon; all too often, in the early volumes of *Heart*, the unusual extrasystole or episode of paroxysmal tachycardia will be explained. The early tracings, obtained photographically with cumbersome apparatus, were often of very high quality (Figure 1), indeed superior to many recordings made in casualty departments today.

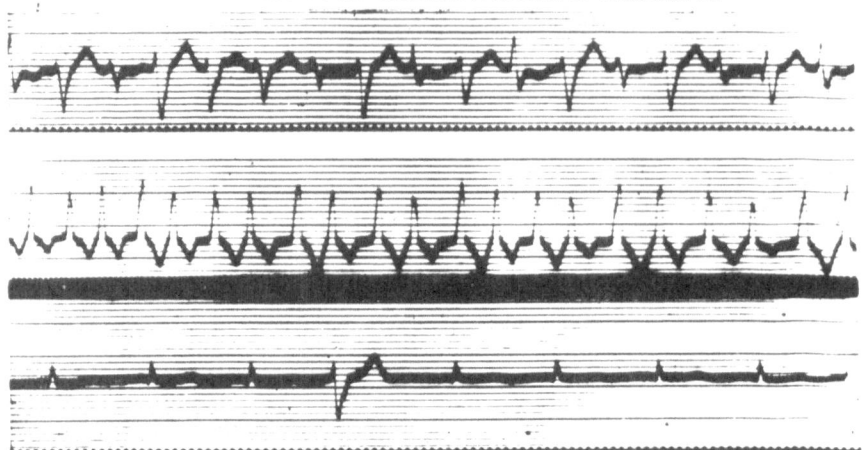

Figure 1 ECG recorded by Sir Thomas Lewis and Dr Alfred Goodman Levy in 1912: tracing kindly provided by Dr Arthur Hollman

The electrocardiograph came on the scene at just the right time. While in this country MacKenzie was trying to classify arrhythmias on the basis of pulse tracings[4], Wenckebach was similarly occupied in the Netherlands. The first edition of his book[5] appeared in 1903; it contains excellent descriptions of many arrhythmias and useful deductions derived from clinical observations and pulse tracings. Eleven years later[6], he had moved to Vienna, and his descriptions were now based on the electrocardiograph. In this decade the whole face of arrhythmia analysis was changed by the availability of the instrument conceived by Waller, developed by Einthoven and applied by Lewis. Also, myocardial infarction could now be diagnosed in life, providing another timely use for the electrocardiograph[7]: Figure 2 shows the features that now enable us confidently to diagnose this disorder. However, we must recall that multiple chest leads were yet to come[8] and that it took many years before their use percolated through into general clinical application, together with the advent of the direct-writing ECG machine.

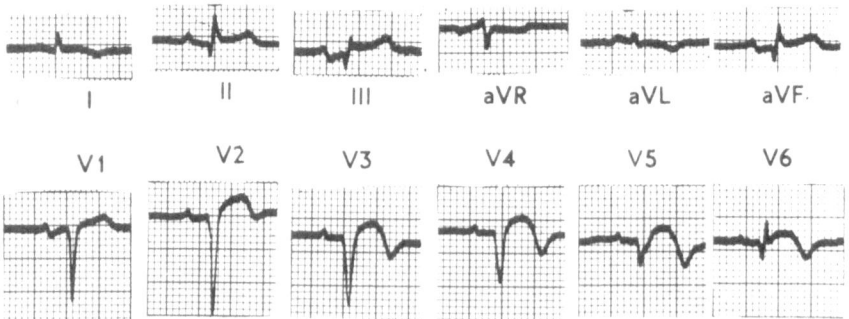

Figure 2 ECG showing extensive anterior myocardial infarct, recorded on the third day after the onset of symptoms. Note the QS-waves in V1–5 as well as a small Q in V6, with ST segment elevation in V2–6 and T-wave inversion in leads I, aVL and V3–6

Among the dedicated experts was W. H. Craib, whose monograph, published by the Medical Research Council in 1929[9] contained the first systematized description of depolarization in terms of the dipole theory or, as he had labelled it, the 'doublet' hypothesis. Craib was a science graduate who took up medicine after the First World War and applied his interests to electrocardiography. During the tenure of a Rockefeller fellowship in the United States, he extended his knowledge, and on his return to Great Britain, worked with Lewis just as that man reached the point where he felt the ECG had yielded its secrets. Craib returned to South Africa, and became a professor of medicine; his interests became more generalized. This country lost a most original thinker and worker, and it is perhaps as a result of this that there was a hiatus in the development of electrocardiographic knowledge in this country. During the subsequent decade many European workers settled in America, and around such men as Louis Katz, Frank Wilson and Emanuel Goldberger, electrocardiography reached the peak of deductive interpretation of arrhythmias and ischaemic disturbances. Further impetus to understanding of the surface ECG was to come from the work described at this meeting by Paul Puech: indeed one of the greatest benefits from intracardiac recording has been the better understanding of conventional surface tracings.

The electrocardiographic pattern does not necessarily tell us the cause of the process. We have already seen a tracing from a patient with acute myocardial infarction (Figure 2). As the infarct heals, the tracing may revert to normal; but, as we well know, sometimes a cardiac aneurysm develops and then shows specific electrocardiographic features (Figure 3). Having seen the evolution we would have no doubt of the aetiology; but a very similar

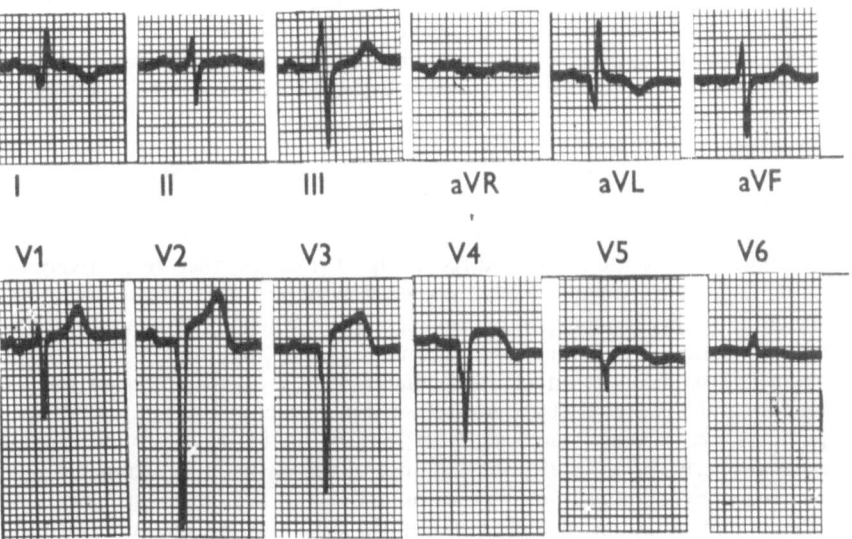

Figure 3 ECG recorded from a patient with a left ventricular aneurysm, 20 years after extensive acute myocardial infarction. The pattern is very similar to that seen in Figure 2

ECG recorded from another patient may well lead to the wrong conclusion. Just these appearances were recorded from a healthy 18-year-old boy who suffered from palpitations. This illustrates how the ECG can be no more than an extension of the clinical senses, for the answer came from the history: 15 years previously he had been kicked by a pony, and had developed a ventricular aneurysm which only manifested itself when ventricular tachycardia occurred when he played football. His clinical condition, but not the ECG appearances, has been rendered normal by resection of the aneurysm.

Let us therefore review the role of the ECG in medical practice in 1978. Earlier this year, in the cardiology course at the Royal Postgraduate Medical School, Professor Frits Meijler of Utrecht spoke of the position of computerized analysis of electrocardiograms. Simple programmes can cope with the vast bulk of tracings recorded in general practice and in non-emergency conditions; those that do not fall into categories should be identified as difficult and analysed by a cardiologist. A somewhat more difficult group of tracings can be analysed by more complex programmes; and there is a third, very small, residue which requires the most careful scrutiny of the dedicated student. One could apply these same principles to the use of the ECG and its reading in practice. In the vast majority of cases the tracings will either be normal or have such gross abnormalities that a definite diagnosis can be made. Difficulties arise with borderline situations on the one hand, and with highly complex and difficult tracings on the other. What, then, are the prerequisites for electrocardiography today?

In the first place, we require recording apparatus of appropriate quality. At the present moment, far too many machines have poor frequency response characteristics. The American Heart Association criteria[10] are stringent and the International Electro-Technical Commission is currently producing specifications which, when they come into general use, will provide a benchmark by which machines can be judged, though it will still take far too long for poor-quality apparatus to fade from the scene. These and other relevant questions were well ventilated at a recent Bethesda conference of the American College of Cardiology[11]. National cardiac societies and our regional and international confederations should exert more pressure to bring about high-quality standards not only of equipment but also in the training of personnel[12]. Currently many tracings are capable of erroneous analysis unless one realizes that one is dealing with inadequate equipment. In Figure 4, we have the sequential recording of tracings taken respectively on an old-fashioned inadequate unit, and on a modern high-quality instrument. The poor-quality machine shows an inadequate height of R-waves, slurring and artifactual broadening of a normal Q-wave that might lead to the erroneous diagnosis of myocardial infarction, and disturbances of the ST segment and T-waves that are not reflected in a machine that has the proper qualities. Even worse, some machines may be unable to cover the area of paper properly, because of poor response of the stylus, and extremely poor low-frequency response may produce artifactual ST segment elevation: patients may be admitted to hospital on the basis of these changes, with the erroneous diagnosis of acute myocardial infarction. Even with accurate machines, such apparently minor changes as different types of paper can

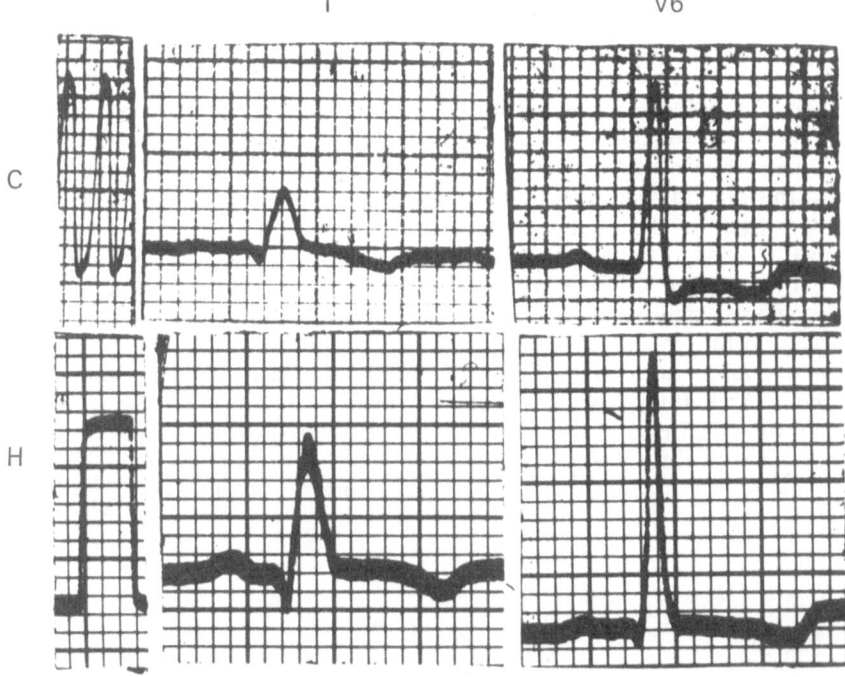

Figure 4 ECG tracings taken successively on an outmoded machine (upper panel, C) and a unit meeting American Heart Association standards (lower panel, H). For details see text

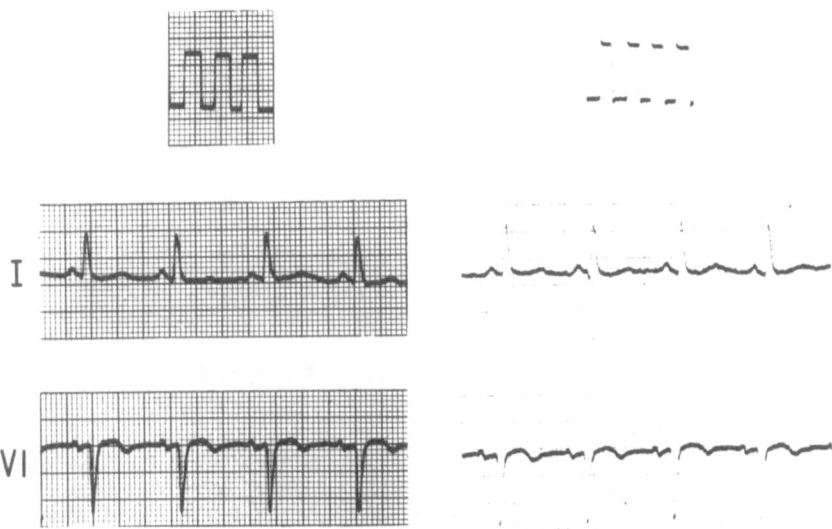

Figure 5 ECG leads taken on the same machine meeting American Heart Association standards, at the same session. The panels on the left were recorded on high-quality paper, those on the right on sub-standard paper. For details see text

109

produce artifacts: Figure 5 shows tracings taken successively from the same patient, the only change being to remove the roll of high-quality paper and replace it with a cheaper one. Even in the standardization complex overshoot is induced by the swing of the stylus across the poorly coated paper, and this is reflected in the poor writing quality and change in the appearances of the leads. Furthermore, wax tends to be burnt off and deposited on the stylus and this may introduce further artifacts.

It is equally vital for the physician who will read the tracing to know as much relevant detail as possible about the patient. This is well known with regard to digitalis, but it is also essential to know whether the patient is taking drugs that may, for example, prolong the QT interval. Thus diuretics, which do this by producing hypokalaemia, antidepressants, phenothiazines and quinidine and similar substances may all have this effect, and may thereby produce arrhythmias; if drugs and electrolyte disturbances can be excluded as possible causes, one must think of other syndromes, sometimes familial, that may produce ventricular tachycardia[13]. The patient's ethnic background is also of considerable importance. An ECG like Figure 6 may cause

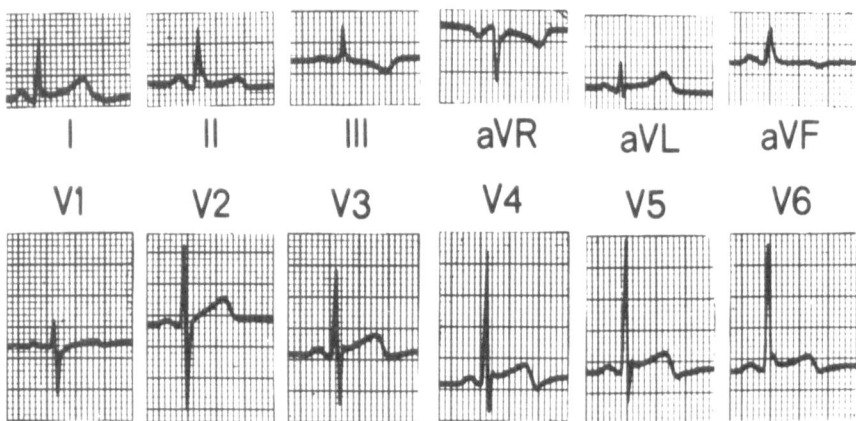

Figure 6 ECG recorded from a 50-year-old Nigerian male with no cardiac disease. Note the relatively tall R-waves, ST elevation and biphasic T-waves seen in mid- and left-precordial leads; the ST elevation is also apparent in leads I and aVL

considerable concern if it emanated from a middle-aged Caucasian; the ST segment changes may suggest acute pericarditis or, under certain circumstances, myocardial ischaemia; but when, as in this case, the recording was taken from a middle-aged Nigerian man, it is entirely consistent with what is normal in this population, as in younger people of other origins, and in some Asians and Africans from other parts[14,15]. Standard criteria for left ventricular hypertrophy may have to be modified when assessing such ECGs as tall R- and deep S-waves over the precordium are common normal findings in such individuals[15].

A conventional ECG provides but a brief recording and may give only a poor reflection of events taking place on a much longer time-scale. This is particularly so in the case of transient arrhythmias, and this is where an important advance has developed from the introduction of ambulatory ECG monitoring. The unit can be worn comfortably concealed within the clothing and recordings may reveal the nature of symptoms of which the patient may have complained, but which may not have been revealed on standard ECGs. In a patient who had experienced syncope an ambulatory recording shows the sudden transformation from normal AV conduction to complete heart block, with a 7-second episode of ventricular asystole during which he felt faint (Figure 7). These episodes have disappeared since a cardiac pacemaker

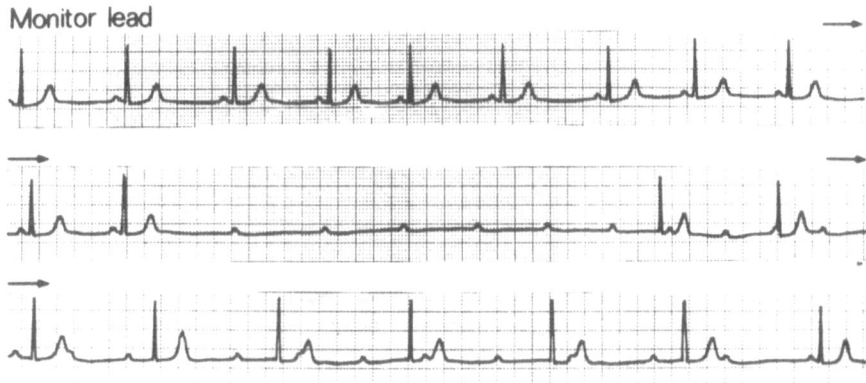

Figure 7 Continuous recording of an ECG by ambulatory monitoring. Sinus rhythm is present throughout; there is normal AV conduction in the upper panel and the first two QRS complexes of the second panel, after which there are six successive P-waves but no QRS complexes. Thereafter high idioventricular rhythm is established and complete atrioventricular block is seen

was implanted. On the other hand, we may discover arrhythmias whose significance is uncertain, e.g. brief runs of ventricular tachycardia of which the patient may be quite unaware. This is a growing problem as ambulatory monitoring becomes more widely used, and we will have to rethink many of our ideas about what is normal and what reflects disease.

It will be from a combination of basic research and the lessons of intra-cardiac recordings that progress will be made. An example of this is the understanding of the ECG appearances in left atrial rhythm, previously the source of much debate and little light. From intracardiac recording and localized stimulation of the left atrium we have learned, as Puech has shown us, what to expect on the surface ECG. As he has also pointed out previously, this can be applied to the sophisticated diagnosis of arrhythmias, e.g. the finding of P-wave inversion following QRS complexes, in reciprocating atrioventricular tachycardia, in lead I (Figure 8). On the intracardiac electro-gram, this was associated with precocious activation of the left atrium in the retrograde direction. The left atrium has been depolarized retrogradely, but

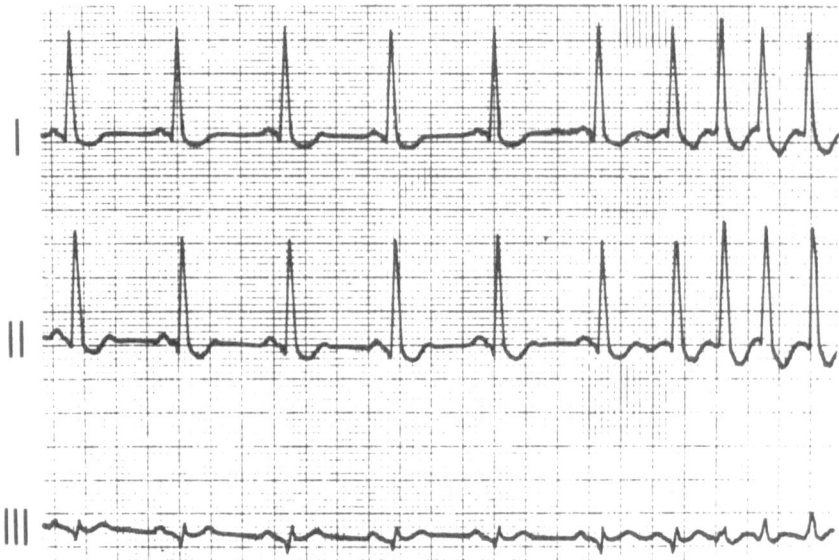

Figure 8 ECG from a patient with a concealed left-sided accessory atrioventricular pathway. The first six complexes show normal sinus rhythm; the seventh represents an atrial extrasystole that induces reciprocating atrioventricular tachycardia and the last four QRS complexes are succeeded by retrograde P'-waves that are inverted in lead I

not via the AV node: the only way that the impulse could have reached it was through an accessory atrioventricular pathway. In cases where there is no evidence of anterograde pre-excitation in sinus rhythm, this may be a most useful clue pointing to the presence of a concealed left-sided accessory pathway[16], and concealed pre-excitation is a far more important cause of reciprocating atrioventricular tachycardia than has been appreciated[17].

This development reinforces the fact that we know very much more about the electrocardiographic interpretation that can be made of atrial and ventricular depolarization than repolarization. As Noble and Cohen[18] have pointed out, the initial physiological interpretation of the T-wave as corresponding to ventricular repolarization is correct, and its polarity is related to differences in the durations of action potentials in various parts of the ventricle; but the U-wave is still an enigma even though it probably reflects repolarization within the Purkinje network[19]. We spend much time, electrocardiographically, analysing T-wave changes yet devote relatively less of our attention to the U-waves; yet here we have, if this is correct, a simple non-invasive index present on many electrocardiograms, that could be compared with the signal-averaging computerized techniques that offer us promise of being able to identify His potentials consistently from the surface of the chest[20].

Let us however remember that one of the main clinical indications for electrocardiography is ischaemic heart disease, and review progress in this field. The precise value of exercise electrocardiography in the diagnosis of cardiac ischaemia remains subject to debate. When carried out using an appropriate sub-maximal exercise test, either graded or continuous, a tread-mill or a bicycle ergometer are equally useful methods of stressing the myocardium, increasing the heart-rate and increasing the need for oxygen[21]. When ischaemia is produced, ST segment depression characteristically results (Figure 9); but unfortunately the test is not yet sufficiently precise to be entirely specific and sensitive. There are a number of patients in whom ST depression develops without there being ischaemia, and false negative tests also arise. Most false positive tests reflect a different type of ST segment depression, as exemplified in Figure 10, but even the strictest criteria, long thought diagnostic of ischaemia, may not be accompanied by abnormalities demonstrable at coronary arteriography[22].

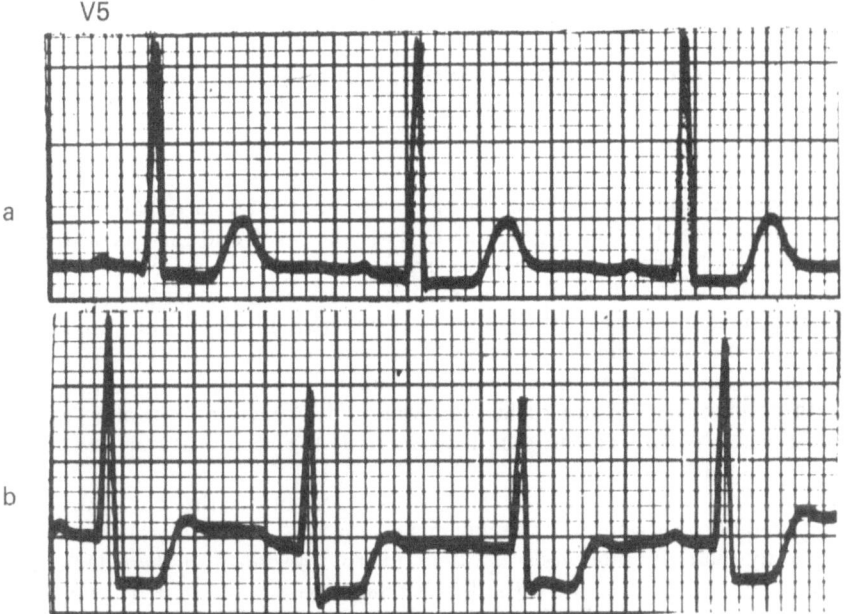

Figure 9 ECG recordings of lead V5 in a patient with angina: (a) was taken at rest and shows no significant ST depression; (b) was recorded after effort and shows plane ST depression of 3 mm persisting for 0.2 s after the onset of the QRS complex (the patient had developed typical angina)

Two other electrocardiographic techniques are currently being evaluated for the assessment of the extent of cardiac damage due to ischaemia. Pre-cordial mapping allows of the serial measurement of quantitative changes in ST segment elevation and other indices and may prove helpful in evaluating therapy for acute myocardial infarction[23]; it also shows promise in exercise electrocardiography for ischaemia[24]. Another example of the way in which one can see improved use of the data visible for so long on the standard

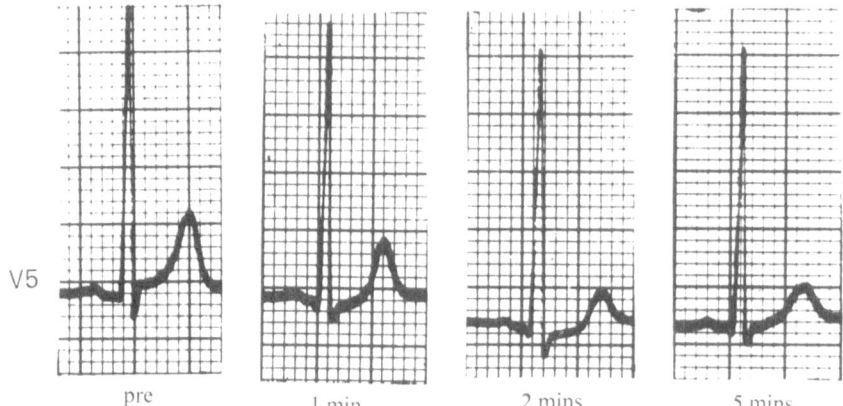

V5

pre   1 min   2 mins   5 mins

Figure 10 ECG recordings of V5 in a patient with hypertension and mild non-specific left chest pain. The resting recording (pre) shows slight ST elevation; 1 and 2 min after exercise there is depression of the junction between the QRS complex and the ST segment, the latter sloping upwards. At 5 min the ST segment no longer showed junctional depression

electrocardiogram is the recent study that showed good correlation between the sum of the R-waves in leads aVL, aVF and V1-6 and the ejection fraction[25]. While the correlation was particularly good between the angiographically demonstrated ejection fraction as seen after premature ventricular contractions, it was also satisfactory when compared with that of sinus beats. This has the great merit of giving a numerical value to the electrocardiographic changes seen after myocardial infarction, permitting comparison with graphic signs of diminished left ventricular function, and offers scope for the use of this classic non-invasive tool, the electrocardiograph, in a more refined fashion.

The electrocardiograph is a relatively old tool but one that has undergone considerable development and refinement. However, the quality of recordings made by the early pioneers was often superb, and much of their deductive reasoning and analysis of arrhythmias, made within the first decade after the development of the ECG, stands up well to the further knowledge acquired through intracardiac recording and other physiological techniques. Another source of progress will be computerized analysis, but this is beyond the scope of the present review. There is still much to be done by careful, thoughtful physicians, using high-quality apparatus currently available.

References

1. Waller, A. D. (1887). A demonstration on man of electromotive changes accompanying the heart's beat. *J. Physiol.*, **8**, 229
2. Snellen, H. A. (1977). *Selected Papers on Electrocardiography of Willem Einthoven, with Bibliography, Biographical Notes and Comments.* (Leiden: Leiden University Press)

3. Lewis, T. (1925). *The Mechanism and Graphic Registration of the Heart Beat.* (London: Shaw & Sons)
4. MacKenzie, J. (1908). *Diseases of the Heart.* (London: Henry Frowde and Hodder & Stoughton)
5. Wenckebach, K. F. (1903). *Die Arythmie als Ausdruck bestimmter Funktionsstörungen des Herzens.* (Leipzig: Wilhelm Engelmann)
6. Wenckebach, K. F. (1914). *Die Unregelmassige Herztätigkeit und ihre Klinische Bedeutung.* (Leipzig: Wilhelm Engelmann)
7. Pardee, H. E. B. (1920). An electrocardiographic sign of coronary artery occlusion. *J. Am. Med. Assoc.*, **26**, 244
8. Wilson, F. N., Johnston, F. D., Rosenbaum, F. F., Erlanger, H., Kossman, C. E., Hecht, H., Cotrim, N., Menezes de Oliveira, R., Scarsi, R. and Barker, P. S. (1944). The precordial electrocardiogram. *Am. Heart J.*, **27**, 19
9. Craib, W. H. (1930). The Electrocardiogram. Medical Research Council Special Report Series, No. 147. (London: His Majesty's Stationery Office)
10. American Heart Association Committee on Electrocardiography (1967). Recommendations for standardization of leads and specifications of instruments in electrocardiography and vectorcardiography. *Circulation*, **35**, 583
11. Tenth Bethesda Conference: Optimal Electrocardiography (1978). *Am. J. Cardiol.*, **41**, 111
12. Krikler, D. M. and Macfarlane, P. W. (1974). Standards for electrocardiographs. *Br. Heart J.*, **36**, 945
13. Krikler, D. M. and Curry, P. V. L. (1976). Torsade de pointes in atypical ventricular tachycardia. *Br. Heart J.*, **38**, 117
14. Littmann, D. (1946). Persistence of the juvenile pattern in the precordial leads of healthy adult Negroes, with support of electrocardiographic survey on 300 Negro and 200 White subjects. *Am. Heart J.*, **32**, 370
15. Krikler, D. M. (1974). The electrocardiogram. In A. G. Shaper, M. S. R. Hutt and Z. Fejfar (eds.). *Cardiovascular Disease in the Tropics*, pp. 160–170. (London: British Medical Association)
16. Puech, P. and Grolleau, R. (1977). L'onde P rétrograde négative en D1, signe du faisceau de Kent posterolateral gauche. *Arch. Mal. Coeur*, **70**, 49
17. Krikler, D. and Rowland, E. (1978). Concealed pre-excitation. *J. Electrocardiol.*, **11** (In press)
18. Noble, D. and Cohen, I. (1978). The interpretation of the T wave of the electrocardiogram. *Cardiovasc. Res.*, **12**, 13
19. Watanabe, Y. and Toda, H. (1978). The U wave and aberrant intraventricular conduction. Further evidence for the Purkinje repolarization theory on genesis of the U wave. *Am. J. Cardiol.*, **41**, 23
20. Vincent, R., Stroud, N. P., Jenner, R., English, M. J., Woollons, D. J. and Chamberlain, D. A. (1978). Noninvasive recording of electrical activity in the PR segment in man. *Br. Heart J.*, **40**, 124
21. Fortuin, N. J. and Weiss, J. L. (1977). Exercise stress testing. *Circulation*, **56**, 699
22. Redwood, D. R., Borer, J. S. and Epstein, S. E. (1976). Whither the ST segment during exercise? *Circulation*, **54**, 703
23. Muller, J. E., Moroko, P. R. and Braunwald, E. (1978). Precordial electrocardiographic mapping. A technique to assess the efficacy of interventions designed to limit infarct size. *Circulation*, **57**, 1
24. Fox, K. M., Selwyn, A. P. and Shillingford, J. P. (1979). A method for praecordial surface mapping of the exercise electrocardiogram. *Br. Heart J.* (In press)

25. Askenazi, J., Parisi, A. F., Cohn, P. F., Freedman, W. B. and Braunwald, E. (1978). Value of the QRS complex in assessing left ventricular ejection fraction. *Am. J. Cardiol.*, **41**, 494

Part III
The myocardium – aspects of contraction

8
The structure of cardiac muscle

V. NAVARATNAM

Muscular architecture

The arrangement of cardiac musculature, particularly in the ventricles, is bewilderingly complex, and though several descriptions are available there is little in the way of general agreement and thus the significance of the arrangement remains obscure.

The disposition is simpler in the atria where two layers of muscle, both incomplete, can be recognized: (a) superficial fibres which run transversely across both atria while some dip into the septum; (b) deep fibres which are restricted to each atrium and may be annular or looped; annular muscle surrounds the base of each auricle (e.g. underlying the crista terminalis), the venous openings and the fossa ovalis while looped fibres pass towards the atrioventricular rings and towards the auricular appendices (e.g. musculi pectinati).

In the ventricular musculature, it is clear that fibre orientation alters considerably as one passes from epicardium towards endocardium; it is oblique in the superficial layers, transverse in the intermediate layers and vertical in the deepest layers. It is interesting that William Harvey commented on this arrangement but did not speculate on its significance. In later times, however, the view emerged that different bands of muscle are wrapped turban-fashion, with natural cleavage planes between layers. The concept of muscle layers was consolidated by many authors, notably by Mall[1], who produced a series of strikingly beautiful illustrations, but it was taken furthest by Robb and Robb[2] who claimed that the bands were separated from each other by fibrous sheaths preventing interconnection between layers. The inferred significance was that the cardiac impulse spreads through the myocardium along specific anatomical pathways, even after it leaves the atrioventricular bundle system. The details differ in individual accounts but, according to Robb and Robb, the ventricular myocardium comprises four separate muscles; viz.: superficial bulbo-spiral and sino-spiral muscles and deep bulbo-spiral and sino-spiral muscles (Figure 1). The two superficial muscles are said to arise from the fibrous skeleton of the heart and to spiral obliquely towards the apex where they enter a vortex-like arrangement and turn inwards into the trabeculae and papillary muscles; of the two muscles, the bulbo-spiral apparently arises from the aortic annulus and to a lesser extent from the mitral, while the sino-spiral takes origin from the tricuspid and pulmonary rings. The two deep muscles form transversely disposed constrictor-like layers, interposed between the superficial muscles and their inturned continuations (Figure 1), but they are incomplete near the cardiac apex. The deep sino-spiral muscle arises from the tricuspid and pulmonary annuli and encircles both ventricles before turning into the septum at the posterior interventricular sulcus. The deep bulbo-spiral, on the other hand, is restricted to the left ventricle where it forms a particularly robust layer lying deep to its sino-spiral counterpart.

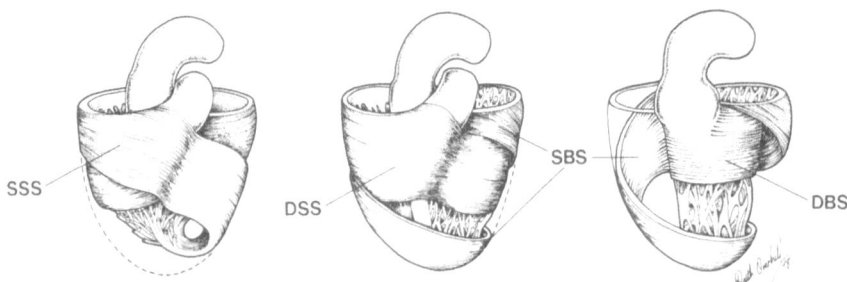

Figure 1 Diagrammatic representation of ventricular musculature of the heart as described by Robb and Robb.[2] SSS – superficial sino-spiral muscle, DSS – deep sino-spiral muscle, SBS – superficial bulbo-spiral muscle, DBS – deep bulbo-spiral muscle

In recent years there has been substantial evidence to refute the traditional interpretation that the myocardium consists of interleaved but separate muscles. Lev and Simkins[3], Grant[4], and Streeter and Bassett[5] have paid attention to muscle fascicles running radially in the heart wall as well as those running tangentially, and they have demonstrated that there are no true cleavage planes in the ventricle wall. While conceding that the orientation of muscle fibres changes systematically through the thickness of the heart wall, it is more realistic to consider the ventricular myocardium as a single muscle mass dividing and subdividing into interconnecting fasciculi. Streeter and Bassett, in particular, demonstrated that the angles of helix at various depths in the myocardium are continuous with each other and show a gradual transition from epicardium to endocardium. The lack of abrupt change in orientation argues strongly against the view of myocardial architecture proposed by Robb and Robb.

STRUCTURE OF CARDIAC MUSCLE CELLS
Typical ventricular myocardium is built up of more or less cylindrical, branching muscle cells each about 100 μm long and 15 μm wide. The nucleus is

centrally placed and the cytoplasm is crowded with organelles, prominent among which are the contractile elements or myofibrils, numerous mito-chrondria and an extensive sarcoplasmic reticulum (SR). The plasma cell membrane or sarcolemma is infolded into the cytoplasm to form a complex T-system (Figure 2) which is coupled closely with SR. A prominent feature of the mitochondria is the close packing of their cristae.

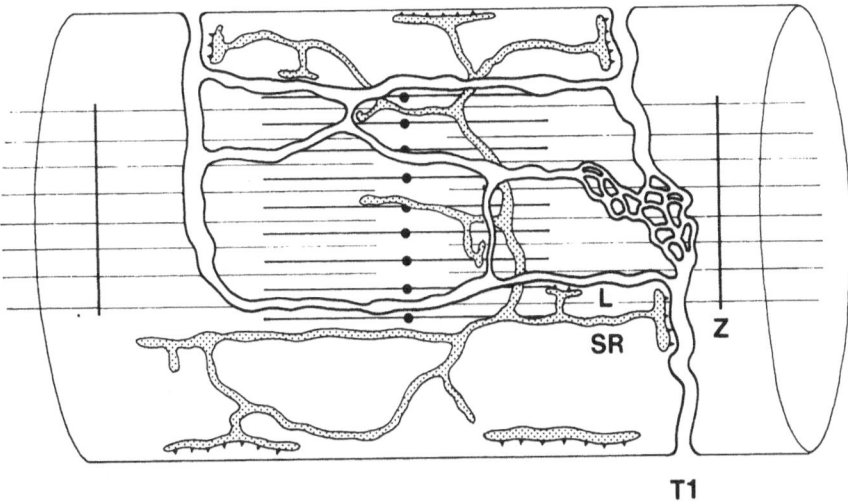

Figure 2 Diagrammatic representation of some cytoplasmic features of a typical ventri-cular myocardial cell. The T-tubule system comprises primary invaginations (T1) of the sarcolemma which give off secondary transverse tubules as well as longitudinal branches (L). The longitudinal branches are further linked by narrow tertiary transverse tubules at A-band level. At all levels of the T-system there occur couplings with cisterns of sarco-plasmic reticulum (SR). Superficial couplings of SR with the surface sarcolemma are also found

The intercalated discs represent sites at which the sarcolemma of adjacent muscle cells are apposed and thickened (Figure 3). Four types of contact can be recognized along a typical disc: (1) nexuses or gap junctions; (2) des-mosomes or adhesion plaques; (3) interfibrillar zones for insertion of myo-fibrils; and (4) unspecialized regions. Over most of the intercalated disc, the gap between the apposed membranes is about 20 nm, but it is reduced to about 2 nm along the nexus components. Electron micrographs, after infiltration with exogenous tracers, such as horseradish peroxidase, and freeze–fracture studies (Figure 4) have revealed that the nexus zone consists of hexagonally packed structures about 2–2½ nm in diameter. Some investi-gators believe that this mosaic-like configuration represents minute inter-cellular channels which may provide the basis for rapid cell-to-cell conduction of the cardiac impulse[6,7].

The contractile apparatus of muscle cells is contained within myofibrils, each of which consists of longitudinally repeating sarcomeres measuring about 2 μm under normal conditions. The sarcomeres are demarcated by Z

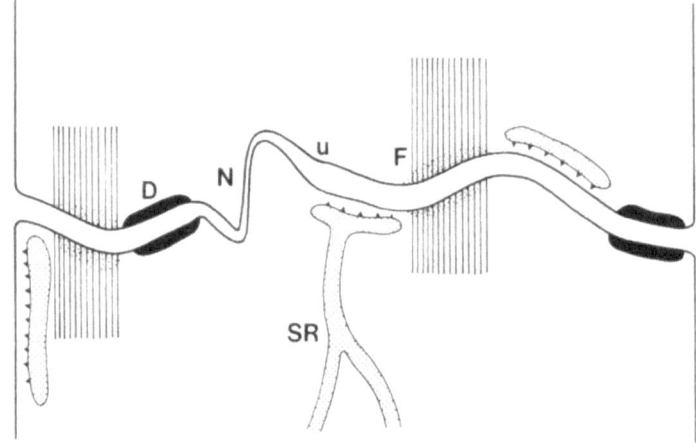

Figure 3 Diagram illustrating the features of a typical intercalated disc in the general myocardium, D – desmosome, N – nexus, F – interfibrillar region, U – so-called unspecialized region which is not infrequently coupled with a cistern of sarcoplasmic reticulum (SR)

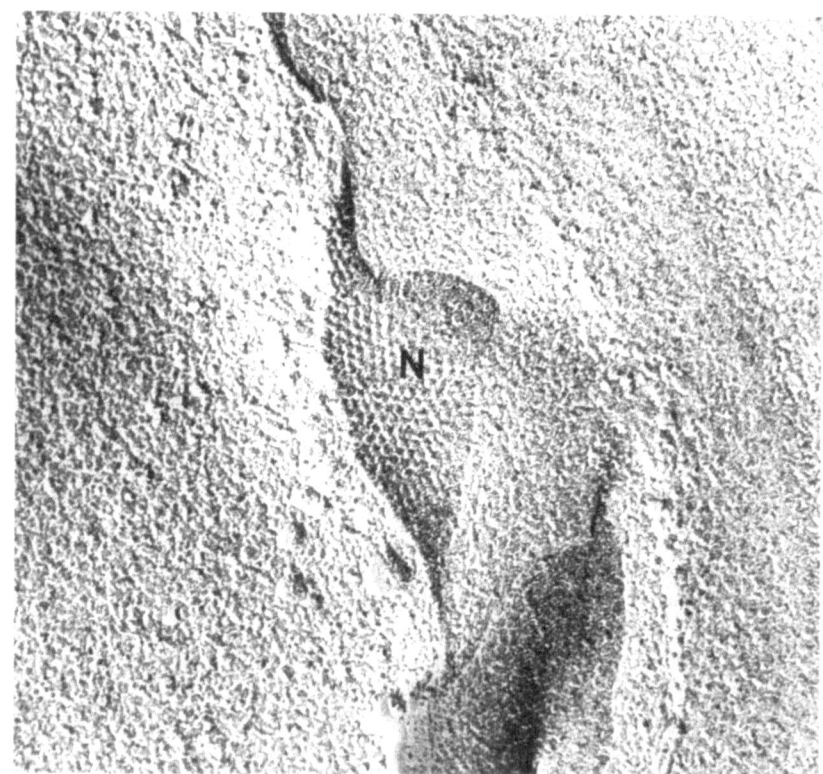

Figure 4 Freeze-fracture preparation of ventricular myocardium showing the mosaic-like arrangement in the nexus region (N) of an intercalated disc (× 80 000)

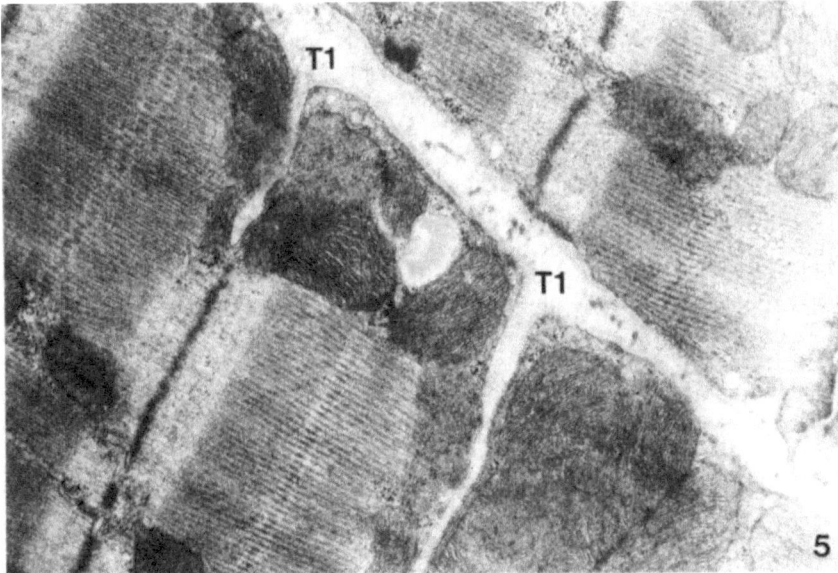

Figure 5 Electron micrograph of a typical ventricular myocardial cell showing wide primary T-tubules (T1) which are invaginations of the surface sarcolemma at I band level of myofibrillae near the Z line ($\times$ 21 000)

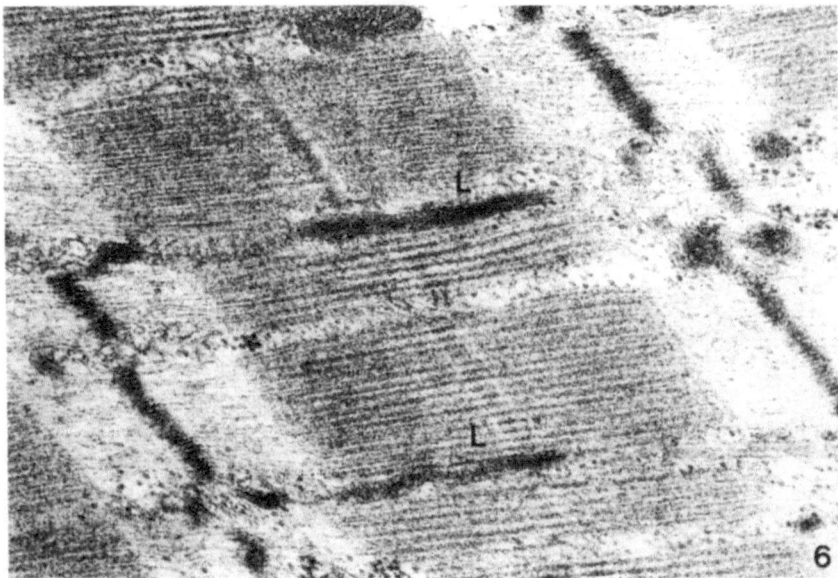

Figure 6 Electron micrograph of a typical myocardial cell after horseradish peroxidase infiltration. Shows labelled longitudinal branches (L) of the T-system running alongside myofibrillae (36 000)

lines and attached to each Z line is an array of thin actin filaments which project towards the middle of the sarcomere (Figure 2). In the middle of the sarcomere is an array of thicker myosin filaments which interdigitate with the actin filaments. There are at least two other proteins related to the actin strands, viz. tropomyosin and troponin. These latter proteins prevent reaction between actin and myosin which would occur spontaneously if actin and myosin were mixed with ATP. When calcium ions bind to troponin, the inhibition is released and cross-bridges can be formed between the thin and thick filaments which slide and shorten the sarcomere.

Interest in the T-system has been boosted by its probable involvement in excitation–contraction coupling and in recent years it has become possible to demonstrate the extensive ramifications of the system by means of horse-radish peroxidase infiltration. In typical ventricular myocytes, there are wide invaginations (primary T-tubules) of the sarcolemma at I band level near the Z line (Figure 5). Several branches arise from the primary T-tubules both in the transverse (secondary T-tubules) and longitudinal axes. The longitudinal branches run alongside the myofibrillae (Figure 6), without transgressing the limits of a single sarcomere, and they are occasionally linked together by narrow tertiary transverse tubules at A band level (Figure 2). All levels of the T-system are closely coupled with cisterns of SR which

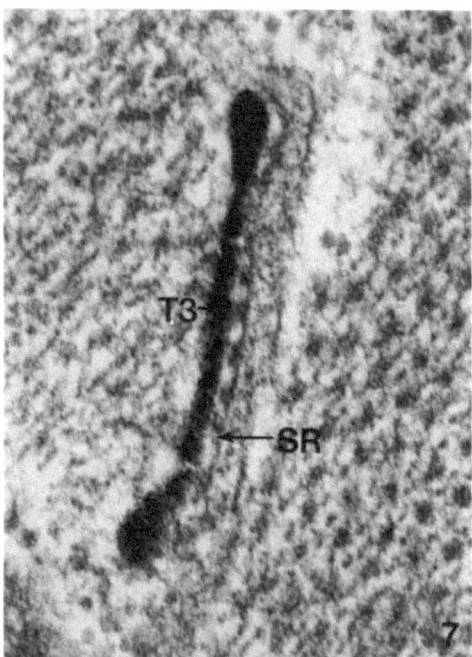

Figure 7 Electron micrograph of a ventricular myocardial cell after horseradish peroxidase labelling, showing a typical coupling arrangement between T-tubule element (in this instance a tertiary transverse tubule – T3) and a cistern of SR. Note the electron-dense spicules in the cytoplasmic gap at the coupling and the granules on the luminal face of the SR ($\times$ 140 000)

contain a high concentration of calcium ions. At these coupling sites (Figure 7), the T-tubule and SR membranes are separated by a cytoplasmic gap of 10–12 nm which lodges dense spicules extending from the SR membrane towards, but not quite reaching, the T-tubule; in addition there are characteristic granules on the luminal aspect of the SR at these couplings, a feature which is not seen elsewhere in the SR. There is considerable physiological evidence to suggest that depolarization of the sarcolemma is channelled by way of the T-system to release calcium ions from the SR, thus activating the myofibrils[8,9].

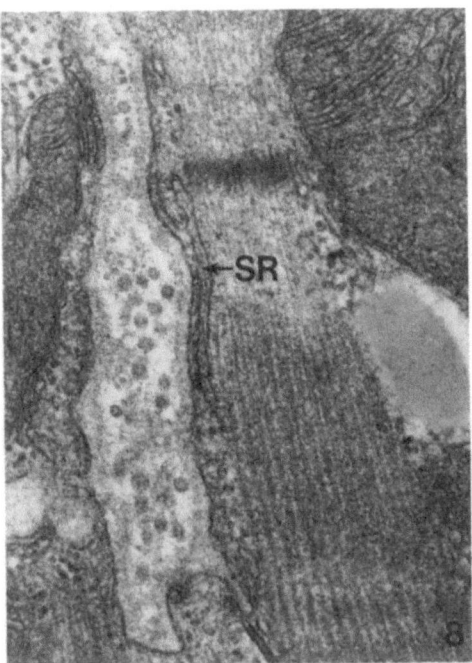

Figure 8 Electron micrograph of a ventricular myocardial cell showing a superficial coupling between a SR cistern and surface sarcolemma (× 70 000)

The SR itself is very extensive in cardiac muscle cells, and a feature not shared with skeletal muscle is the presence of typical SR couplings at the surface sarcolemma (Figure 8), including the unspecialized parts of intercalated discs (Figure 3). The significance of these superficial couplings is not clear, but it is worth noting that they occur frequently in specialized myocardium, including the nodal regions, where the T-system is poorly differentiated and hence deeper couplings are not numerous.

Atrial myocardial cells are generally similar to those in the ventricles. They are slightly more elongated and the T-system is less elaborate, but the most conspicuous difference is the presence of numerous round, osmiophilic, membrane-bound granules (300–400 nm in diameter) in the cytoplasm especially near the nuclear poles (Figure 9); they probably arise from the

Golgi apparatus. These granules have been extensively investigated[10-12] and several functions, including catecholamine storage[11] and calcium storage[12], have been suggested; but these have not been definitely proved. It is worth emphasizing that cells in the specialized nodal regions lack such granules, and this feature has been a useful criterion in distinguishing specialized musculature from the general atrial myocardium.

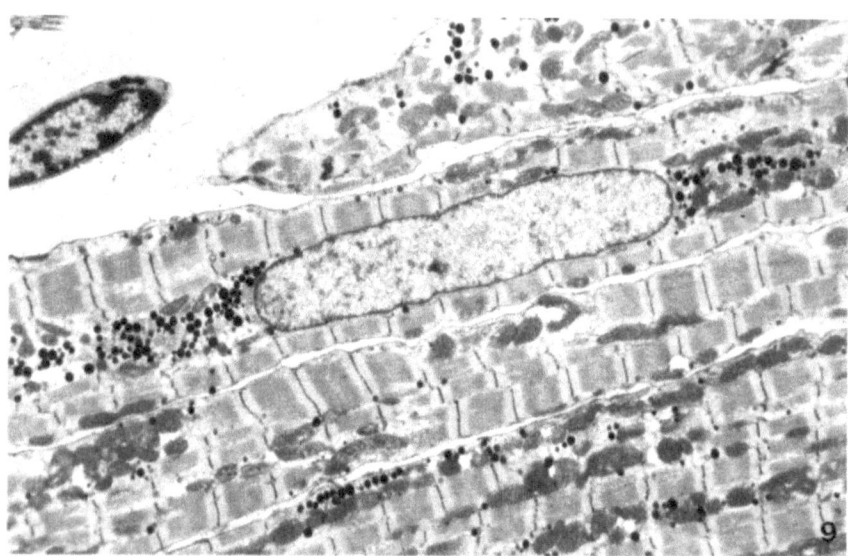

Figure 9 Electron micrograph of a typical atrial myocardial cell showing accumulations of specific atrial granules near the nuclear poles ($\times$ 4200)

SPECIALIZED MUSCULATURE OF THE HEART

There is a certain amount of confusion in the literature about the precise distribution of the specialized impulse-generating and conducting system, particularly in the atrial wall, because the structural criteria for identification are not always clearly appreciated. However, using the absence of specific atrial granules as the principal ultrastructural criterion to distinguish specialized cells from general atrial myocytes, it has been possible to confirm that the system does indeed comprise a sinoatrial (SA) node, atrioventricular (AV) node, AV bundle and bundle branches. There is no convincing ultrastructural evidence for the existence of specialized tracts between the SA and AV nodes, though several have been claimed in the early literature.

The SA node, which lies in the right atrial wall near its junction with the superior vena cava, is a tadpole-shaped structure with the head lying in front of the caval inlet and the tail extending about halfway down the crista terminalis. The node consists of small irregularly arranged cells (Figure 10) and the intercalated discs are indistinct with few or no nexus regions. The cells contain relatively few myofibrillae which, moreover, are irregularly disposed and the T-system is poorly differentiated, comprising only a few

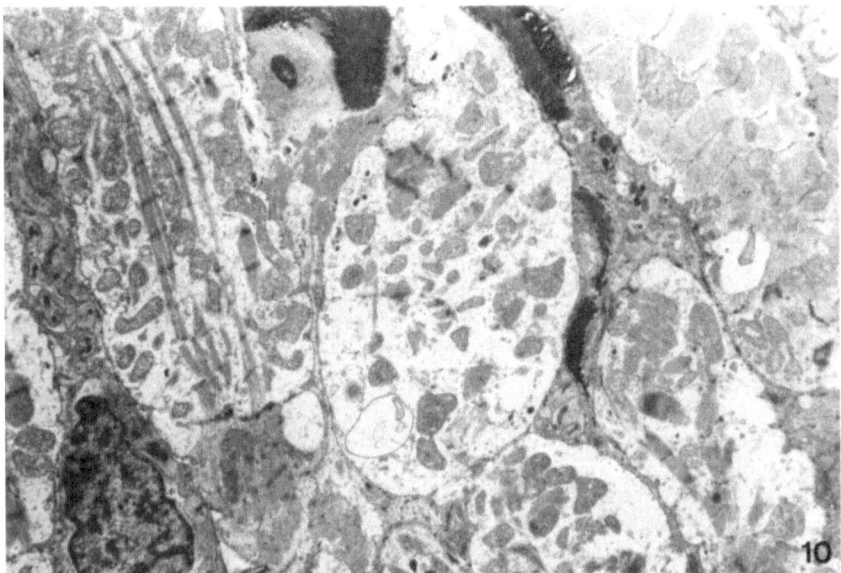

Figure 10 Electron micrograph of sinoatrial node, showing typical small cells with sparse irregular myofibrillae. Intercalated discs are rarely seen ($\times$ 3000)

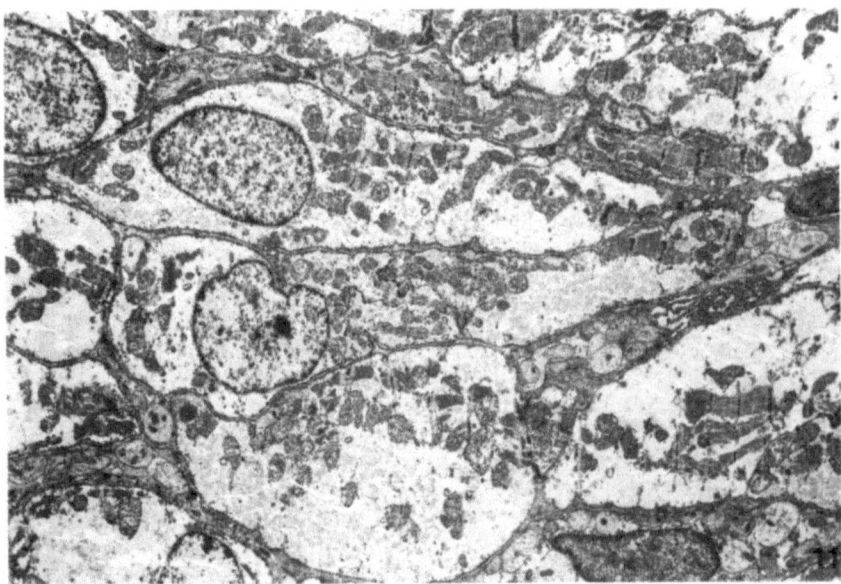

Figure 11 Electron micrograph of atrioventricular node which has a structure similar to that of the sinoatrial node. The cells are small and contain irregularly arranged myofibrillae. Intercalated discs are rare ($\times$ 3000)

primary tubules. The SR is also poorly developed but superficial couplings are present; indeed the proportion of sarcolemma coupled with superficial SR appears to be higher in these cells than in the general myocardium. There are no atrial granules.

The AV node, the ultrastructure of which is very similar to that of the SA node (Figure 11), lies in the right atrial wall just in front of the coronary sinus orifice and above the septal cusp of the tricuspid valve. It continues into the AV bundle which pierces the fibrous trigone and extends into the interventricular septum between the membranous and muscular parts. The bundle then divides into right and left bundle branches which extend into the corresponding ventricles and ramify beneath the endocardium near the cardiac apex. The bundle is made up of slender cells, but in the terminal ramifications the cells are generally thicker than those in the general myocardium, though nowhere in the human heart are these cells comparable to Purkinje fibres of the sheep. As one passes along the bundle system, the myofibrils, T-system and SR become better differentiated and the intercalated discs become prominent. A feature of the bundle branches and their ramifications is the occurrence of extensive nexuses which correlates well with the rapid conduction rate in these regions.

References

1. Mall, F. P. (1911). On the muscular architecture of the ventricles of the human heart. *Am. J. Anat.*, **11**, 211
2. Robb, J. S. and Robb, R. C. (1942). The normal heart. Anatomy and physiology of the structural units. *Am. Heart J.*, **23**, 455
3. Lev, M. and Simkins, C. S. (1956). Architecture of the human ventricular myocardium. *Lab. Invest.*, **5**, 396
4. Grant, R. P. (1965). Notes on the muscular architecture of the left ventricle. *Circulation*, **32**, 301
5. Streeter, D. D. and Bassett, D. L. (1966). An engineering analysis of myocardial fiber orientation in pig's left ventricle in systole. *Anat. Rec.*, **155**, 503
6. McNutt, N. S. and Weinstein, R. A. (1970). The ultrastructure of the nexus. A correlated thin section and freeze-cleave study. *J. Cell Biol.*, **47**, 666
7. Vassalle, M. (1976). Cardiac automaticity. In Mario Vassalle (ed.). *Cardiac Physiology for the Clinician.* (New York: Academic Press)
8. Endo, M. (1977). Calcium release from the sarcoplasmic reticulum. *Physiol. Rev.*, **57**, 71
9. Fabiato, F. (1977). Calcium release from the sarcoplasmic reticulum. *Circ. Res.*, **40**, 119
10. Jamieson, J. E. and Palade, G. E. (1964). Specific granules in atrial muscle cells. *J. Cell Biol.*, **23**, 151
11. Sosa-Lucero, J. C., del le Iglesia, F. A., Lumb, G., Berger, J. M. and Bencosome, S. (1969). Subcellular distribution of catecholamines and specific granules in the rat heart. *Lab. Invest.*, **21**, 19
12. Blaineau-Peyretti, S. and Nicaise, G. (1976). Strontium accumulation in atrial muscle cells. *J. Microsc. et Biol. Cell.*, **26**, 127

9
The physiology of cardiac muscle contraction

B. R. JEWELL

'for when muscles are moving and in action,
they gain strength and become tense,
from soft they become hard,
they are lifted up and thickened,
and so likewise the heart'

William Harvey, 1628

In this passage Harvey likened the contraction of the heart to that of skeletal muscle, but it was not until 1958 that any detailed comparisons of the mechanical properties of the two types of muscle were attempted by physiologists[1,2]. During the period 1958–68 the techniques and conceptual framework developed by A. V. Hill and his school for examining the mechanical properties of skeletal muscle were applied very successfully to the study of isolated preparations of cardiac muscle, mainly by E. H. Sonnenblick and his collaborators[3,4]. These studies explored the complex interactions among four important variables in muscle physiology—the tension produced by the muscle, its velocity of shortening or lengthening, muscle length, and time from the onset of contraction—and they showed that the mechanical properties of cardiac muscle are essentially the same as those of skeletal muscle[5,6].

The pattern of length and tension changes recorded externally when an isolated muscle contracts depends on the mechanical constraints introduced by the experimenter. Figure 1 shows typical data obtained from a cat papillary muscle during isometric and afterloaded isotonic contractions[3]. The isometric contraction appears to be the least complicated mechanical response because only the tension in the muscle is changing, but it must be remembered that internal shortening occurs in a preparation held at constant overall length. The central part of the muscle shortens and stretches the damaged or weaker regions at the ends of the preparation[7,8]. This greatly complicates the

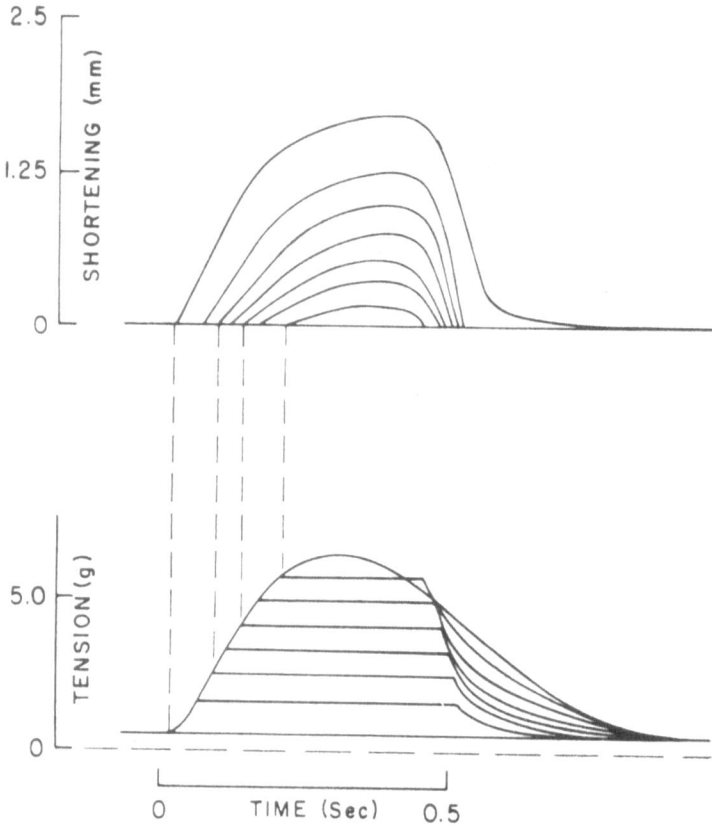

Figure 1 Simultaneous records of length and tension changes during isometric and afterloaded isotonic contractions of a cat papillary muscle (length 7.0 mm, diameter 0.7 mm, temperature 29 °C)[3]. Maximum *shortening* occurred when the muscle contracted against the preload alone (horizontal line at 0.4 g in tension records), and maximum *tension development* occurred when the muscle contracted under isometric conditions (horizontal line at zero in shortening records). The other traces show the length and tension changes when the afterload was incremented in steps of 0.8 g

interpretation of mechanical and energetic studies on isolated preparations and it could invalidate completely the extrapolation of such measurements to the intact heart.

FACTORS DETERMINING MYOCARDIAL PERFORMANCE

Cardiac muscle differs from skeletal muscle in that its contractile response is very sensitive to changes of muscle length and to inotropic interventions. An example of this is given in Figure 2, which shows how tension production in isometric contractions varies with muscle length at different frequencies of stimulation[9]. Similar families of length–tension curves were obtained when maximum rate of rise of tension was used instead of peak tension as an index of myocardial performance[9], and when variation of the bathing calcium concentration was used instead as the inotropic intervention[10,11].

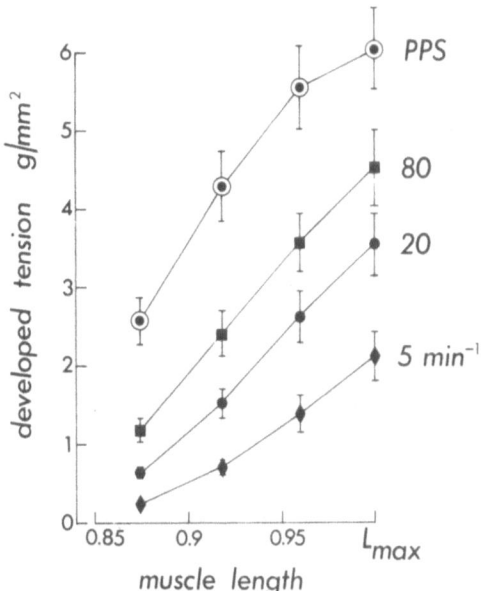

Figure 2 Length–tension curves showing how peak tension developed in isometric contractions varied with muscle length during stimulation at various frequencies (5, 20 and 80/min) and during paired pulse stimulation (PPS)[9]. Muscle length is expressed as a fraction of L_{max}, the length at which maximum tension was developed. Each point shows the mean ±SEM for pooled data from eight to twelve preparations

The dependence of the contractile response on 'external' influences is of vital importance in the intact animal because the heart is a functional syncytium and is therefore denied the possibility of having its contractile strength regulated by variation in the proportions of active and inactive muscle fibres. Adjustments of myocardial performance are possible only because the contractile response of each muscle fibre can be varied by the sympathetic nervous system. Similarly the dependence of myocardial performance on diastolic size (Starling's 'Law of the Heart') appears to arise largely because the contractile strength of cardiac muscle varies steeply over a narrow range of muscle lengths[12].

Until recently it had been generally assumed that inotropic interventions and changes of muscle length are independent regulators of myocardial performance (Figure 3A)[5], but there is now increasing evidence that both inotropic interventions and changes of muscle length act primarily by altering the inotropic state of the muscle (Figure 3B)[13]. Further examination of the possible mechanisms involved in this interaction requires consideration of the events linking the action potential to the mechanical response, because the explanation for the particular sensitivity of cardiac muscle to inotropic interventions and to changes of muscle length seems to lie in special features of excitation–contraction coupling in this type of muscle.

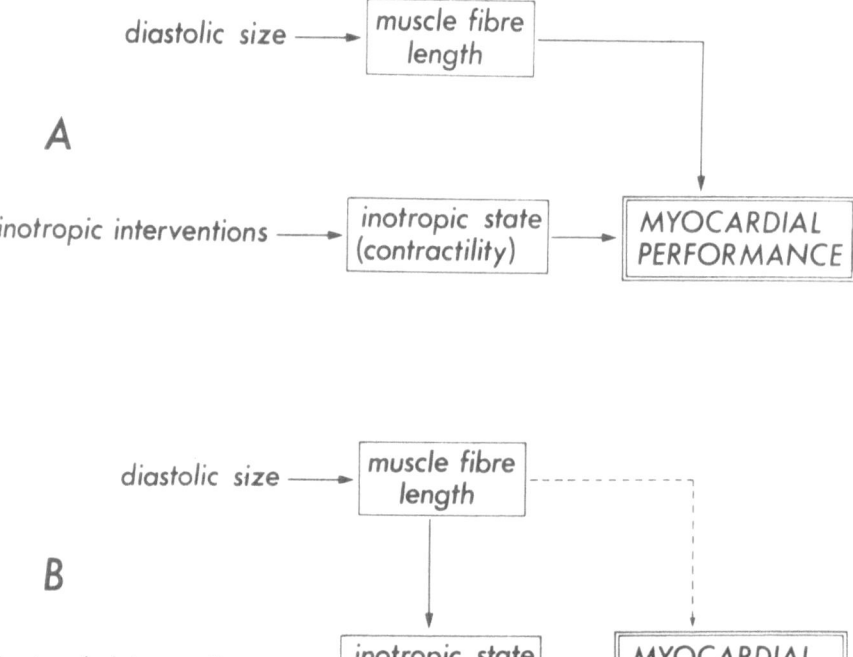

Figure 3 Diagrams summarizing the traditional view that inotropic state and muscle length are independent regulators of myocardial performance (panel A) and the view more recently put forward that inotropic interventions and changes of muscle length both act primarily by altering the inotropic state of the muscle (panel B)

EXCITATION–CONTRACTION COUPLING IN CARDIAC MUSCLE

The chain of events involved in excitation–contraction coupling is shown diagrammatically in Figure 4, which gives an indication of the relative time-courses of the main events. This sequence is essentially the same as in skeletal muscle, but some of the steps appear to be much more susceptible to external influences. The key event is the rise in sarcoplasmic Ca^{++} concentration, $[Ca^{++}]_s$, though there was no *direct* evidence for this in cardiac muscle until recently when Allen and Blinks succeeded in the difficult task of using the photoprotein aequorin as an intracellular indicator of calcium concentration in cardiac muscle[14]. The timing of the rise and fall of $[Ca^{++}]_s$ relative to that of tension in Figure 4 is based on their findings in frog atrial trabeculae. The time-course of the calcium transient relative to the twitch response in mammalian ventricular muscle is likely to be even faster than this, as it is in skeletal muscle[15].

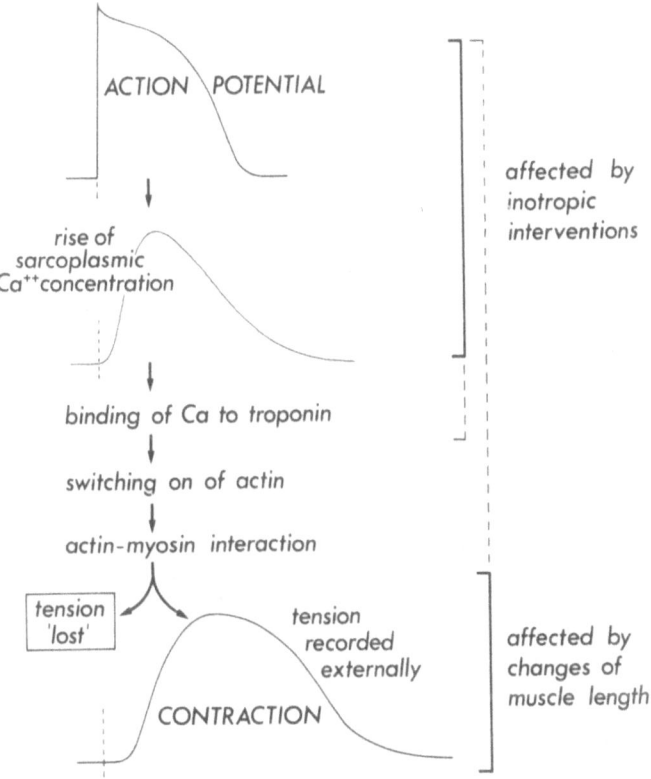

Figure 4 Schematic diagram to show the main events in excitation–contraction coupling in cardiac muscle. The solid brackets on the right indicate events that are generally considered to be influenced by inotropic interventions and changes of muscle length. These have been extended with broken lines to take account of the recent discoveries described in the text

Figure 4 shows that there are several steps between the rise of $[Ca^{++}]_s$ and the development of tension[16]. The switching on of the contractile system in skeletal and cardiac muscle is brought about by the action of Ca^{++} on the thin filaments, though a complementary effect of Ca^{++} on the thick filaments cannot be excluded at the present time. The reactivity of the actin molecules with respect to myosin is controlled by troponin and tropomyosin, which are regulatory proteins found in association with actin in the thin filaments. The rise in $[Ca^{++}]_s$ results in the binding of calcium to troponin, and this leads in turn to the removal of the inhibitory influence of tropomyosin on neighbouring actin molecules. These are then free to interact with myosin molecules in the adjacent overlapping parts of the thick filaments and a shearing force is generated which results in tension development and/or shortening of the muscle. The generation of this shearing force is generally[17], but not universally[18], believed to be due to the formation of cross-bridges between the thick and the thin filaments, and the slow time-course with which these make and break under isometric conditions probably accounts for most of the delay between the rise and fall of $[Ca^{++}]_s$ and the rise and fall of tension shown in Figure 4[19].

The rise in $[Ca^{++}]_s$ is due to entry of calcium into the sarcoplasm from two sources:

1. The 'plateau' of the cardiac action potential is due to a slow inward current across the sarcolemma; this is carried mainly by Ca^{++} and the amount crossing the cell membrane is sufficient to produce a significant rise in $[Ca^{++}]_s$ because of the small size of the cardiac muscle fibre[20]. Activation of the contractile system in frog heart muscle is thought to result almost entirely from this trans-sarcolemmal flux of Ca^{++}, but in mammalian ventricular muscle most of the calcium entering the cell seems to be trapped at storage sites close to the cell membrane (perhaps the subsarcolemmal cisternae of the sarcoplasmic reticulum or the inner surface of the sarcolemma itself)[21].

2. The action potential triggers off a release of calcium from intracellular storage sites; this could be a direct consequence of depolarization of the membrane, or it could result from 'calcium-induced calcium release' which is triggered off by Ca^{++} entering the cell during the action potential[22]. Calcium released from intracellular storage sites is thought to play a minor role in the activation of contraction in frog heart muscle, but in mammalian ventricular muscle these sites appear to be the main source of activator calcium[21].

ACTIVATION OF THE CONTRACTILE SYSTEM IN 'SKINNED' FIBRES

'Skinning' techniques which remove or damage the cell membrane can be used to eliminate early events in excitation–contraction coupling. The sarcoplasm is then brought into contact with the bathing solution and $[Ca^{++}]_s$ can be controlled directly by the experimenter with the aid of suitable chemical buffers such as EGTA. It is possible by microdissection to remove the sarcolemma from single cardiac muscle cells (produced by mechanically homogenizing rat ventricles)[23], but there are also chemical 'skinning' methods which remove or damage cell membranes and produce varying degrees of damage to the internal membrane systems (T-tubules and sarcoplasmic reticulum); these include treatment with glycerol which probably works by osmotic disruption of the cell membrane[24]; treatment with non-ionic detergents such as Brij 58 or Triton-X, which destroy the cell membranes by detergent action[25]; and treatment with powerful chelating agents such as EDTA and EGTA which are thought to render the membrane highly permeable to calcium and other ions[26], though this interpretation has recently been challenged[27]. What preparations have in common after being 'skinned' in one or other of these ways is that they can be brought into a state of contraction by raising the bathing Ca^{++} concentration to micromolar levels. Tension is maintained at a steady level at a given bathing Ca^{++} concentration and it is possible to obtain log dose–response curves of the kind illustrated by Figure 5[28]. The tension produced by the muscle is expressed as a fraction of the maximum value obtained, and the Ca^{++} concentration is given as pCa, where pCa $= -\log_{10}[Ca^{++}]$. The tension–pCa curve shows how the degree

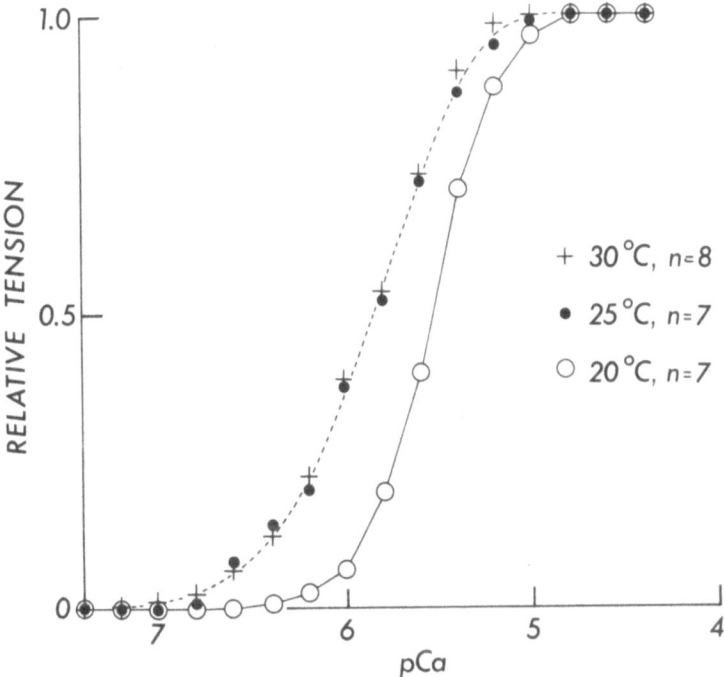

Figure 5 Tension–pCa curve showing how the tension produced in tonic contractions of 'skinned' preparations of cat ventricular muscle varies with the bathing Ca^{++} concentration[28]. Tensions have been expressed as a percentage of the maximum value observed and the Ca^{++} concentration is given as pCa where pCa $= -\log_{10}[Ca^{++}]$

of activation of the contractile system varies with $[Ca^{++}]_s$, and its S-shape is presumed to reflect the binding of calcium by troponin, which reaches saturation at Ca^{++} concentrations above about 10^{-5} mol/l (i.e. pCa 5).

Figure 5 was chosen to illustrate the dependence of activation on the bathing Ca^{++} concentration because it includes the only published results for cat ventricular muscle at 25 and 30 °C[28]. Much of what is known about cardiac muscle mechanics has come from studies of cat papillary muscles at these temperatures, and in Figures 6 and 8 the tension–pCa curve shown by the broken line in Figure 5 will be combined with length–tension data from Figure 2 to illustrate possible explanations for the dependence of tension production on inotropic state and muscle length in cat papillary muscle.

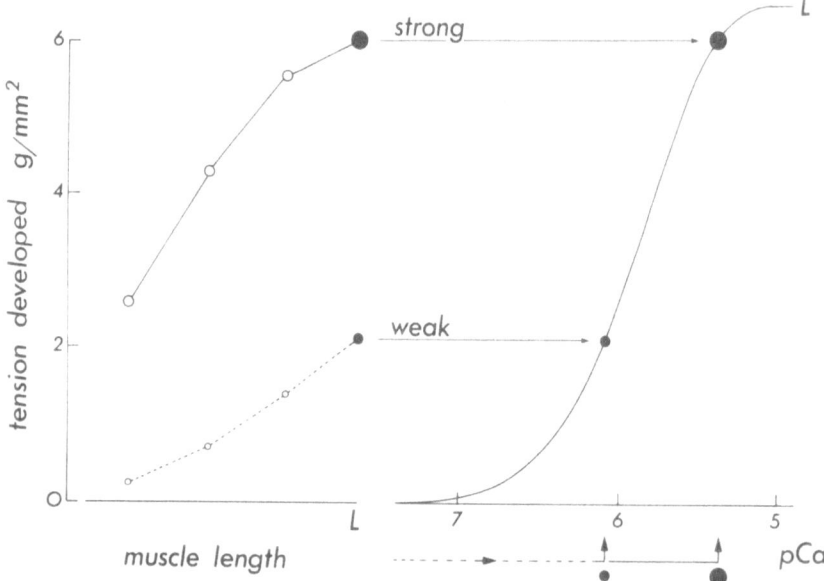

Figure 6 Diagram to illustrate the relationship between inotropic state and activation of the contractile system. The tension–length curves in the left-hand panel are those shown for paired pulse stimulation ('strong' contractions) and for stimulation at 5/min ('weak' contractions) in Figure 2. The tension–pCa curve in the right-hand panel is the broken curve from Figure 5, scaled so that paired pulse stimulation at muscle length L (L_{max}) produces 95% of the maximum possible tension. The horizontal lines show projections of the tensions produced in strong and weak contractions on to the tension–pCa curve, and the arrows below the abscissa show the corresponding levels to which $[Ca^{++}]_s$ would have to rise to produce these tensions

EFFECT OF INOTROPIC INTERVENTIONS ON ACTIVATION

The left-hand panel in Figure 6 shows length–tension curves obtained during paired pulse stimulation ('strong' contractions) and during low frequency stimulation ('weak' contractions), as previously displayed in Figure 2. The right-hand panel is the tension–pCa curve at 25/30 °C from Figure 5, and it has been scaled so that the tension produced by paired pulse stimulation at L_{max} (denoted by L in Figure 6) gives 95% of the maximum possible tension. The justification for this is that paired pulse stimulation is generally thought to produce almost complete activation of the contractile system in ventricular muscle[29]. The horizontal lines linking the two panels show projections of the tensions observed in 'strong' and 'weak' contractions at L_{max} on to the tension–pCa curve, and the arrows below the abscissa on the right-hand panel show estimated values for the $[Ca^{++}]_s$ required to produce these tensions. They are of course the concentrations that would be required to produce these tensions under steady-state conditions (i.e. in tonic contractions) and they cannot be regarded as exact predictions of what might be expected as the peak values of $[Ca^{++}]_s$ under non-steady-state conditions (i.e. twitches). However they do in fact agree quite well with the peak values observed in frog atrial trabeculae as determined by the aequorin technique[14], though this agreement may be fortuitous in view of the difference in species.

All the results reported by Allen and Blinks support the general concept embodied in Figure 6 that variations in inotropic state can be equated with variations in the degree of activation of the contractile system. The inotropic effects of catecholamines, cardiac glycosides, and increases in either stimulus frequency or bathing Ca^{++} concentration were accompanied by greater peak

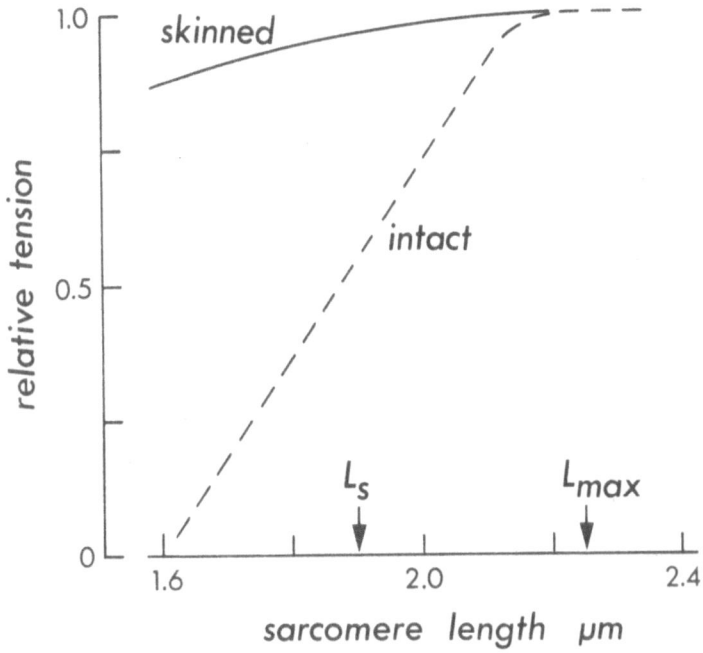

Figure 7 Length–tension curves obtained from skinned and intact preparations of rat ventricular muscle[13,23,33] L_{max} is the sarcomere length at which maximum tension is developed, and L_s is the slack length of the muscle – i.e. the sarcomere length to which the muscle returns spontaneously after passive stretching or after active shortening against zero load

values of $[Ca^{++}]_s$ during contraction, but equal inotropic effects were not necessarily accompanied by equal increases in the Ca^{++} transient[14]. This suggests that there may be other factors involved, and in the case of catecholamines there is some evidence for an alteration in the sensitivity of the contractile system to calcium which is thought to be a consequence of the phosphorylation of troponin by a cyclic AMP-activated protein kinase[30,31]. The bracket on the upper right-hand side of Figure 4 has been extended downwards with a broken line to include this possibility, but it seems safe to assume that inotropic interventions act only on early events in excitation–contraction coupling.

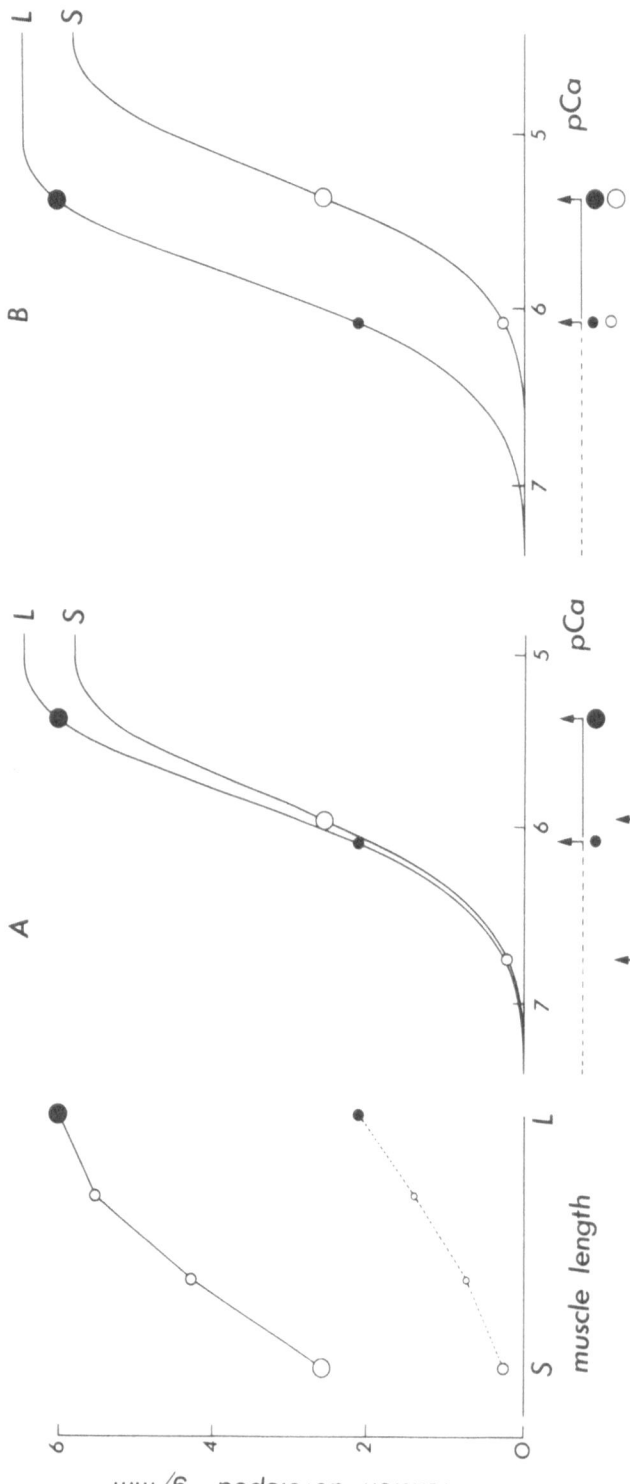

Figure 8 Diagram to illustrate two possible explanations for length-dependence of activation. The approach is the same as in Figure 6, but it now includes the tensions produced in strong and weak contractions at a shorter muscle length S (0.87 L_{max}). In panel A the tensions observed at this length (open circles) have been projected on to a tension–pCa curve for length S, which is the curve for length L scaled down to 90 % for reasons given in the text. The corresponding values of $[Ca^{++}]_s$ that would be needed to produce these tensions are shown by the arrows below the abscissa. In panel B it has been assumed that the Ca^{++} concentrations reached during weak and strong contractions at length S are the same as at length L, and the tension–pCa curve for the short length has been shifted sufficiently to the right to make the tensions observed at this length (open circles) fall on the curve

DEPENDENCE OF ACTIVATION ON MUSCLE LENGTH

The basis for the traditional view that length and inotropic state are independent regulators of myocardial performance (Figure 3A) is that a decline of tension production would be expected at short muscle lengths according to the sliding filament hypothesis[32]. At muscle lengths below L_{max} a fall in the tension recorded externally would be expected because tension is 'lost' internally in bringing about double overlap of the thin filaments in the central region of each sarcomere and because the double overlap results in interference with normal cross-bridge formation. In terms of Figure 4 myocardial performance is altered because a change of muscle length affects the final stage in excitation–contraction coupling, as indicated by the solid bracket on the lower right of that Figure.

In fact tension production in cardiac muscle falls off much more steeply at muscle lengths below L_{max} than would be expected according to the sliding filament hypothesis[13]. This has been shown most convincingly in studies of rat ventricular muscle in which the sarcomere length was measured instead of muscle length. The dashed line in Figure 7 shows the ascending limb of the length–tension relation observed in a rat papillary muscle preparation in which sarcomere length was held constant in the central part of the muscle during contractions at each sarcomere length[33]. There is a plateau of tension production over the range of sarcomere lengths from 2.35 μm down to 2.2 μm, and then a steep decline towards zero at a sarcomere length of about 1.6 μm. The solid line shows the length–tension relation observed in skinned fibres in which the contractile system was maximally activated at each sarcomere length[23]. It is essentially the same as the curve obtained from living and skinned frog skeletal muscle fibres[32,34] and it shows the decline in tension production at muscle lengths below L_{max} that would be expected as a result of the tension 'losses' predicted by the sliding filament hypothesis. The curve obtained from the intact muscle is clearly much steeper than this, and there is now an increasing body of evidence of various kinds that the steepness of the length–tension relation results mainly from length-dependence of activation processes in cardiac muscle[13].

In Figure 4 the lower right-hand bracket has been extended with a dashed line to indicate that earlier events in excitation–contraction coupling may be affected by changes of muscle length, and Figure 8 illustrates two possible explanations for length-dependence of activation. The approach used is the same as in Figure 6 and the assumption made in constructing these graphs is that if the intact muscle could be fully activated at length S (0.87 L_{max}) tension production would be about 90% of that at length L (L_{max})—i.e. a tension loss of about 10% over this range of lengths is what would be expected from the sliding filament hypothesis[32]. A tension–pCa curve for length S has therefore been drawn by scaling down the curve for length L (Figure 7) to 90%.

The explanation for length-dependence of activation illustrated by Figure 8A is that the tension produced at length S is less than at length L because the peak value of $[Ca^{++}]_s$ reached in a twitch is less at the shorter muscle length. The arrows below the abscissa of Figure 8A show estimated values obtained by projecting the tensions observed in 'strong' and 'weak' contractions at length S on to the tension–pCa curve for that length: these values for $[Ca^{++}]_s$ are less than the corresponding values at length L. The explanation for length-dependence of activation illustrated by Figure 8B is that the tension produced at length S is less than at length L because the contractile system is less sensitive to calcium at the shorter muscle length. In the construction of Figure 8B it has been assumed that the peak values of $[Ca^{++}]_s$ reached in 'strong' and 'weak' contractions at length S are the same as at length L, and the tension–pCa curve for length S has been shifted to the right until the tensions observed at length S fall on the curve. If the tension–pCa curve directly reflects the binding of Ca^{++} to troponin, then a shift to the right can be interpreted as showing a reduction in the affinity of troponin for calcium at the shorter length.

Evidence for the first of these explanations has come from the work of the Fabiatos on skinned fibres from rat ventricles[23]. Figure 9 shows length–

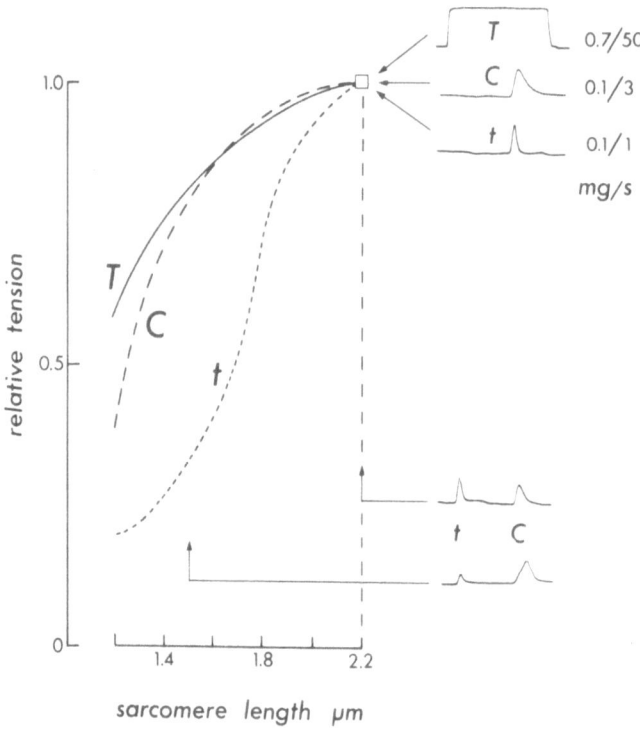

Figure 9 Tension–length curves obtained from skinned rat ventricular muscle during tonic contractions (T) and during phasic contractions induced by caffeine (C) or triggered by a small increase in the bathing Ca^{++} concentration (t)[23]. The numbers alongside the upper traces show the magnitude (tension in mg) and duration (seconds) of typical contractions. The lower traces show the tensions produced at long and short sarcomere lengths when a Ca^{++}-triggered response (t) was immediately followed by a caffeine-induced response (C). Adapted from published data[14]

tension curves obtained from three different types of contraction: *tonic* contractions (T) produced by clamping the bathing Ca^{++} concentration at selected values with the aid of calcium buffers, and *phasic* contractions resulting from the release of Ca^{++} from intracellular stores, which can be induced by caffeine (C) or by a small increase in bathing Ca^{++} concentration in a weakly buffered solution (calcium-induced calcium release, t). There is evidence that the normal mechanism of calcium release from intracellular stores in the intact muscle may involve calcium-induced calcium release[22] and the third type of contraction studied may therefore be a realistic model of the normal contractile response. The strengths and durations of these tonic and phasic contractions are very different, as indicated by the typical data included in Figure 9, and the length–tension curves for the different types of contraction have been normalized so that all tensions are expressed as a fraction of that observed at L_{max}.

The length–tension curve for tonic responses (T in Figure 9) shows the least decline of tension at lengths below L_{max} and this is regarded as the length–tension relation for a muscle that is maximally activated at each muscle length. (This curve has already been used in Figure 7 for comparison with that obtained from intact muscle.) The length–tension curve for caffeine-induced phasic responses (C) is similar to curve T at lengths close to L_{max} but it becomes steeper at shorter lengths. Finally the length–tension curve for calcium-triggered phasic responses (t) is steeper than either of these and it is more like the curve obtained from intact rat ventricular muscle, as shown in Figure 7.

The authors have argued that the steep decline of curve t occurs because less calcium is released at short lengths, and their evidence for this is also shown in Figure 9. When caffeine was used to induce a phasic response immediately after a calcium-triggered response (i.e. before significant reloading of the intracellular calcium stores could have occurred) the contraction produced was greater at short muscle lengths than at long lengths. The simplest interpretation of this finding is that there was more calcium left in the stores to be released by caffeine at short lengths because less had been released in the previous Ca^{++}-triggered contraction.

There is also evidence from work with aequorin in intact frog skeletal muscle fibres that less calcium is released at short muscle lengths[15], but comparable studies in frog atrial trabeculae do not support this hypothesis[14]. Figure 10 shows the data obtained by Allen and Blinks at four different muscle lengths, all on the ascending limb of the length–tension curve for frog atrial muscle, and it is clear from this that greater tension production at longer muscle lengths is accompanied by *smaller* calcium transients.

The only published evidence for the second explanation illustrated by Figure 8 comes from the work of Endo on skinned skeletal muscle fibres from *Xenopus laevis*[35]. He showed that the sensitivity of this preparation to Ca^{++} concentrations which give submaximal tonic contractions was greater at a sarcomere length of 2.8 μm than it was at shorter lengths, and this finding has been interpreted as showing that the affinity of troponin for calcium may be length-dependent[35,36]. In my laboratory we have been trying similar experiments on skinned fibres from rat ventricular muscle over the range of

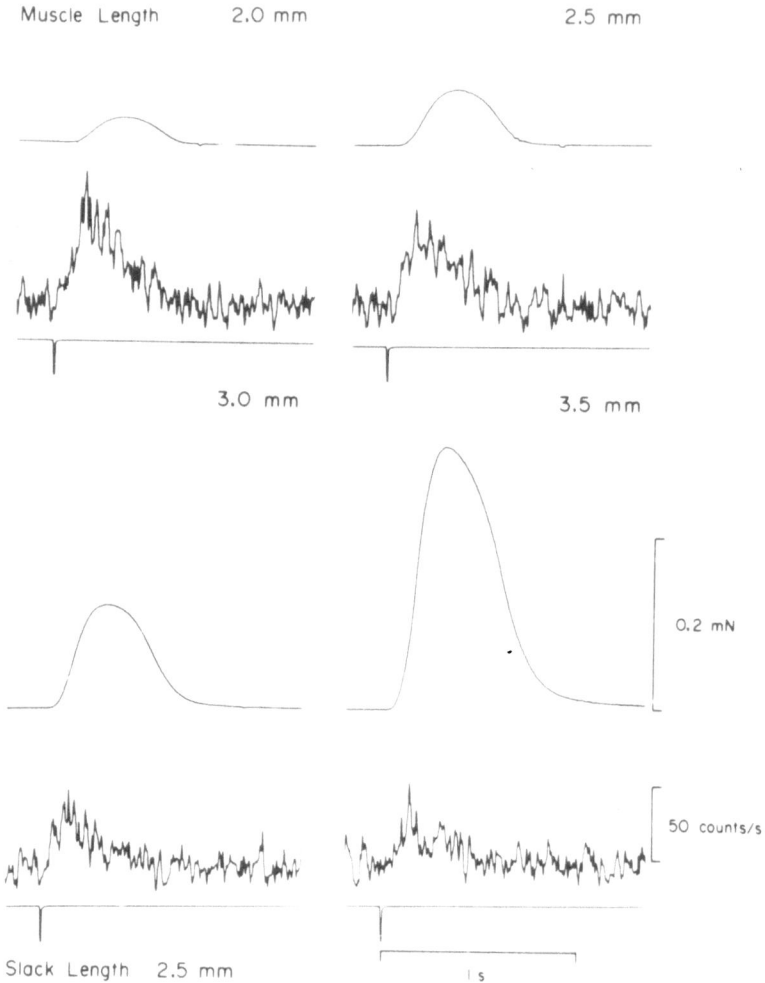

Figure 10 Records of tension production and the light response from aequorin in contractions of a frog atrial trabecula at the muscle lengths indicated (slack length 2.5 mm)[14]. The calibration bars show the tension produced (0.2 mN ≈ 20 mg) and the light output recorded by the photomultiplier (counts/s)

sarcomere lengths covered by the ascending limb of the length–tension relation[25]. Although our preliminary results show a shift of the tension–pCa curve to the left when the preparation is stretched, the shift is only of the order of 0.1–0.2 of a pCa unit, and this would not be sufficient by itself to account for the steepness of the length–tension relation observed in the intact muscle.

The present situation is therefore rather tantalizing. The available evidence from studies with aequorin, at least according to current interpretations of the light responses obtained, does not support the hypothesis illustrated by Figure 8A, and it appears that the affinity of troponin does not change enough when the muscle is stretched to make Figure 8B a satisfactory alternative hypothesis. If these results are confirmed by further work, then it will be necessary to look for another explanation for length-dependence of activation in cardiac muscle, and this remains a field of continuing interest to cardiac muscle physiologists, particularly in view of its importance in understanding the physiological basis of Starling's Law of the Heart.

CONCLUSION

I began with a quotation from *De motu cordis* in which Harvey drew our attention to similarities between the action of the heart and muscular contraction. In my lecture I have assumed that the molecular mechanism of contraction is the same in the two types of muscle (though that has not yet been demonstrated conclusively), and I have concentrated on recent advances in our understanding of how inotropic interventions and changes of muscle length alter myocardial performance. The argument has been put forward that all changes in contractility result primarily from alterations in the degree of activation of the contractile system and that inotropic state and muscle length should not be regarded as independent regulators of myocardial performance.

References

1. Trendelenburg, U. and Lüllman, H. (1958). Uber die Messung des 'Active State' am Herzmuskel des Frosches. *Biochem. Biophys. Acta*, **29**, 13
2. Abbott, B. C. and Mommaerts, W. F. H. M. (1959). A study of inotropic mechanisms in the papillary muscle preparation. *J. Gen. Physiol.*, **42**, 533
3. Sonnenblick, E. H. (1962). Force–velocity relations in mammalian heart muscle. *Am. J. Physiol.*, **202**, 931
4. Sonnenblick, E. H. (1966). In S. A. Briller and H. L. Conn (eds.). *The Myocardial Cell*, pp. 193–250. (Philadelphia: Univ. Pennsylvania Press)
5. Blinks, J. R. and Jewell, B. R. (1972). The meaning and measurement of myocardial contractility. In D. H. Bergel (ed.). *Cardiovascular Fluid Dynamics*, vol. 1, pp. 225–260. (London: Academic Press)
6. Simmons, R. M., and Jewell, B. R. (1974). Mechanics and models of muscular contraction. *Recent Adv. Physiol.*, **9**, 87
7. Krueger, J. W. and Pollack, G. H. (1975). Myocardial sarcomere dynamics during isometric contractions. *J. Physiol. (Lond.)*, **251**, 627
8. Julian, F. J. and Sollins, M. R. (1975). Sarcomere length–tension relations in living rat papillary muscle. *Circ. Res.*, **37**, 299
9. Lakatta, E. G. and Jewell, B. R. (1977). Length-dependent activation. Its effect on the length–tension relation in cat ventricular muscle. *Circ. Res.*, **40**, 251
10. Allen, D. G., Jewell, B. R. and Murray, J. W. (1974). The contribution of activation processes to the length–tension relation of cardiac muscle. *Nature*, **248**, 606
11. Huntsman, L. L. and Stewart, D. K. (1977). Length-dependent calcium inotropism in cat papillary muscle. *Circ. Res.*, **40**, 366
12. Ford, L. E. (1976). Heart size. *Circ. Res.*, **39**, 297
13. Jewell, B. R. (1977). A reexamination of the influence of muscle length on myocardial performance. *Circ. Res.*, **40**, 221
14. Allen, D. G. and Blinks, J. R. (1978). Calcium transients in aequorin-injected frog cardiac muscle. *Nature*, **273**, 509

15. Blinks, J. R., Rüdel, R. and Taylor, S. R. (1978). Calcium transients in isolated amphibian skeletal muscle fibres: detection with aequorin. *J. Physiol. (Lond.)*, **277**, 291
16. Ebashi, S., Endo, M. and Ohtsuki, I. (1969). Control of muscle contraction. *Quart. Rev. Biophys.*, **2**, 351
17. Huxley, A. F. (1957). Muscle structure and theories of contraction. *Prog. Biophys.*, **7**, 257
18. Noble, M. I. M. and Pollack, G. H. (1977). Molecular mechanisms of contraction. *Circ. Res.*, **40**, 333
19. Julian, F. J. and Moss, R. L. (1976). The concept of active state in striated muscle. *Circ. Res.*, **38**, 53
20. Bassingthwaighte, J. B. and Reuter, H. (1972). Calcium movements and excitation-contraction coupling in cardiac cells. In W. C. de Mello (ed.). *Electrical Phenomena in the Heart*, pp. 353–395. (London and New York: Academic Press)
21. Morad, M. and Goldman, Y. (1973). Excitation–contraction coupling in heart muscle: membrane control of development of tension. *Prog. Biophys. Mol. Biol.*, **27**, 257
22. Fabiato, A. and Fabiato, F. (1977). Calcium release from the sarcoplasmic reticulum. *Circ. Res.*, **40**, 119
23. Fabiato, A. and Fabiato, F. (1975). Dependence of the contractile activation of skinned cardiac muscle cells on the sarcomere length. *Nature*, **256**, 54
24. Reiermann, H. J., Herzig, J. W. and Rüegg, J. C. (1977). Ca^{++} activation of ATPase activity, ATP-P_1 exchange, and tension in briefly glycerinated heart muscle. *Basic Res. Cardiol.*, **72**, 133
25. Hibberd, M. G. and Jewell, B. R. Unpublished observations
26. Winegrad, S. (1971). Studies of cardiac muscle with a high permeability to calcium produced by treatment with ethylenediaminetetraacetic acid. *J. Gen. Physiol.*, **58**, 71
27. Miller, D. J. (1978). Chemical 'skinning' of cardiac muscle: a reinvestigation. *J. Physiol. (Lond.)*, in press
28. Brandt, P. W. and Hibberd, M. G. (1976). Effect of temperature on the pCa–tension relation of skinned ventricular muscle of the cat. *J. Physiol. (Lond.)*, **258**, 76P
29. Fisher, V. F., Lee, R. J., Marlon, A. and Kavaler, F. (1967). Paired electrical stimulation and the maximal contractile response of the ventricle. *Circ. Res.*, **20**, 520
30. Solaro, R. J., Moir, A. J. G. and Perry, S. V. (1976). Phosphorylation of troponin I and the inotropic effect of adrenaline in the perfused rabbit heart. *Nature*, **262**, 615
31. Ray, K. P. and England, P. J. (1976). Phosphorylation of the inhibitory subunit of troponin and its effect on the calcium dependence of cardiac myofibril adenosine triphosphatase. *FEBS Letters*, **70**, 11
32. Gordon, A. M., Huxley, A. F. and Julian, F. J. (1966). The variation in isometric tension with sarcomere length in vertebrate muscle fibres. *J. Physiol. (Lond.)*, **184**, 170
33. Pollack, G. H. and Krueger, J. W. (1976). Sarcomere dynamics in intact cardiac muscle. *Eur. J. Cardiol.*, **4**, 53
34. Schoenberg, M. and Podolsky, R. J. (1972). Length–force relation of calcium-activated muscle fibres. *Science*, **176**, 52
35. Endo, M. (1972). Stretch-induced increase in activation of skinned muscle fibres by calcium. *Nature New Biol.*, **237**, 211
36. Fuchs, F. (1974). Striated muscle. *Ann. Rev. Physiol.*, **36**, 461

10
Metabolism of the normal and ischaemic myocardium

M. F. OLIVER

It has been shown by reason and experiment that blood by the beat of the ventricles flows through the lungs and heart and is pumped to the whole body. . . .

(WILLIAM HARVEY, 1628)

INTRODUCTION

Cardiac muscle cells comprise complex systems which are able to adjust and control the pumping action of the heart to meet the constantly changing demands of the body. These self-regulatory systems are mostly biochemical in nature and are complemented by other self-regulatory systems, including myocardial coronary arterial perfusion and the excitatory activation of the myocardium.

In this chapter, an outline will be given of the production and utilization of the energy required for the pump; of the influence of ischaemia on normal biochemical and metabolic pathways; of some biochemical consequences leading to tissue damage and changes in the co-ordinated electrophysiological function of the heart; and some protective effects of metabolic intervention.

Details of the complex pathways of intermediary metabolism which provide the source of chemical energy required for normal cardiac contraction will not be discussed and can be found in most standard textbooks of biochemistry.

ENERGY PRODUCTION AND UTILIZATION IN THE NORMAL MYOCARDIUM

High-energy phosphates

Adenosine triphosphate (ATP) is the essential source of energy for the processes which lead to the liberation of mechanical energy by the heart

145

muscle. This is accompanied by the breakdown of phosphocreatine, a labile compound of creatine and phosphoric acid. In the normal heart, a decrease in phosphocreatine is proportional to the work done. The overall reaction describing the production of energy from adenine nucleotides is:

$$ADP + phosphocreatine = ATP + creatine$$
$$ATP \rightarrow ADP + inorganic\ phosphate + energy$$

ATP is synthesized in exchange for the energy derived from a number of different chemical processes, such as the metabolism of fats and carbohydrates. It is used for a variety of energy-consuming processes, such as muscular contraction, oxidative metabolism and membrane transport. The following sections will describe some of the reasons why ATP is essential for the sustained action of the pump. But the relations between contractile proteins (actin and myosin) and regulatory proteins (troponin and tropomyosin) and their dependence on Ca^{++} are beyond the scope of this chapter, except to say that essential aspects of the physiological control of the interactions between actin and myosin are that the regulatory proteins are inhibited in the absence of Ca^{++} and that the ability of Ca^{++} to initial contraction results from the reversal of this inhibitory effect.

Controlling mechanisms

Fat in the form of fatty acids is the principal source of energy comprising about 75% of the substrates in the fasting state. Glucose, which contributes about 15% in the fasting state, can contribute as much as 40–50% in the fed state. Lactate contributes approximately 5% physiologically, with amino acids and ketones providing the remainder.

There are three general types of controlling mechanisms which permit the heart to make optimal use of the substrates delivered to it in the coronary arterial blood. They influence substrate uptake, intermediary metabolism and substrate utilization. One is hormonal, which acts mainly to regulate the entry rates of substrates, both fats and carbohydrate, into the pathways of intermediary metabolism. A hormonal signal is able to augment the availability of chemical energy in the heart at the same time as it increases the rate of energy utilization through its effects in increasing the strength and frequency of cardiac contraction. Another is a homeostatic control which responds to the cellular requirements of high-energy phosphates. This mechanism serves to match the rate of production of the adenine nucleotide— ATP—with that of ATP utilization. In this way, cellular levels of this critical source of chemical energy remain constant and the rate of energy production does not fall behind that of energy utilization. A third is the relative states of oxidation and reduction of the various enzymes which are responsible for integrating the oxidative and anaerobic steps of intermediary metabolism.

Fat metabolism

The myocardium derives its chief source of energy from fat in the coronary arterial blood (Figure 1). This is present principally in the form of triglycerides,

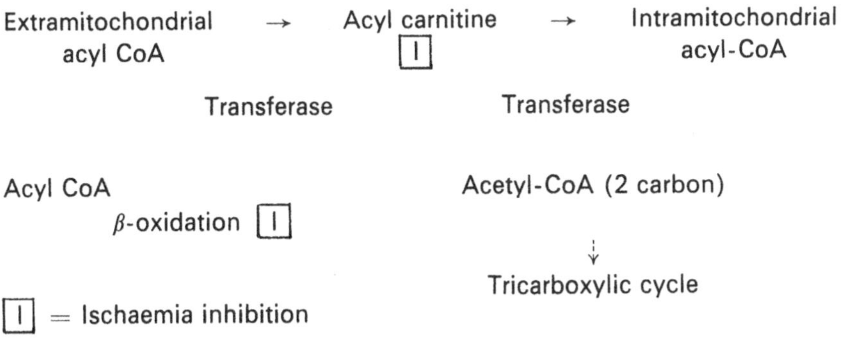

Extramitochondrial   →   Acyl carnitine   →   Intramitochondrial
acyl CoA $\boxed{\text{I}}$ acyl-CoA

        Transferase   Transferase

Acyl CoA   Acetyl-CoA (2 carbon)
    β-oxidation $\boxed{\text{I}}$

                        ↓
                Tricarboxylic cycle
$\boxed{\text{I}}$ = Ischaemia inhibition

Figure 1   Fat transport into the cell

either as chylomicra (in the post-absorptive state) or as triglyceride-rich, very low-density lipoproteins. These lipoprotein complexes contain glycerol, a three-carbon sugar to which are esterified various fatty acids. Progressive hydrolysis of the triglyceride component of these lipoproteins takes place in the plasma as a result of the action of various lipoprotein lipases with release of free (unesterified) fatty acid (FFA) which is instantly bound to albumin. The action of these lipoprotein lipases (LPL) is influenced by various acid mucopolysaccharides, secreted at endothelial cell level, and by cyclic AMP. The most striking example of the former is heparin which releases activated LPL. Adrenaline appears to transfer inactive LPL to an active form at the endothelial surface.

FFA are transported in the plasma bound to albumin. They are very rapidly taken up by tissues and have a plasma half-life of less than 2 min. Increases in plasma concentration of FFA can lead to increased fatty acid uptake, and this is dependent upon the molar-binding ratio with albumin. When high concentrations of fatty acids exceed the capacity of high-affinity fatty acid binding sites of albumin, there is less restraint on the diffusion of fatty acids into cells. This process probably involves very rapid exchange with fatty acids esterified with phospholipids in the sarcolemma membrane. Esterified fatty acids do not enter the cell.

Another source for intracellular fatty acids is the store of myocardial triglyceride. The balance between hydrolysis of stored triglyceride, which is activated by a cyclic-AMP-dependent protein kinase, and esterification of triglyceride from fatty acid, which is dependent upon the presence of adequate a-glycerophosphate, will determine the contribution of this intracellular source of intracellular fatty acid.

Once in the cell, fatty acids form a complex with co-enzyme A (CoA). The resulting fatty acid ester, acyl-CoA, carries fatty acids into the mitochondria, but this process requires ATP. Different fatty acids are complexed with CoA in different regions of the myocardial cell. Extramitochondrial acyl-CoA, the 'activated' fatty acid, cannot be transferred into the mitochondria unless the acyl groups are first linked to carnitine, a 7-carbon acid, that can replace the CoA to which the fatty acid is esterified. The formation of acyl carnitine is therefore an essential step in this transport process. The role of carnitine is probably that of a carrier and can be inhibited when fatty acids are present in excess. The transport of fatty acids into mitochondria requires the participation of two membrane-bound transferring enzymes or transferases. One is associated with the mitochondrial outer membrane and the other with the inner membrane.

Finally, the entry of fatty acids into the tricarboxylic acid cycle, which is the major oxidative pathway of the myocardium, occurs through the formation of acetyl-CoA. This step is dependent upon β-oxidation, the rate of which is regulated by the available oxygen, the concentrations of fatty acids within the cell and the availability of certain adenine co-enzymes. β-oxidation is absolutely dependent upon a continuing supply of oxygen so that when coronary flow is interrupted, ATP cannot be produced from fats. In this way, fatty acid metabolism, like that of glucose, leads to the formation of the 2-carbon end-point, acetyl-CoA. These steps are illustrated in Figure 2. It

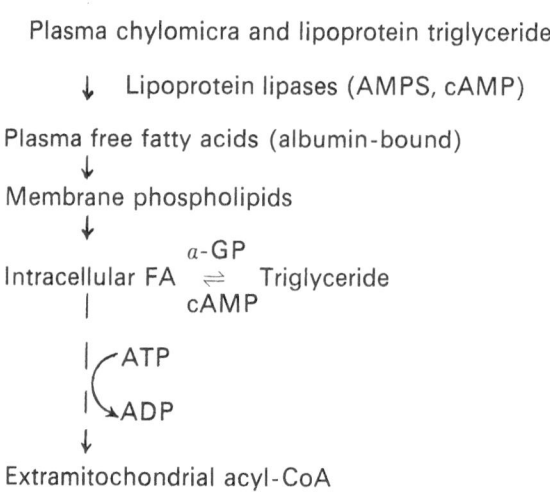

Figure 2   Fat metabolism in the cell

differs from carbohydrate metabolism, however, because there is no alternative pathway through which metabolism can proceed in the absence of oxygen; i.e. the formation of lactate from pyruvate.

Carbohydrate metabolism

ATP can be generated in the myocardium by glycolysis with a net production of 2 ATP moles per mole of glucose. Control of glycolysis is complex and there are at least five rate-limiting steps which require mention, because they are sensitive to hypoxia and ischaemia (Figure 3).

Glucose is transported into the myocardial cell from the plasma. This process does not require energy, as the sugar moves in from a region of high concentration outside the cell to one of low concentration in the cytosol. It combines with a glucose carrier in the sarcolemma during this process. The transport can be accelerated by oxygen lack, insulin and adrenaline. Stimulation of glucose transport in the hypoxic myocardium serves to increase the availability of carbohydrate substrate for anaerobic glycolysis under conditions where oxidative metabolism is inhibited. Insulin lack slows this process.

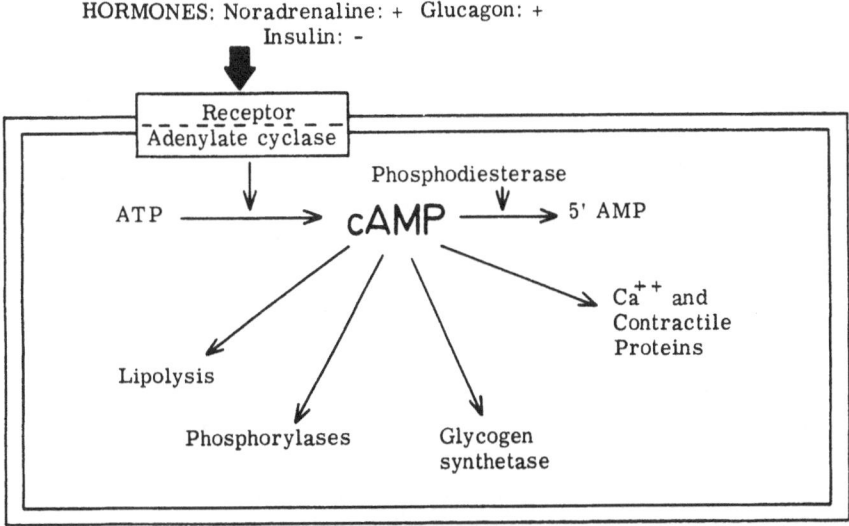

Figure 3 Overall reaction scheme of glycolysis. Major control points are: (1) glucose transport; (2) the hexokinase reaction (glucose phosphorylation); (3) the phosphofructokinase reaction (fructose-6-phosphate phosphorylation); (4) the glyceraldehyde-3-phosphate dehydrogenase reaction (glyceraldehyde-3-phosphate oxidation); and (5) the lactate dehydrogenase reaction (pyruvate reduction). ATP is utilized at two steps at the beginning of the scheme. Two moles of ATP are generated at each of two steps towards the end of the scheme, giving a net yield of 2 moles of ATP per mole of glucose[24]

A second rate-limiting step is the hexokinase reaction which catalyses glucose phosphorylation. Glycolysis occurs through the action of soluble enzymes on soluble substrates in the cytosol. It is necessary that neither leaks out of the cell. Phosphorylation achieves this because it converts non-polar sugars into negatively charged ions, to which the sarcolemma is impermeable. A second reason why phosphorylation in the cytosol is necessary is that it provides the intra-molar forces to permit high-energy phosphate bonds to be formed. The hexokinase reaction is ATP-dependent and results in the 'loss' of one ATP mole per mole of glucose. It is influenced by many regulatory factors, of which the most important is that mediated by glucose-6-phosphate, which in high concentrations inhibits the ability of hexokinase to catalyse glucose phosphorylation. Thus, inhibition of glycolysis lower in the catalytic pathway could inhibit this reaction.

A third important rate-limiting step in glycolysis is the phosphofructokinase reaction, which forms fructose-1-6-diphosphate. This also involves the investment of ATP with the 'loss' of a further mole ATP per mole of glucose. The phosphofructokinase reaction is stimulated by an increase in ADP, inorganic phosphate, cyclic-AMP and fructose-1-6-diphosphate, and inhibited by an increase in ATP, hydrogen ion concentration, phosphocreatine and citrate.

A fourth step is the oxidation of glyceraldehyde-3-phosphate where an oxidative reaction (in which NAD is reduced to NADH) leads to the formation of a diphosphosugar containing one high-energy phosphate bond. Under conditions of ischaemia, the ability to oxidize NADH is remarkably impaired, and this becomes a crucial step in inhibiting glycolysis.

Finally, ischaemia can increase the reduction of pyruvate to lactate, helping the cell to regenerate oxidized NAD. In the well-oxygenated heart this reaction, which is catalysed by the enzyme dehydrogenase, is not utilized and NAD is regenerated from NADH in the mitochondria. Usually, pyruvate is converted to acetyl-CoA, the two-carbon fragment which is subsequently oxidized into the tricarboxylic acid cycle. In the ischaemic heart, where pyruvate concentrations can be very high, lactate is produced and pyruvate is not utilized as a source of energy.

Hormones and cyclic-AMP

The principal mechanism through which hormones influence myocardial cellular metabolism is the activation in cell membranes of a receptor-system which increases adenylate cyclase activity. This enzyme converts ATP to cyclic-AMP in the presence of Mg^{++}. In its turn, cyclic-AMP activates one or more cyclic-AMP-dependent protein kinases. These are stimulatory of various enzyme systems which have regulatory effects over lipases, phosphorylases, glycogen synthesis and contractile protein function. Another group of enzymes, phosphodiesterases, convert cyclic-AMP into the physiologically inactive 5-AMP. Yet another group of enzymes, the phosphoprotein phosphatases, can terminate through protein dephosphorylation the effects of hormones mediated by cyclic-AMP. Some hormones may exert their action by using cyclic-AMP as a secondary mediator, or even act independently of cyclic-AMP. The secondary messenger role of cyclic-AMP is fundamental to the adrenergic control of myocardial function (Figure 4). The membrane receptor is also activated by glucagon. Insulin inhibits adenylate cyclase activity.

EFFECTS OF ISCHAEMIA ON MYOCARDIAL SUBSTRATE UTILIZATION

Nutritional insufficiency in the ischaemic myocardium occurs mainly in regions of the most extreme reductions in flow or increases in demand[1]. The degree of ischaemia varies in severity and is determined by many factors, including non-uniform distribution of collateral flow and metabolic demands. These in turn are regulated by the contractile state, heart rate, perfusion

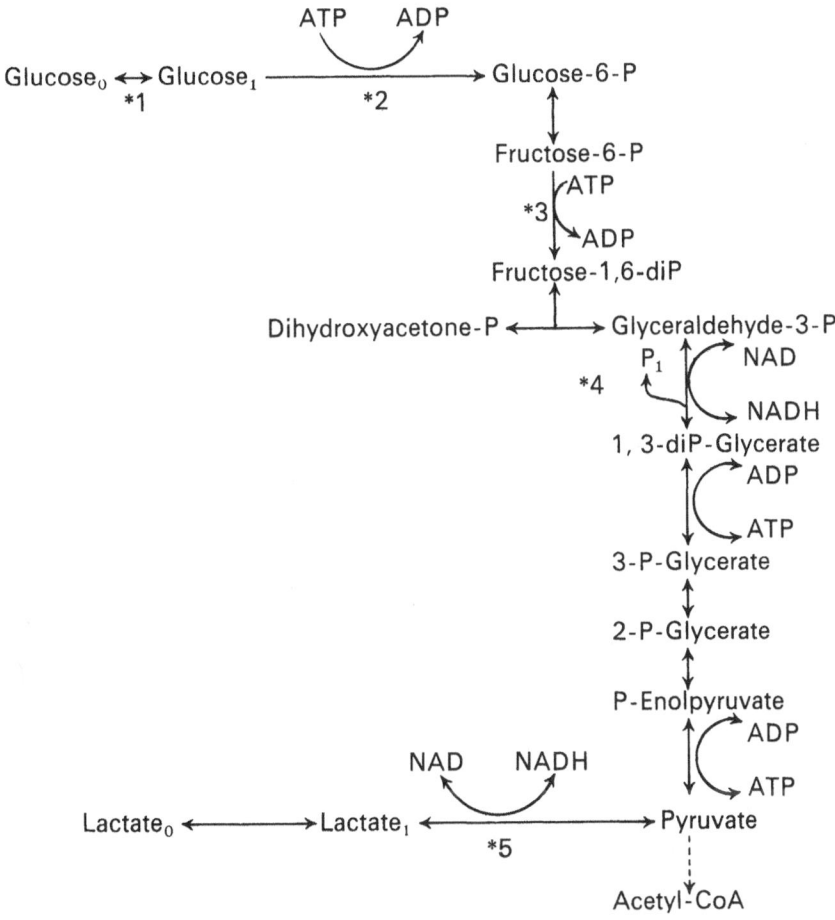

Figure 4 Hormonal and cyclic-AMP regulation of metabolism

pressure or by hormonal influences. Thus, it is an intermittent cellular phenomenon of regional distribution and probably never global. The heterogeneity of myocardial ischaemia may be the most important determinant of survival and death.

The concept of areas of partial ischaemia is important in understanding some of the complications. It is likely that both the chest pain and the arrhythmias associated with ischaemic heart disease arise in partially ischaemic regions of the myocardium. Once cell death occurs, the ability to initiate pain and generate arrhythmias is probably lost. Sharp differences in substrate and ionic gradients are probably responsible for local viability, and lead to impaired contractility and re-entry arrhythmias.

Although artificial in concept, it is easier perhaps to understand the effects of ischaemia by considering the intracellular and extracellular (peripheral) responses separately.

The intracellular response

The substrate, the lack of which is felt most promptly by the ischaemic myocardium, is *oxygen*. Within a minute after the blood supply to the heart is interrupted, intramyocardial oxygen tension falls to extremely low levels. Soon after coronary artery blood flow has been interrupted, there is a significant and rapid fall in cellular ATP content. The fall in phosphocreatine content, however, exceeds this.

The hypothesis has been proposed that during myocardial ischaemia a decrease in tissue oxygenation prevents optimum oxidation of *fatty acids* and permits a critical increase of intracellular long-chain acyl-CoA esters. β-oxidation is inhibited, with a decrease in acetyl-CoA in the mitochondrial matrix. The accumulation of long-chain acyl derivatives may have severe consequences on the metabolism of ischaemic hearts. Long-chain acyl-CoA is known to inhibit a number of enzymes, including adenine nucleotide transferases. Most of the accumulation of acyl-CoA in ischaemic hearts occurs outside the mitochondrial matrix. There is an associated increase in levels of long-chain acyl carnitine in the cytosol with low levels of carnitine available as an acyl acceptor in the transferase reaction. The resultant inhibition of adenine nucleotide translocase causes an immediate interruption of energy production and disturbance of the ATP/ADP ratio responsible for the phosphate potential of the cell[2]. Fatty acid amines may also combine with intracellular cations and produce 'soaps'. Fatty acids may also have marked non-specific detergent effects on membranes and enzymes[3]. This detergent effect of unbound FFA can be demonstrated during infusion when the blood pH falls very rapidly and red cells undergo severe haemolysis: accumulation of FFA within the ischaemic myocardial cells may have a similar lytic effect. If esterification of intracellular fatty acids to triglyceride also becomes impaired due to inadequate glucose uptake and a reduction of a-glycerophosphate, unoxidized FFA will accumulate even more.

Initially, there is an increased rate of *glycolysis* notably as a result of stimulation of the reaction catalysed by phosphofructokinase. This is due to increased cellular levels of ADP, AMP and inorganic phosphate which activate this enzyme and to reduced concentrations of ATP and phosphocreatine, both of which are inhibitory at normal cellular levels[4]. Glycogenolysis occurs also with an early increase in glucose flux. Unfortunately, the increase of glycolysis in the ischaemic heart is only transient. The maintenance of glycolysis is critically important as a source of ATP. In the presence of accumulated unoxidized FFA or long-chain acyl-CoA, glucose may be the only external source of energy and glycogen the principal intracellular source[5]. The metabolism of a single mole of glucose leads to the production of 36 moles of ATP, and all but 2 require that the cell be provided with oxygen. Thus, ischaemia can inhibit the pathways responsible for producing almost 95% of the ATP from carbohydrate. During ischaemia, the glycolytic flux is particularly limited at the level of glyceraldehyde-3-phosphate dehydrogenase. Lactate and pyruvate block glycolysis during anaerobic conditions, probably by acting on this enzyme and also phosphofructokinase. The exact mechanisms are not clear.

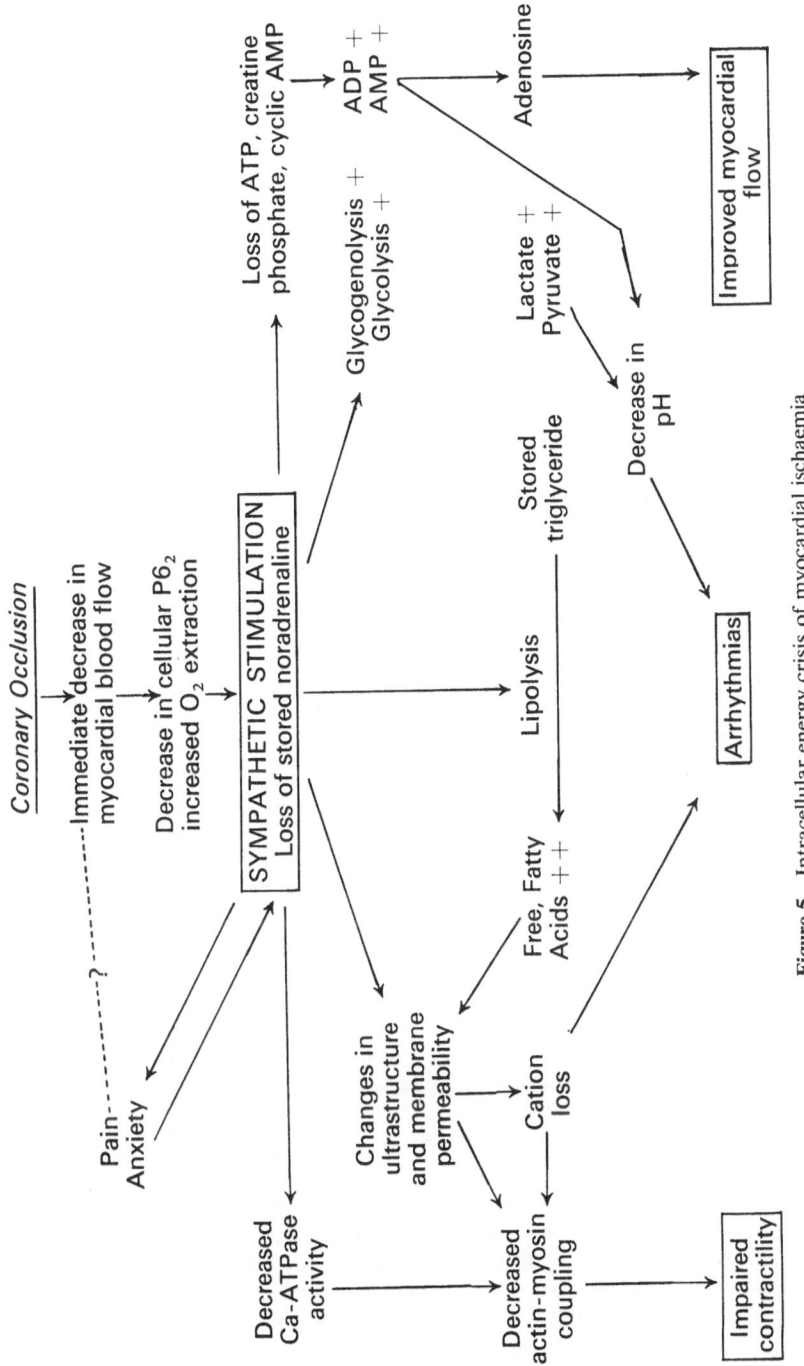

Figure 5 Intracellular energy crisis of myocardial ischaemia

Hydrogen ion concentrations increase during ischaemia. This slows glycolysis by effecting phosphofructokinase activity. It also reduces coronary blood flow. Reduction in coronary flow reduces glycolysis in the presence of anoxia, regardless of whether or not substrates are being oxidized. With decreased coronary flow and reduced oxygen delivery, accumulation of carbon dioxide and lactate occurs with a decrease in intracellular and coronary effluent pH. A specific negative inotropic effect has been attributed to a fall in intracellular pH, and this is independent of the degree of hypoxia in the tissue. These changes are coincident, experimentally, with depletion of high-energy phosphate compounds and the development of heart failure.

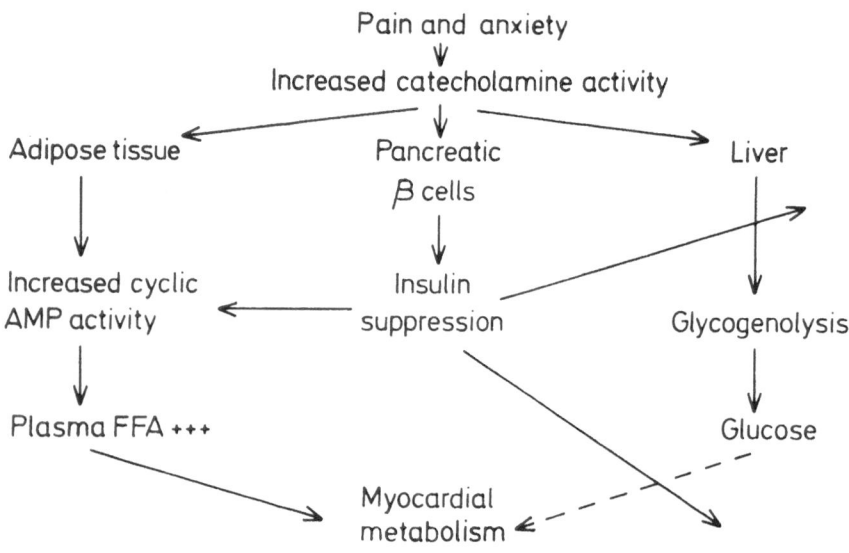

Figure 6   Peripheral response to ischaemia

An increase occurs in myocardial *cyclic-AMP* consequent upon stimulation of postganglionic sympathetic nerve endings and release of noradrenaline intracellularly, and on the effect of increased concentrations of plasma catecholamines acting on β-agonist receptor sites in the sarcolemma. Experimentally, increased concentrations of cyclic-AMP decrease ventricular fibrillation thresholds in the ischaemic myocardium, and this may be an important mechanism through which ischaemia adversely affects electrical stability[6].

Lysosomal enzyme release occurs early after the induction of ischaemia in the myocardium[7]. These acid hydrolases lead to cell injury and death. The stimulus to their release is not really understood, but lysosome membrane stability can be enhanced by glucocorticoids reducing enzyme release.

These changes are summarized in Figure 5. It is understandable how devastating the effects of ischaemia can be on myocardial contractility and electrical stability.

The peripheral response

Comparatively little attention has been given to changes which occur in the concentrations and activities of hormones during the stress and pain associated with acute myocardial ischaemia (Figure 6)[8]. While these are probably the chief stimuli to the peripheral changes, myocardial injury itself may have an effect in increasing adrenaline output through a spinal reflex.

In man, plasma catecholamines are known to be raised within 10 min of the onset of symptoms[9]. In dogs, an efflux of noradrenaline occurs in the coronary sinus within 1 min of the onset of ischaemia[10]. There is prompt and often very marked stimulation of post-sympathetic ganglionic activity. This leads to adipose tissue lipolysis with release of FFA and free glycerol into the plasma compartment, and also to hydrolysis of stored triglyceride in the myocardium. Starvation is another factor which will increase plasma FFA concentrations. An increase in plasma cortisol concentrations occurs very early[9]. Adrenaline and cortisol are major stimuli to an increase in glucose in the plasma. Growth hormone and glucagon activity are not clearly defined in the first 2 h after the onset of symptoms, but both may also contribute to an increase in plasma glucose. Usually, this increase is proportionately less than that of plasma FFA. Glucose uptake by the myocardium is dependent upon the availability of insulin, and the adrenaline response to the stress of myocardial infarction suppresses pancreatic β-cell activity and reduces plasma insulin concentrations[11]. In contrast, the uptake of FFA from the plasma compartment is mostly determined by the degree of saturation of the high-affinity binding sites of albumin and any excess beyond the two principal binding sites (this amounts in man to approximately 1200 μEq/l) is associated with an exponential increase in FFA in tissues[12]. Increases in plasma FFA are associated with an increase in myocardial oxygen consumption.

The combination of high noradrenaline concentrations, a relatively small increase in plasma glucose concentrations, peripheral mobilization of FFA in excess of their albumin binding in the plasma and adrenaline suppression of insulin production can lead to an imbalance of the concentrations of substrates presented to the ischaemic myocardium. Even if the intracellular metabolic response is not severely impaired in regions which are relatively well perfused, a moderate degree of ischaemia could be worsened by an excessive peripheral response leading to the need to catabolize an excess of oxygen-wasting FFA[13] in the presence of a paucity of glucose.

ISCHAEMIC METABOLISM, MYOCARDIAL DAMAGE AND VENTRICULAR ARRHYTHMIAS

Myocardial blood flow

To a considerable extent, the consequence of ischaemic myocardial metabolism will depend upon the self-regulatory aspects of myocardial blood flow. If regional perfusion recovers rapidly, there may not be any adverse effects. In contrast, complete occlusion of blood supply will lead to myocardial damage, loss of contractility and vulnerability to arrhythmias. The key to these two extremes would appear to be the small arterioles, particularly in the subendocardial region[1]. The regulation of arteriole resistance is primarily carried out at local level, although both alpha- and beta-adrenergic and cholinergic receptors participate. The most attractive hypothesis concerning local regulation is that, in the presence of a low-oxygen environment, high-energy phosphate compounds degrade by reduction and finally stabilize in the form of adenosine. Adenosine freely diffuses out of cells, and in so doing acts as a highly potent dilator of the adjacent arterioles[14]. Restitution of blood supply turns off the mechanism by reconstitution of the cell reservoir of high-energy phosphate. This mechanism would seem to provide a sensitive means by which blood flow can be regulated and adjusted to the requirements of segments within the myocardium where there are different metabolic demands. By some mechanism not understood, the arterioles auto-regulate to a degree of resistance which will produce the optimum cellular Po_2 for ordinary metabolic activity.

Ionic basis for cardiac action potential (see 'Bibliography').

The maintenance of normal cardiac action potential is dependent upon the selective permeability of the cell membrane to certain ions and also normal transmembrane ionic gradients.

At rest a transmembrane potential difference of around 85 mV is maintained due to the preferential permeability of the membrane to K^+ and to the maintenance of higher intracellular than extracellular K^+ concentrations. This K^+ gradient is energy-dependent and determined by a Na^+- and K^+-activated membrane ATPase.

Excitation results in a rapid reversal of transmembrane potential or depolarization initiating the cardiac action potential. A propagated wave of depolarization initiating cardiac contraction is then carried from cell to cell by regenerative action potential. Action potential characteristics differ between atrial, ventricular, nodal and conducting tissue and are dependent upon sequential time and voltage-dependent variations in selective permeability of the membrane to Na^+, K^+, Ca^{++} and Cl^- ions.

Changes in the pattern of ionic fluxes throughout the period of a single ventricular muscle action potential are shown in Figure 7. The initial very rapid phase of depolarization is associated with a rapid influx of Na^+ ion due to a voltage-dependent opening of a special 'sodium channel' across the lipoprotein structure of the cell membrane. Ca^{++} ion may also contribute to this rapid inward current.

The most distinctive feature of the cardiac action potential, however, is the 'plateau' phase which confirms on it the unique property of prolonged refractoriness. The maintenance of this plateau is related to a slow inward flux of Ca^{++} ion commencing during phase 0 and continuing during the plateau phase. Repolarization is then initiated probably from a balance between a time-dependent decrease in this slow inward calcium current and a time-dependent increase in outward K^+ current carried by several complex channels.

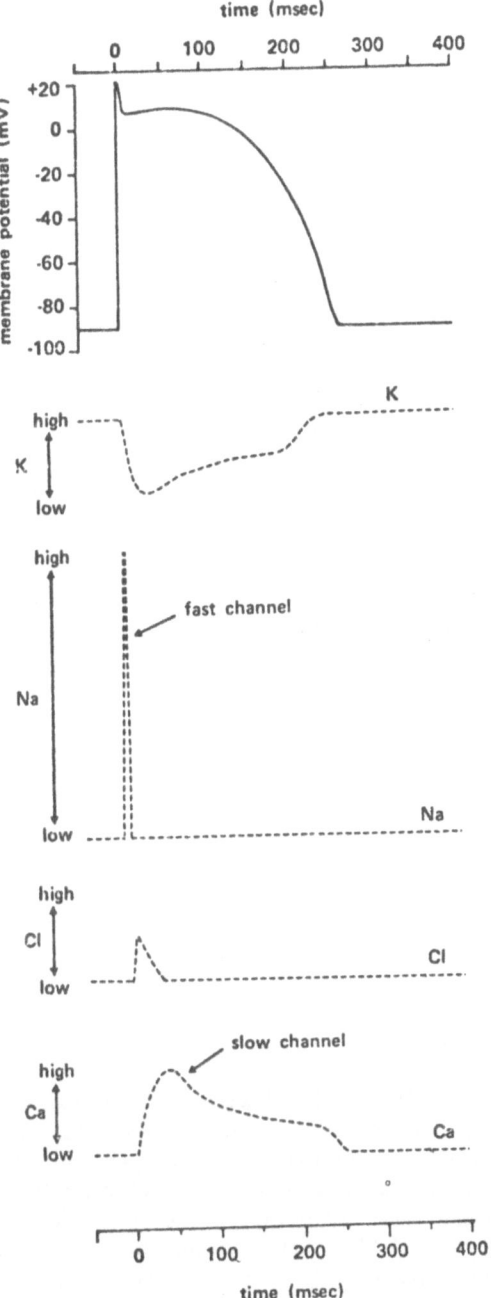

Figure 7 Changes in ions during the action potential in a Purkinje fibre

Myocardial ischaemia is associated with shortening of the action potential plateau. It is likely that this is related to a modification of the slow inward current largely carried by Ca^{++} ion. There is evidence that, unlike ionic fluxes of Na^+ or K^+ ion, this inward flux of Ca^{++} ion may be at least in part dependent upon metabolic processes and intracellular cytoplasmic ATP availability. The rapid accumulation of lactate and lowering of intracellular pH may in addition alter the affinity of the membrane for Ca^{++}. The direct depression of contractility due to decreased ATP production may therefore be augmented by a further depression resulting from shortening of plateau duration.

Multiple factors are operative upon the ischaemic cell *in vivo*. Inhibition of the sodium pump may be directly responsible for a fall in intracellular potassium. This, combined with accumulation of extracellular K^+, has a depolarizing effect on the resting transmembrane potential. The rapid inward current which permits normal rapid propagation of the cardiac impulse may be totally inactivated by this process leading to the appearance of slowly conducting 'slow-response' potentials mediated largely by ionic Ca^{++} ion flux through the 'slow channels'. Local release of catecholamines may have additional effects.

Ventricular arrhythmias may appear as a result of impulse propagation through so-called re-entrant circuits. Some requirements for such re-entry to occur are: (1) slowing of conduction; (2) unidimentional conduction block; (3) inhomogeneities of refractoriness. All such criteria are fulfilled in the ischaemic myocardium but the relative importance of the various determinants of re-entry remain unclear. Re-entry may under certain conditions not relate to re-excitation on repolarization due to the appearance of post-repolarization refractoriness. In addition, the role of automatic activity arising in conducting tissue or ventricular myocardium itself in initiating arrhythmias remains ill-defined.

It is not, however, within the scope of this chapter to discuss the complex electrophysiological inter-relationships thought to be responsible for re-entry arrhythmias and the details of these can be obtained from standard textbooks of electrophysiology.

METABOLIC INTERVENTION

The emphasis of this chapter has been on the critical importance of the balance of energy production and utilization in the ischaemic myocardium. It should be the biochemical aim, from what has been said, to increase glucose availability and glycolysis and decrease FFA uptake and the accumulation of long-chain acyl-CoA. Either or both approaches should form the basis for metabolic intervention. Additionally, curtailment of the hormonal response to acute ischaemia—particularly increased catecholamine and decreased insulin activity—should enhance survival of ischaemic tissue. Maintenance of the slow inward Ca^{++} current and decrease in K^+ loss should overcome some of the inhomogeneity of action potential in different areas of the myocardium.

There is encouraging evidence that it is possible to achieve these metabolic aims. One example is that inhibition of catecholamine-induced lipolysis by nicotinic acid derivatives not only reduces plasma concentrations of FFA but also ST segment elevation in patients with acute myocardial ischaemia and infarction[15,16]. It is possible, by using the same anti-lipolytic treatment, to reduce the degree of ST depression induced by exercise in patients with angina. These clinical studies are amply backed up by extensive evidence showing that there is a positive correlation between changes in free fatty acid/albumin concentrations and ST segments in dogs with induced myocardial ischaemia (Figure 8). Thus, when FFA are elevated by catecholamines,

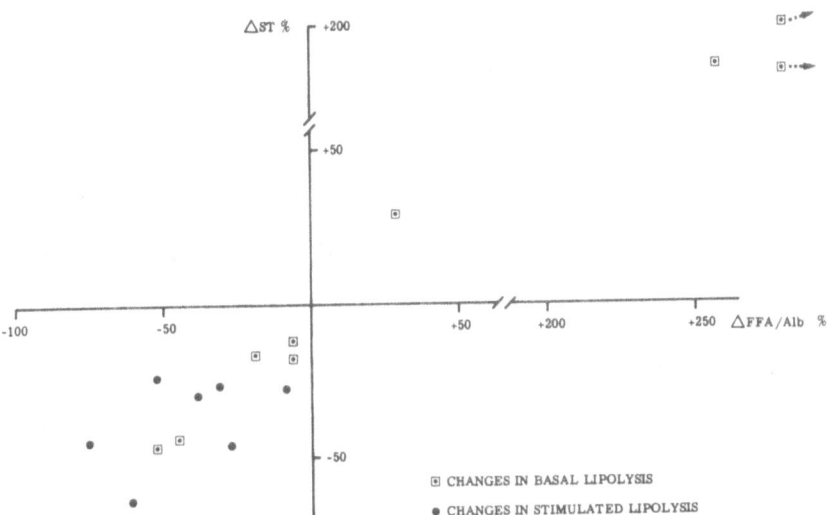

Figure 8 Relation between epicardial ST segment change (12 lead map over ischaemic area) to FFA/albumin ratio in dogs with experimental coronary artery occlusion. Each point represents the mean of eight dogs. Substances used to elevate plasma FFA were isoprenaline, adrenaline, noradrenaline and nicotine. Substances used to lower plasma FFA were glucose, dichloroacetate, lipid-free albumin, clofibrate, prostaglandin β and a β-blocker

ST segments are increased in such dogs; when FFA are lowered by such methods as glucose infusions, dichloroacetate[17], anti-lipolytic treatment, lipid-free albumin infusions[18], prostaglandin E1[19] or β-blockers, ST segments are lowered. The release of creatine kinase as an index of myocardial damage in man is too late to be of much value as a means of assessing the effectiveness of metabolic intervention in acute myocardial ischaemia, but its release in isolated perfused rat hearts with coronary arterial ligation has been shown to be several times greater with palmitate in the perfusate compared with glucose. Complementary results have been obtained by using glucose alone, or glucose and insulin, in patients with acute myocardial ischaemia and reduction of ST segment elevation has been observed. β-adrenergic blockers have a similar effect.

The effects of changing FFA concentrations on ventricular arrhythmias are also striking. Clinically, there is a correlation between the incidence of serious ventricular arrhythmias and plasma FFA in patients with myocardial infarction[20]. A positive correlation also exists between free glycerol concentrations[21], which are a less evanescent measure of catecholamine-induced lipolysis, and ventricular arrhythmias in patients with infarction. Also, diabetic patients on oral hypoglycaemic drugs have higher FFA concentrations and a higher incidence of ventricular fibrillation when compared with diabetic patients receiving insulin. These observations are also backed up by animal evidence, although this is somewhat conflicting according to the models used, that ventricular tachycardia follows the injection of a triglyceride–heparin solution in dogs with coronary occlusion. One of the difficulties about this experimental work is that plasma FFA are raised very high by infusion of triglyceride–heparin solutions and that the substrate usually used does not release a physiological spectrum of fatty acids.

Recent electrophysiological findings are also of particular interest. It has now been shown that the action potential shortening and conduction delay induced by ischaemia in dogs can both be brought back towards normal by glucose infusion and less strikingly by anti-lipolytic treatment. Ischaemic changes produced in action potential as a result of occlusion in a branch coronary artery with a small area of regional ischaemia can be completely rectified by glucose (Figure 9). In contrast, a higher occlusion with larger areas of ischaemia does not respond in this way, and action potential shortening remains unchanged. The positive effects of glucose in small areas of regional ischaemia and the negative effects in large areas would be consistent with biochemical changes likely to be present. Thus, the larger the area of ischaemia the greater the extent of anaerobic metabolism in the centre and the less likely it will be that raising glucose concentrations in perfusing coronary blood (if it actually penetrates to that area) will make much difference. On the other hand, small areas may be very critically dependent upon raising the concentration of glucose and glycolytic intermediates in the cytosol.

The measurement of gradients of refractoriness from the ischaemic to the normal ventricle is a method of studying ventricular vulnerability to arrhythmias—the greater the gradient the more the incidence of ventricular fibrillation. They can be strikingly reduced by raising the molar concentration of glucose[22]. Ventricular fibrillation thresholds have also been used for assessing myocardial vulnerability. This is an unsatisfactory index in metabolic terms, because of the biochemical changes which must occur in the cell during such an arrhythmia and during the electrical defibrillation which is necessary to allow the experiment to proceed. But using a system which stimulates ventricular premature beats, glucose has been shown to increase the threshold at which they are produced and is therefore 'protective'.

The differential effect of glucose according to the size of regional ischaemia may explain some of the confusion which exists in clinical studies using glucose, insulin and potassium. Some report a decrease in arrhythmias, failure and mortality rates, while others have been negative in outcome. This might be expected in view of the heterogeneity of the extent of myocardial damage in patients admitted to hospital and our inability clinically to measure the extent of the damage with precision. The most positive clinical report in recent years has suggested fairly convincingly that patients with the least coronary artery disease and with few complications of myocardial infarction received the greatest benefit from glucose–insulin–potassium[23].

The goals for metabolic intervention are to improve oxygenation, increase the supply of glucose, decrease the intracellular accumulation of fatty acids and contain the catecholamine response. If these can be achieved in patients with small regional areas of ischaemia, it is to be expected that there will be less myocardial damage and fewer potentially lethal ventricular arrhythmias. This approach has a sound biochemical basis and requires more intensive study. Furthermore, it might be adapted to prevent complications in patients with impending ischaemia. Maintenance of an adequate and balanced supply of energy for the pump should be the prime consideration during ischaemia.

At present, we have however a therapeutic impasse. How can metabolic intervention be made available immediately before or at the time of onset of acute myocardial ischaemia, when it is impossible to identify patients about to have a heart attack and impossible to get medical aid to the majority at this most critical moment.

This is just the kind of riddle which would have challenged William Harvey —for there is much more to learn about the best method of providing the optimum energy for the continued beat of the ventricles.

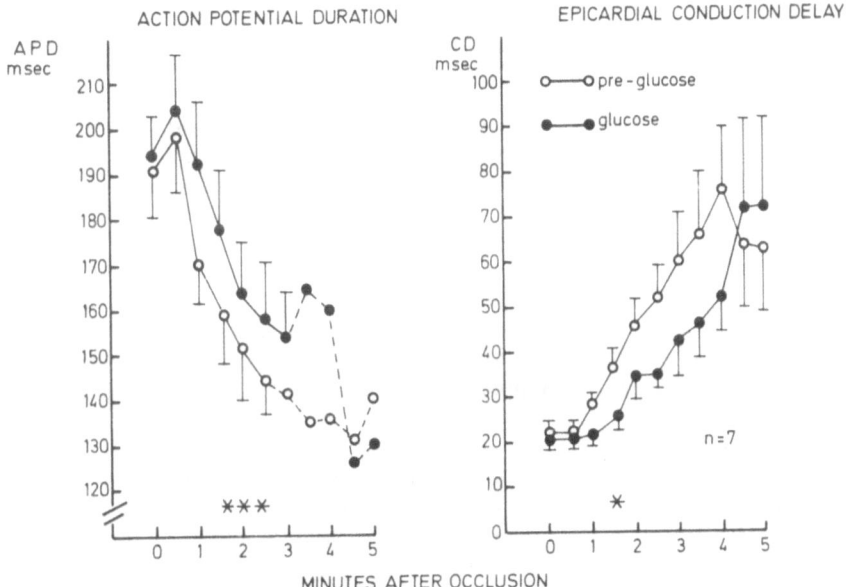

Figure 9 Changes in action potential and epicardial conduction delay during experimental coronary artery occlusion in dogs and the effects of a glucose infusion which raised plasma concentrations from 5 to 12 mmol/l[22]

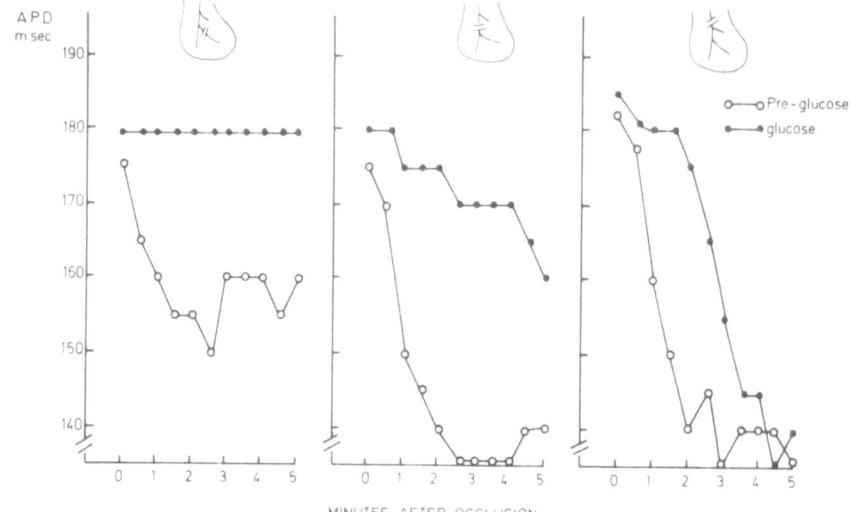

Figure 10 Glucose infusions which raised plasma concentrations from 5 to 12 mmol/l were effective in restoring shortened action potential to normal only in dogs in which a branch coronary artery was occluded with a small resultant area of ischaemia (left). They were less effective when moderate ischaemia had been induced, and not effective in the presence of a high coronary occlusion and major myocardial ischaemia (right)[25]

SUMMARY

Fat and glucose are the principal substrates for normal myocardial metabolism, and lactate contributes a small percentage. The availability and utilization of each is influenced by several controlling mechanisms. These include hormonal activity, the cellular requirements for high-energy phosphates and the redox state of intermediary enzymes.

The oxidation of fatty acids is wholly dependent on adequate oxygenation, and myocardial ischaemia causes accumulation of long-chain acyl-CoA with reduction of the transference of high-energy phosphates into the mitochondria. Ischaemia also slows or inhibits glycolysis: lactate and hydrogen ions increase. An energy crisis may occur.

The catecholamine-induced peripheral response to a heart attack leads to a rapid and early increase in plasma-free fatty acids with proportionately less rise in plasma glucose, and suppression of insulin, the ischaemic myocardium has too much fatty acid and too little glucose to metabolize. The energy crisis may be worsened.

Although the self-regulatory mechanisms of coronary arterial flow may be protective, these biochemical changes can lead, in areas of inhomogeneous myocardial ischaemia, to the development of damage, alteration in the ionic currents governing myocardial cellular action potential sufficient to cause re-entry arrhythmias, and impairment of the normal regulation of contractile proteins leading to pump failure.

Metabolic intervention aimed at decreasing the intracellular accumulation of fatty acids, increasing the supply of glucose and containing the catecholamine response has been shown to decrease myocardial damage, the vulnerability to induced arrhythmias and the incidence of ventricular arrhythmias during myocardial ischaemia, experimentally, and in patients.

Bibliography

Braunwald, E. (1976). Protection of the ischaemic myocardium. *Circulation*, **53** (Suppl. 1)

Gettes, L. S. (1976). Possible role of ionic changes in the appearance of arrhythmias. *Pharmacol. Ther.*, **2**, 787

Gorlin, R. (1976). *Coronary Artery Disease*. (Philadelphia: W. B. Saunders)

Lefer, A. M., Kelliher, G. J. and Rovetto, M. J. (1977). *Pathophysiology and Therapeutics of Myocardial Ischaemia*, pp. 227–238. (New York: Spectrum Publications)

Moret, P. and Fejfar, Z. (1972). Metabolism of the hypoxic and ischaemic heart. (Basel: S. Karger)

Nayler, W. G. (1975). *Contraction of Relaxation in the Myocardium*. (London: Academic Press)

Neilly, J. R., Rovetto, M. J. and Oram, J. F. (1972). Myocardial utilisation of carbohydrate and lipids. *Progr. Cardiovasc. Dis.*, **15**, 239

Newsholme, E. A. and Stark, C. (1973). *Regulation in Metabolism*. (London: John Wiley & Sons)

Oliver, M. F. (1973). The metabolic response to acute myocardial infarction. In L. E. Meltzer and A. J. Dunning (eds.). *Textbook of Coronary Care*, p. 231. *Excerpta Medica*. (Amsterdam)

Oliver, M. F., Julian, D. G. and Donald, K. W. (1972). *Effect of Acute Ischaemia on Myocardial Function*. (Edinburgh: Churchill Livingstone)

Opie, L. H. (1968, 1969). Metabolism of the heart in health and disease. *Am. Heart J.*, **76**, 685; **77**, 100, 383

Trautwein, W. (1962). Membrane currents in cardiac muscle fibres. *Physiol. Rev.*, **53**, 793

References

1. Hoffman, J. I. E. and Bookverd, G. D. (1978). The myocardial supply : demand ratio—a critical review. *Am. J. Cardiol.*, **41**, 327
2. Shug, A. L., Shrago, E., Dittar, M., Folts, J. D. and Cokes, J. R. (1975). Acyl-CoA inhibition of adenine nucleotide translocation in the ischaemic myocardium. *Am. J. Physiol.*, **228**, 689
3. Kurien, V. A. and Oliver, M. F. (1970). A metabolic cause for arrhythmias during acute myocardial hypoxia. *Lancet*, **1**, 813
4. Kubler, W. and Katz, A. M. (1977). Mechanism of early pump failure of the ischaemic heart: Possible role of adenosine triphosphate depletion and inorganic phosphate accumulation. *Am. J. Cardiol.*, **40**, 467
5. Opie, L. H. (1975). Metabolism of FFA, glucose and catecholamines in acute myocardial infarction. *Am. J. Cardiol.*, **36**, 938
6. Lubbe, W. F., Podzuweit, T., Daries, P. S. and Opie, L. H. (1978). The role of cyclic adenosine monophosphate in adrenergic effects on ventricular vulnerability to fibrillation in the isolated perfused rat heart. *J. Clin. Invest.*, **62**, 1260
7. Hoffstein, S., Weissmann, G. and Fox, A. C. (1976). Lysosomes in myocardial infarction: studies by means of cytochemistry and subcellular fractionation, with observations on the effects of methylprednisolone. *Circulation*, **53**, 1

8. Oliver, M. F. (1972). Metabolic response during impending myocardial infarction. *Circulation*, **45**, 491

9. Vetter, N. J., Strange, R. C., Adams, W. and Oliver, M. F. (1974). Initial metabolic and hormonal response to acute myocardial infarction. *Lancet*, **2**, 284

10. Shahab, L., Wollenberger, A., Krause, E. G. and Geinz, S. (1972). The effect of acute ischaemia on catecholamines and cyclic AMP levels in normal and hypertrophied myocardium. In M. F. Oliver, D. G. Julian and K. W. Donald (eds.). *Effect of Acute Ischaemia on Myocardial Function*, p. 97. (Edinburgh: Churchill Livingstone)

11. Porte, D., Graber, A. L., Kuzuya, T. and Williams, R. H. (1968). The effect of epinephrine on immunoreactive insulin levels in man. *J. Clin. Invest.*, **45**, 228

12. Spector, A. A. (1968). The transport and utilization of free fatty acid. *Ann. N Y Acad. Sci.*, **149**, 768

13. Mjos, O. D. (1971). Effect of free fatty acids on myocardial function and oxygen consumption in intact dogs. *J. Clin. Invest.*, **50**, 1386

14. Rubio, R. and Berne, R. N. (1969). Release of adenosine by the normal myocardium in dogs and its relationship to regulation of coronary resistance. *Circ. Res.*, **25**, 407

15. Luxton, M. R., Miller, N. E. and Oliver, M. F. (1976). Antilipolytic treatment in angina pectoris. *Br. Heart J.*, **38**, 1204

16. Russell, D. C. and Oliver, M. F. (1978). Effect of antilipolytic therapy on ST segment elevation during myocardial ischaemia in man. *Br. Heart J.*, **40**, 117

17. Mjos, O. D., Miller, N. E., Riemersma, R. A. and Oliver, M. F. (1976). Effects of dichloracetate on myocardial substrate extraction, epicardial ST-segment elevation, and ventricular blood flow following coronary occlusion in dogs. *Cardiovasc. Res.*, **10**, 427

18. Miller, N. E., Mjos, O. D. and Oliver, M. F. (1976). Relationship of epicardial ST-segment elevation to the plasma free fatty acid/albumin ratio during coronary occlusion in dogs. *Clin. Sci. Mol. Med.*, **51**, 209

19. Riemersma, R. A., Talbot, R. C., Ungar, A., Mjos, O. D. and Oliver, M. F. (1977). Effects of prostaglandin E on ST-segment elevation and regional myocardial blood flow during experimental myocardial ischaemia in dogs. *Europ. J. Clin. Invest.*, **7**, 515

20. Oliver, M. F., Kurien, V. A. and Greenwood, T. W. (1968). Relation between serum free fatty acids and arrhythmias and death after myocardial infarction. *Lancet*, **1**, 710

21. Carlstrom, S. and Christensson, B. (1971). Plasma glycerol after acute myocardial infarction. *Br. Heart J.*, **33**, 884

22. Russell, D. C. and Oliver, M. F. (1978). The effect of intravenous glucose on ventricular vulnerability following acute coronary artery occlusion in the dog. *J. Mol. Cell. Cardiol.* (in press)

23. Rogers, W. J., Stanley, Jr. A. W., Breinig, J. B., Prather, J. W., McDaniel, H. G., Moraski, R. E., Mantle, J. A., Russell, Jr. R. O. and Rackley, C. E. (1976). Reduction of hospital mortality rate of acute myocardial infarction with glucose-insulin-potassium infusion. *Am. Heart J.*, **92**, 441

24. Katz, A. M. (1977). *Physiology of the Heart.* (New York: Raven Press)

25. Russell, D. C., Smith, H. J. and Oliver, M. F. (1978). Metabolic and electrophysiological effects of glucose in acute myocardial ischaemia in dogs. *Europ. J. Clin. Invest.*, **8**, Abstr. 182, p. 14

11
Aspects of cardiac contraction from the radiologist's point of view

R. E. STEINER

Many radiological techniques have been used for years to study cardiac function; for example fluoroscopy, the plain chest film, kymography and in later years cine-angiography. To these well-established techniques isotope imaging of the myocardium has only recently been added. There can be no doubt that the various methods of investigation have made a significant contribution to the understanding of cardiac function. The majority lend themselves well to a visual display of cardiac contraction. In some instances the visual images can be translated into a numerical form, thus providing absolute values of end-systolic and end-diastolic volumes or ejection fractions of the left ventricle.

Two methods of investigation have been chosen to illustrate the potential of these new imaging techniques; firstly cine-angiocardiography of the left ventricle and secondly, [81m]Krypton myocardial perfusion scanning.

LEFT VENTRICULAR ANGIOCARDIOGRAPHY

By this technique it is possible to outline the left ventricle with a contrast medium and study it during the cardiac cycle, so that contour and volume changes of the left ventricle can be recorded. The individual cine frames can be accurately analysed and so provide a clear visual picture of chamber contraction during the various phases of the cardiac cycle. There are a number of techniques available to assess left ventricular volume from cine angiographic studies[1-3]. In our investigations we have used the method described by Kasser and Kennedy[4], measuring left ventricular volume by single-plane cine-angiography.

The different appearances of left ventricular function in ischaemic heart disease provide an ideal model to demonstrate some of the results obtained by cine left ventriculography. We have studied 125 patients with definite

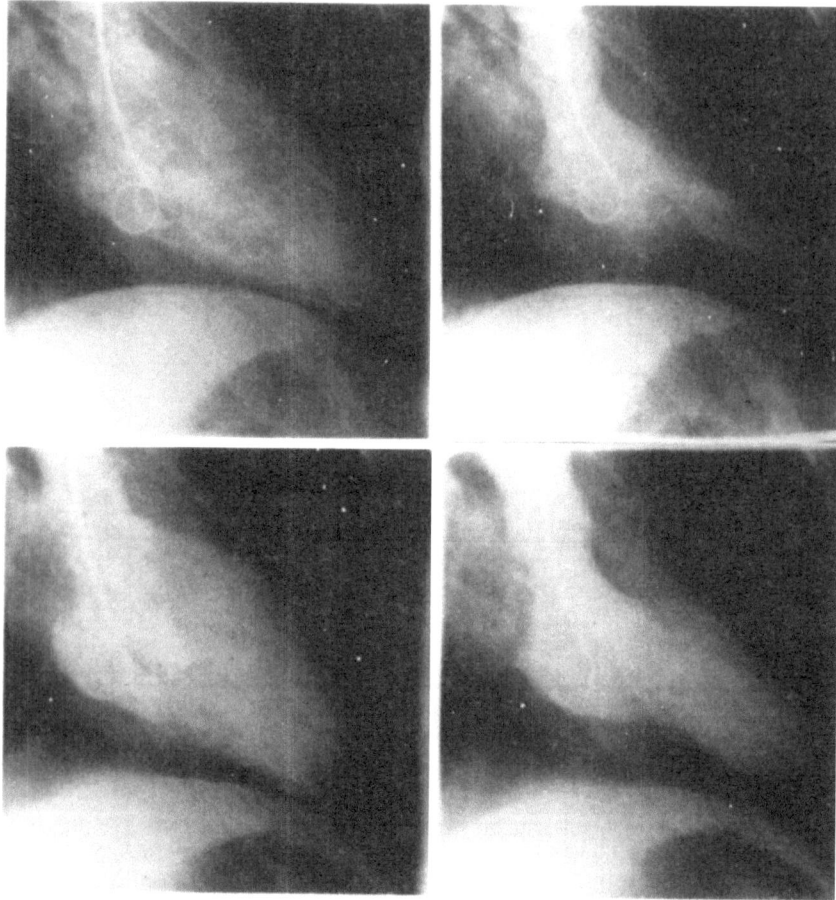

Figure 1 Cine angiogram of a patient with ischaemic heart disease. Normal left ventriculogram at rest. Top left diastole, top right systole. At the bottom left ventriculogram after exercise, left diastole, right systole. Note the slightly larger left ventricular size in diastole after exercise and the change in the systolic appearances with dyskinesia of the anterior wall and the apex of the ventricle

angina[5]; in this group of patients there were twenty-five with definite cardiac aneurysm, forty-nine with localized dyskinesia and fifty with a normal left ventricular study at rest. In the patients with cardiac aneurysm there was no doubt about the angiographic evidence of this lesion. The common features were gross dilatation of the left ventricular cavity with marked dyskinesia of the dilated segment, involving more than half of the chamber. By contrast there was good contraction of the proximal part of the ventricle just below the aortic valve and close to the mitral valve. The transitional area from the vigorously contracting subvalvar zone to the aneurysmal sac was clearly

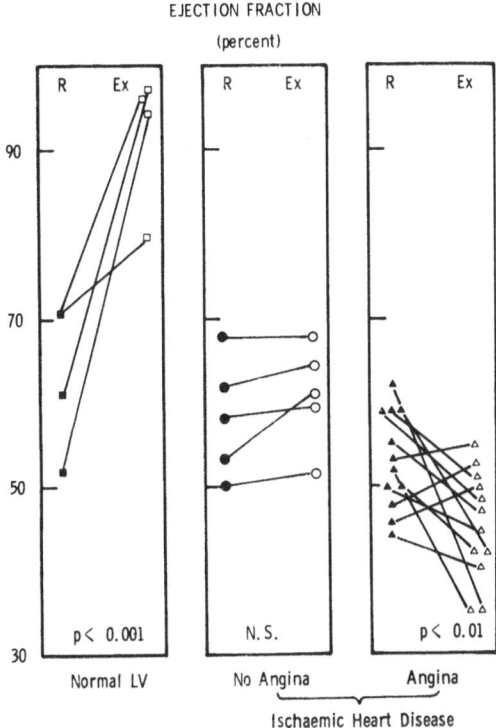

EJECTION FRACTION
(percent)

Figure 2 Ejection fractions at rest and after exercise. In the first column are four patients with normal left ventricular function; in the second and third columns are patients with ischaemic heart disease. (By permission of the *British Heart Journal*)

defined on the cine-angiogram, even in the absence of an obvious anatomical neck. In the majority of patients with cardiac aneurysm there was total obstruction of the left anterior descending branch of the coronary artery.

In the forty-nine patients with dyskinesia only, this usually affected one or more areas of the left ventricular wall; only one patient had diffuse impairment of left ventricular contraction.

The relationship of the severity of coronary artery disease to local dyskinesia was assessed in 125 patients. There were none with dyskinesia who had a normal coronary arteriogram; all had either single-, two- or three-vessel disease. Of the fifty patients who had a normal left ventricular study at rest twelve had a normal coronary arteriogram, but the remainder had either significant single-, two- or three-vessel disease. Dyskinesia demonstrated at rest provides objective evidence of myocardial ischaemia and is definitely associated with previous infarction at the site of abnormal left ventricular contraction. There is good correlation between abnormal function and obstruction of the regional coronary artery supply.

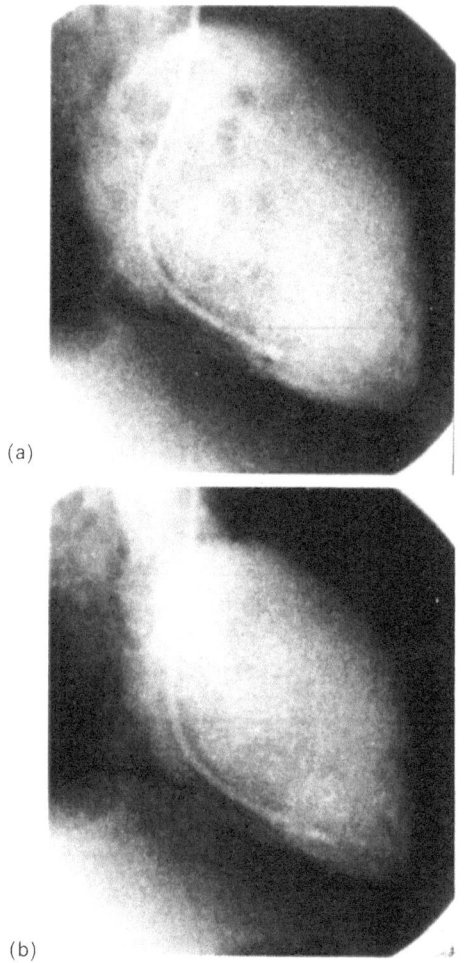

(a)

(b)

Figure 3 (a) Left ventricular angiogram RAO projection. Patient with congestive cardio-myopathy. Diastolic film. Note the very large distended left ventricle. (b) Same patient, systole. Note very inadequate systolic contraction of the ventricle

The striking absence of abnormal left ventricular contraction in fifty patients with symptomatic proven coronary artery disease who had normal left ventricular contraction at rest led us to study a further group of patients with similar symptoms at rest and following exercise[6,7]. Sharma and Taylor[8] showed that of seven patients with normal left ventricular contraction at rest six developed dyskinesia on exercise. This lesion was associated with an obstructed anterior descending coronary artery in five; one patient developed inferior dyskinesia, and he had an obstructed right coronary artery. These findings suggested that acute ischaemia led to reversal of localized impairment of left ventricular contraction. We therefore investigated seventeen patients using the same technique of exercise left ventricular angiography as described

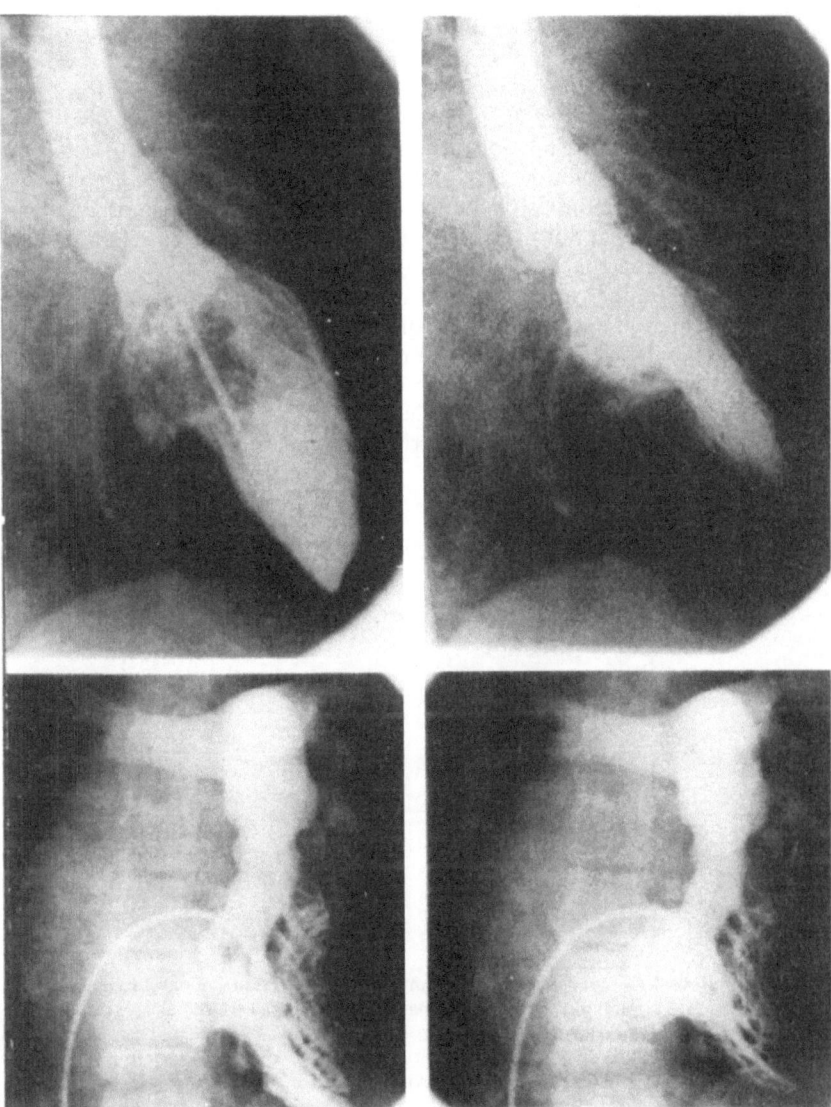

Figure 4 Patient with hypertrophic cardiomyopathy. At the top cine-angiogram of left ventricle, left diastole. Note the inadequate expansion of the chamber, 'reduced compliance'. Right systole. Note good ejection and left ventricular contraction. The two figures at the bottom represent cine-angiograms of the right ventricle in diastole and systole. Note the marked bulge of the hypertrophied interventricular septum into the right ventricular cavity

by Sharma and Taylor[8] with special reference to the relationship of the rest and exercise angiocardiogram, and compared some of these patients with other haemodynamic parameters, such as left ventricular end-diastolic pressures, end-systolic and end-diastolic volumes and ejection fractions. The patients with ischaemic heart disease were also compared with four normal patients. After exercise in the supine position, following leg raising for 2 min, the left ventricular end-systolic and end-diastolic volume in the patients with normal left ventricular function decreased. In the patients with ischaemic heart disease who did not develop angina within 2 min of exercise no change in end-systolic and end-diastolic volumes was noted, whereas in the patients who developed angina during exercise a very significant increase in both end-systolic and end-diastolic volumes was observed (Figure 1).

Angiocardiographic studies of this nature demonstrated very clearly that ventricular function can be assessed, and the data can separate patients with normal left ventricular function from those who developed angina after exercise (Figure 2).

A further group of patients who clearly demonstrated the value of cine-angiography for the study of left ventricular function are those with various forms of cardiomyopathy.

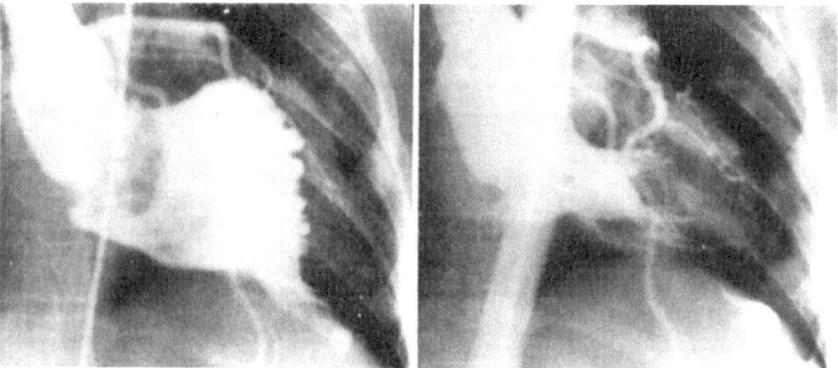

Figure 5 Patient with hypertrophic cardiomyopathy. Left ventriculogram; left-diastole. There is adequate compliance of the proximal portion of the left ventricle which is well-distended, the apical portion of the ventricle hardly fills. Right-systole. The ventricle has virtually emptied itself, very good ejection. Note the small sequestrated amount of contrast at the apex of the heart, completely cut off from the rest of the ventricle

In congestive cardiomyopathy the examination will demonstrate uniform dilatation of the left ventricle during diastole and the very inadequate contraction during systole (Figures 3a and b). By contrast in patients with hypertrophic cardiomyopathy the cine-angiogram will show the inadequate compliance of the left ventricle in diastole and the forceful and extreme ejection during systole (Figure 4), sometimes producing quite bizarre contour changes of the ventricle due to the grossly hypertrophied ventricular muscle (Figure 5).

ISOTOPE STUDIES OF THE MYOCARDIUM

Myocardial imaging with radioactive isotopes is now a well-established technique. In the last 2 years we have used a new short-lived isotope, [81m]Krypton ([81m]Kr) to study myocardial perfusion (Figures 6a, b, c). Fifteen patients with a history of angina had routine cardiac catheterization and coronary angiography, and after completion of this study the specially designed cardiac

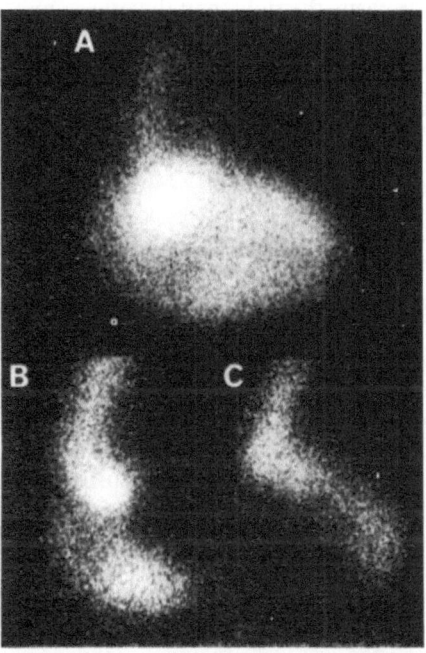

Figure 6 Anterior projection of a [81m] Kr perfusion scan of the myocardium. Normal appearances. Note the area of greatest activity at the infusion site into the aortic root. (A) Uniform perfusion of the left ventricular myocardium. (B) The catheter has been slightly withdrawn; scintographic activity can only now be seen in the aortic root and the myocardium only perfused by the right coronary artery. (C) The catheter has been repositioned in such a way that only the myocardium supplied by the left coronary artery is now perfused

catheter[9] was placed into the aortic root. Through this catheter [81m]Kr was continuously infused into the right and left coronary artery. At intervals gamma camera images were obtained from the patient at rest, during cardiac pacing and after recovery. These perfusion studies of the myocardium permit a continuous imaging and recording of moment-to-moment changes of visual myocardial perfusion[10]. Other scintographic techniques using [201]Thallium, a non-invasive method, have some disadvantages. Due to the low energy emission of this isotope, 80 kV, the heart-to-background ratio of activity and the long life of this tracer, there is a complex relationship between flow and metabolism which makes analysis rather complex[11]. Similarly there are some disadvantages and difficulties with the direct coronary injection of radio-active-labelled microspheres[12] and the much newer techniques of positron emission using transaxial tomography[13].

[81m]Kr is a short-lived isotope with a 13 s half-life. It can be continuously eluted in a sterile 5% dextrose solution from a portable Rubidium generator. This generator is produced by the Hammersmith Cyclotron[14]. [81m]Kr in solution is then infused by a roller-pump at 10 ml/min through the specially shaped cardiac catheter, previously positioned by fluoroscopy so that one loop of the catheter is located opposite the right, and the other opposite the left, coronary ostium. The calculated dose is 5–7 mCi/min. Patients are studied in the anterior, right anterior oblique and left anterior oblique projections. In our studies images were taken with the patient at rest, after pacing up to 140 beats/min, or pacing until the patient developed chest pain, but never exceeding 140 beats/min. Images were then obtained at these higher pacing rates and following recovery.

Before this new technique of [81m]Kr myocardial imaging was used in man the method had been used extensively in the dog and its usefulness established[10]. It has been shown that the delivered arterial concentration of Krypton and the mixing in the aortic root are sufficiently stable and relatively unaffected by changes in heart rate, blood pressure and cardiac output to make the studies meaningful.

In the first fifteen patients studied by this technique, where the coronary arteriogram was normal and the stenosis below 50%, myocardial perfusion was normal at rest and after pacing. In patients with a past history of myocardial infarction a distinction defect of perfusion was noted at rest and during pacing (Figures 7 a and b). In patients who developed angina during pacing, and where the stenosis of the coronary arteries was above 50%, perfusion was normal at rest but became abnormal after pacing.

It appears therefore that continuous infusion of [81m]Kr into the aortic root provides a technique which allows continuous imaging and assessment of moment-to-moment changes of regional myocardial perfusion. These changes can be related to the severity of the coronary artery disease, and there is good correlation between the degree of stenosis and an abnormal perfusion pattern. In patients with minimal coronary artery disease pacing was followed by an increase of perfusion, whereas in patients with significant coronary artery disease perfusion decreased significantly. In some patients this decrease in perfusion was reversible when the heart rate had returned to normal.

CONCLUSIONS

The two radiological imaging techniques briefly described in this review undoubtedly provide a great deal of information about cardiac function.

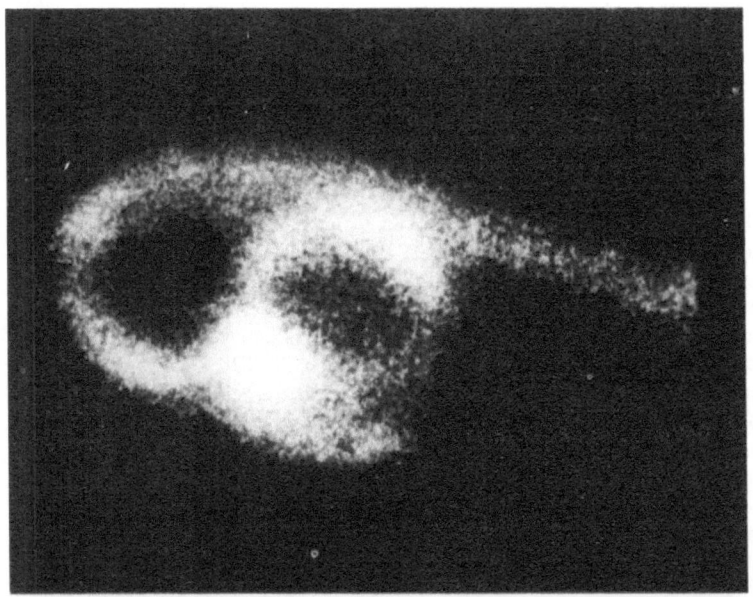

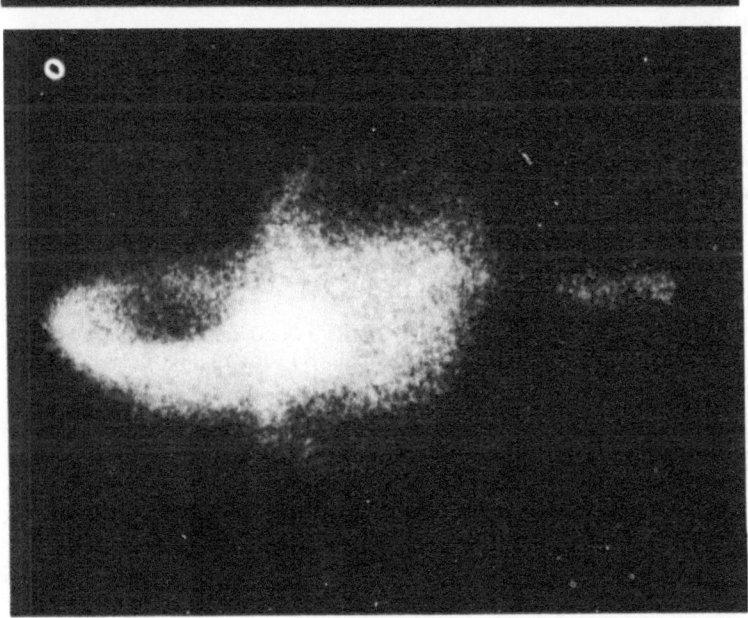

Figure 7 (a) Patient with an anterior myocardial infarct, anterior view. ^{81m}Kr perfusion scan. This shows the area of maximum perfusion in the aortic root. There is an extensive area of the left ventricle, along the anterior wall, which is hardly perfused. (b) Left anterior oblique view of the same patient. This shows the very inadequate perfusion at the apex of the heart and its inferior aspect, extending into the interventricular septum. The posterior aspect of the ventricle is well perfused. The central area of the ventricle, where scintillation counts are relatively low, represents the left ventricular cavity. This area also coincides with the inadequately perfused anterior wall of the chamber, which is superimposed on the left ventricular cavity in this projection

They are complementary methods of investigation, truly physiological tests giving us the opportunity of relating myocardial perfusion with the extent and degree of coronary artery disease and the visual demonstration of normal and abnormal cardiac contraction.

References

1. Dodge, H. T., Hay, R. E. and Sandler, H. (1962). An angiographic method for directly determining left ventricular stroke volume in man. *Circ. Res.*, **11**, 739

2. Dodge, H. T., Sandler, H., Baxley, W. A. and Hawley, R. R. (1966). Usefulness and limitations of radiographic methods of determining left ventricular volume. *Am. J. Cardiol.*, **18**, 10

3. Dodge, H. T. and Baxley, W. A. (1969). Left ventricular volume and mass and their significance in heart disease. *Am. J. Cardiol.*, **23**, 528

4. Kasser, I. S. and Kennedy, J. W. (1969). Measurement of left ventricular volume in man by single-plane cineangiography. *Invest. Radiol.*, **4**, 83

5. Khattri, H. N., Sharma, B., Raphael, M. J., Steiner, R. E. and Goodwin, J. F. (1978). Left ventricular function in ischaemic heart disease. A review. *Postgrad. Med. J.*, **54**, 16

6. Sharma, B., Goodwin, J. F., Raphael, M. J., Steiner, R. E., Rainbow, R. J. and Taylor, S. H. (1976). Left ventricular angiography on exercise. A new method of assessing left ventricular function in ischaemic heart disease. *Br. Heart J.*, **38**, 59

7. Sharma, B., Raina, S., Goodwin, J. F., Raphael, M. J. and Steiner, R. E. (1976). Stress ventriculography in coronary heart disease. A comparative assessment of left ventricular.function and wall motion during angina induced by exercise and atrial pacing. In P. R. Lichtlen (ed.). *Coronary Angiography and Angina Pectoris*, pp. 133–151. (Stuttgart: Georg Thième)

8. Sharma, B. and Taylor, S. H. (1975). Localisation of left ventricular ischaemia in angina pectoris by cineangiography during exercise. *Br. Heart J.*, **37**, 963

9. Selwyn, A. P., Steiner, R. E., Kivisaari, A., Fox, K. and Forse, G. (1978). Krypton 81m in the physiological assessment of coronary artery stenosis in man. (In press)

10. Selwyn, A. P., Jones, T., Turner, J. H., Pratt, T. and Lavender, J. P. (1978). Continuous assessment of regional myocardial perfusion in dogs using Krypton 81m. *Circ. Res.*, **42**, 8

11. Bailey, I. K., Griffith, L. S. C., Strauss, H. W. and Pitt, B. (1976). Detection of coronary artery disease and myocardial ischaemia by electrocardiography and myocardial perfusion scanning with Thallium 201. *Am. J. Cardiol.*, **37**, 118

12. Ashburn, W. L., Braunwald, E., Simon, A. J., Peterson, K. L. and Gault, J. H. (1971). Myocardial perfusion imaging with radioactive labelled particles injected directly into the coronary circulation of patients with coronary artery disease. *Circulation*, **44**, 851

13. Ter-Pogossian, M. M., Hoffman, E. J., Weiss, E. S., Coleman, R. E., Phelps, M. E., Welch, M. J. and Sobel, B. E. (1976). Positron emission reconstruction tomography for the assessment of regional myocardial metabolism by the administration of substrates labelled with cyclotron produced radionuclides. In D. C. Harrison, H. Sandler and H. A. Miller (eds.). *Cardiovascular Imaging*

and Image Processing: Theory and Practice. (Palos Verdes Estates: Society of Photo-optical Instrumentation Engineers)

14. Jones, T. and Clark, J. C. (1969). A cyclotron produced ^{81}RB 81^m Kr. generator and its use in gamma camera studies. *Br. J. Radiol.*, **42,** 237

Part IV
The genesis of oedema in heart failure

12
Mechanisms influencing urinary sodium excretion

H. E. de WARDENER

The control of urinary sodium excretion is an unruly subject. Any attempt to impose some sort of order on the existing data in order to make them more digestible is bound to reflect one's own personal views. I have to confess that I shall be no less guilty in this respect than most of those who have attempted this task before me.

I have to start with a recent interesting finding about the relation of function to structure along the nephron. It appears that the first part of the distal tubule has the same function and structure (EM appearances) as the ascending limb of Henle, while the second half of the distal tubule has the same structure and function as the collecting duct. Functionally therefore, the nephron seems to be divided into four areas: glomerulus, proximal tubule, the loop of Henle, and the collecting duct.

The problem as regards the control of urinary sodium excretion can be considered in the following way. In one hour a normal man filters about 1000 mEq of sodium, reabsorbs 993 and thus excretes around 7. The rotation of these large quantities of sodium in and out of the tubule is the inevitable accompaniment of the high glomerular filtration rates needed to dispose of those materials that can only be excreted in the urine by filtration. One of the most important functions of the kidney therefore, as regards the control of sodium excretion, is to ensure that the bulk of these enormous quantities of sodium are reabsorbed. This takes place in the proximal tubule and the loop of Henle. A second function is to adjust the small amounts of sodium that are excreted in the urine in such a way that sodium balance is maintained. This occurs in the collecting duct. One unifying view of these mechanisms which are responsible for the filtration and subsequent reabsorption of sodium up to the collecting duct, is that they act as a set of buffers that ensure that the amount of sodium that is delivered to the collecting duct shall remain relatively constant. This is a system which must facilitate the fine adjustments which are subsequently made in the collecting duct. In 24 h a normal man will filter approximately 24 000 mEq of sodium and yet can easily make a 10 mEq change in 24 h urinary sodium excretion. Clearly this delicate control would be less precise and perhaps impossible if the collecting duct was not buffered from large oscillations in the amount of sodium delivered into it. Under certain conditions, however, such as pronounced salt loading and salt depletion, this constancy is not achieved, the whole nephron appears to contribute to the alteration in sodium excretion in that there is then a change in the delivery of sodium to the collecting duct which parallels the change in urinary sodium excretion.

The relative constancy of the amount of sodium delivered into the collecting duct under normal circumstances is the end-result of three sets of mechanisms. The first includes those mechanisms which try and maintain a constant glomerular filtration, in other words, a constant load of sodium into the proximal tubule. The mechanisms involved include circulatory autoregulation to changes in hydrostatic pressure[1,2], and haematocrit[3], and the distal tubule to glomerulus feedback mechanism[4,5]. The latter, probably working via the juxtaglomerular apparatus, causes a reduction in filtration rate when there is a sudden surge of tubular fluid emerging out of the ascending limb of Henle.

In the proximal tubule, the constancy of the amount of sodium that emerges from its distal end, and which is thus delivered into the loop of Henle, is ensured by the remarkable phenomenon of glomerulotubular balance. This phenomenon becomes evident when there occurs a spontaneous change in glomerular filtration rate and therefore of sodium delivered into the proximal tubule. There is then a parallel change in sodium reabsorption[6-8]. Before discussing this phenomenon further however, it is necessary to describe briefly the present concepts[9,10] about sodium reabsorption in the proximal tubule (Figure 1). Any hypothesis has to explain how large

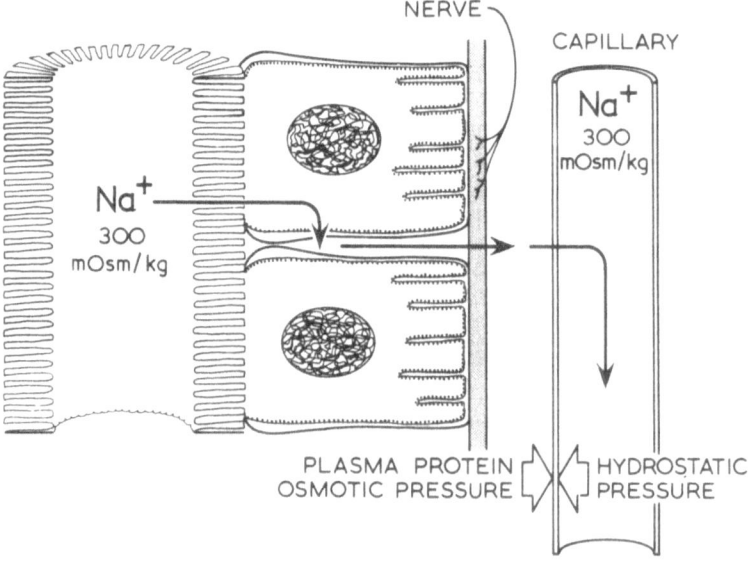

Figure 1 Proximal tubule: schema to illustrate path of sodium reabsorption

quantities of isotonic fluid in the lumen move across the wall of the proximal tubule to another isotonic area on the outside of the tubule which contains the peritubular capillaries. It is proposed that sodium diffuses from the lumen of the tubule into the cell via the vast surface area of the brush border. It is then actively pumped out of the cell by a sodium–potassium–ATPase pump lining the intercellular channel[11] into the channel where it raises the osmolality of the fluid contained therein. This induces a passive movement of water down an osmotic gradient into the channel which increases the volume of fluid in the channel. This in turn must raise the hydrostatic pressure of the fluid in the intercellular channel so that the fluid flows out towards the open end of the channel under the basement membrane. The fluid, which is becoming more isotonic as it travels down, diffuses across the basement membrane into the interstitial space, and then into the peritubular capillary.

Three factors which probably influence this process are the hydrostatic pressure within the peritubular capillary[12-15], the plasma protein osmotic pressure[15-18], and the renal nerves[19]. The evidence suggests that the hydrostatic ·and oncotic pressure influence the rate of reabsorption from the interstitial space into the lumen of the capillary. How the renal nerves influence the movement of sodium is not known. The nerve terminals which have been found appear to end in the peritubular basement membrane, and some have been identified to be adrenergic.

Now to return to the phenomenon of glomerulotubular balance. Figure 2

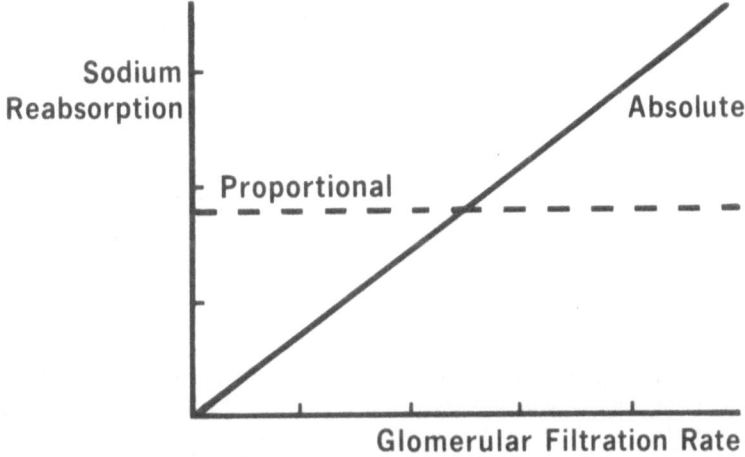

Figure 2 Proximal tubule: relation of sodium reabsorption to sodium delivered into the tubule with spontaneous changes in glomerular filtration rate.

illustrates the phenomenon that when there are changes in the amount of sodium delivered into the proximal tubule produced by spontaneous changes in glomerular filtration rate there is a parallel change in absolute sodium reabsorption (while the proportion reabsorbed remains the same). The mechanism responsible for this phenomenon remains a most contentious issue. The difficulty started with the demonstration that if the delivery of sodium delivered into the proximal tubule is produced artificially with micro-perfusion of saline or Ringer there is no glomerulotubular balance[20-24]. To reconcile the two findings and explain the phenomenon of glomerulotubular balance it has been proposed that this remarkable difference exists because a spontaneous change in glomerular filtration rate tends to change the peritubular environment, whereas microperfusion of the tubular lumen does not. It has been suggested that the most relevant change in the peritubular environment that occurs with a change in glomerular filtration rate is a parallel change in plasma protein concentration in the peritubular capillaries[16]. For instance when plasma flow is constant, a rise in glomerular filtration rate must raise the plasma protein concentration of the plasma flowing from the glomerulus to the peritubular capillaries.

In an attempt to resolve this point the effect on sodium reabsorption from the proximal tubule has been studied while perfusing the peritubular capillaries with fluids of various oncotic pressures. The initial experiments appeared to confirm the hypothesis that changes in peritubular oncotic pressure might be responsible for glomerulotubular balance[16,25-29]. Subsequent experiments however, which have used the same technique but have been technically more satisfactory, have not been able to confirm that changes in plasma protein concentration have any detectable effect on reabsorption of fluid from the proximal tubule[30-32]. The present position is that changes in plasma protein concentration in the peritubular capillaries may at most have a small effect on sodium reabsorption from the proximal tubule but that this is not sufficient to account for glomerulotubular balance.

It seems, therefore, that proximal tubular reabsorption of sodium adjusts itself to the rate of glomerular filtration by some mechanism other than changes in peritubular protein concentration. Earley has suggested that the stimulus for this adjustment is something in the glomerular filtrate itself. Some initial observations by Earley[33] are consistent with such an explanation, but the most convincing evidence has been obtained by Häbeler and Shiigai[34]. Their experiment consists of perfusing a proximal tubule with harvested proximal tubule fluid from another proximal tubule (Figure 3). When the rate of sodium delivery to the proximal tubule is changed in this way there is good glomerulotubular balance in that reabsorption parallels delivery of sodium in the same manner as when sodium delivery is altered by spontaneous changes in filtration (Figure 4). On reflection it seems reasonable to suppose that to perfuse a proximal tubule with harvested proximal tubule fluid is the technique which is most likely to yield the true answer about the nature of glomerulotubular balance. There is thus a body of evidence, which urgently needs confirmation, which suggests that the rate of proximal tubule reabsorption is so perfectly related to the rate of glomerular filtration because the filtrate contains substances which stimulate its own reabsorption. If this hypothesis is correct it follows that the rate of proximal tubule reabsorption might be altered by variations in the concentration of one more of these substances. It also follows that such changes in proximal tubule reabsorption would alter the intraluminal hydrostatic pressure in the proximal tubule, and consequently, glomerular filtration rate. The proposal that significant changes in glomerular filtration rate may be secondary to alterations

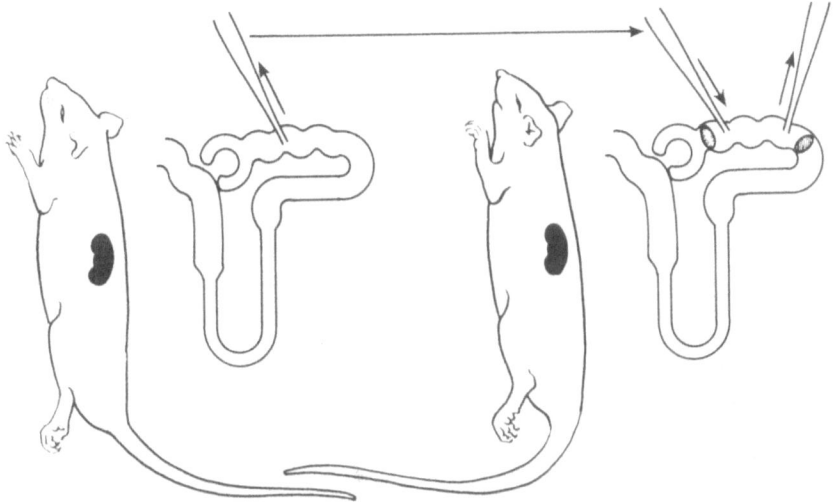

Figure 3 Proximal tubule: technique of perfusing a proximal tubule with fluid obtained from another proximal tubule (Häbeler's experiment)

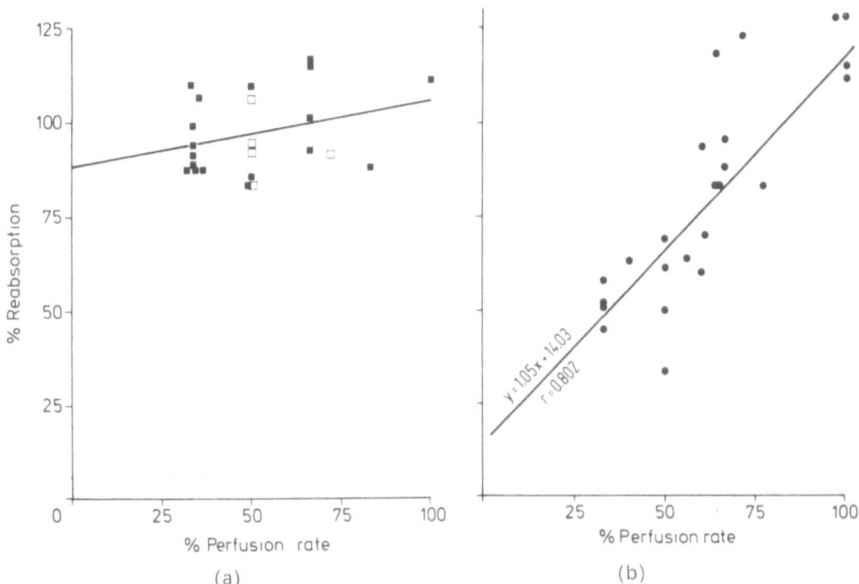

Figure 4 (a) Microperfusion of the lumen of the proximal tubule with either Ringer's solution (closed squares) or the fluid ultrafiltered through an Amicon filter UM05 (open spaces). In each experiment the tubule was perfused at two rates of flow, one between 10 and 20 nl/min and the other between 20 and 30 nl/min. The perfusion rates are expressed as a percentage of the highest perfusion rate used in each experiment. Reabsorption is expressed as a percentage of the reabsorption at the highest perfusion rate in that experiment. Each re-puncture value is corrected for differences in the length of the tubule perfused. (b) Microperfusion of the lumen of the proximal tubule with proximal tubule fluid harvested from late proximal tubules. From Häbeler & Shiigai (1977) (by permission)

in tubular reabsorption was originally put forward many years ago by Bojesen[35] and more recently has been developed by Leyssac[36].

There is one other facet about the proximal tubule and sodium reabsorption which I would like to mention in relation to glomerulotubular balance. There seems little doubt that proximal tubule microvilli (generally known as the brush border), like microvilli elsewhere, contain filaments which have the structural and immunological properties of actin[37]. The implication that the brush border of the proximal tubule might be motile is obviously arresting. Such a property would tend to stir the fluid in the tubule and thus increase the rate of reabsorption by facilitating the permeation of proximal tubule fluid to a greater area of the surface of the microvilli. Such considerations lead one to speculate whether the substance in the glomerular filtrate which may be responsible for glomerulotubular balance might act by controlling the motility of the brush border.

The loop of Henle including the early part of the distal tubule can also be shown to have a form of 'glomerulotubular balance', i.e. reabsorption

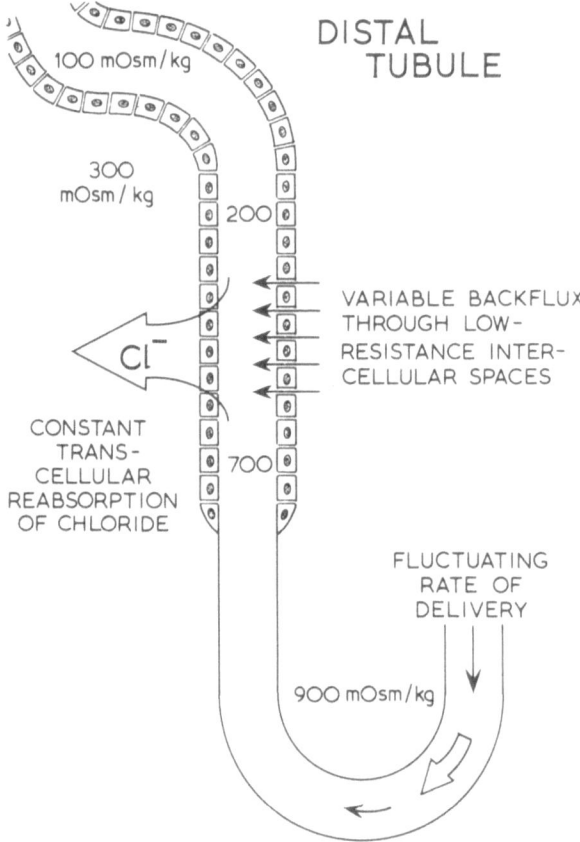

Figure 5 Ascending limb of Henle and early distal tubule. Schema of possible explanation for parallelism between sodium delivered and sodium reabsorption

adjusts itself to the delivery of sodium. The outstanding difference between the proximal tubule and the loop of Henle and early distal tubule, however, is that in the latter absolute reabsorption is directly related to the rate of sodium delivery, whether the sodium is contained in normal tubule fluid delivered in the natural way from the end of the proximal tubule, or whether it is in saline or Ringer's delivered by microperfusion[38,39]. There is another important difference in that the movement of sodium in the ascending limb of Henle is secondary to the active reabsorption of chloride. This suggests that the mechanisms responsible for the parallelism between sodium delivery and absorption in this segment of the nephron is very different from that responsible for glomerulotubular balance in the proximal tubule. It has been pointed out by Morgan[40] that glomerulotubular balance in the ascending limb of Henle and early distal tubule need not necessarily be associated with any change in the absolute amount of ions actively transported out of the lumen of the tubule (Figure 5). He points out that, in contrast to the proximal tubule where there is normally little concentration gradient for sodium between the lumen of the tubule and the interstitial space, in the ascending limb of the loop of Henle and the early distal tubule there is a considerable ionic gradient. This is due to the chloride pump and the counter-current system which reduce the osmolality of the tubule fluid while increasing the osmolality of the interstitial space. The greater ionic gradient means that back-diffusion will be greater, and this likelihood is accentuated by the fact that the inter-cellular channels in this area are particularly leaky. It is this gradient and decreased resistance to back-diffusion which makes it theoretically possible for glomerulotubular balance to occur without any change in active trans-port. For example, assuming an unchanging active reabsorption of chloride, a greater delivery of chloride into the loop of Henle from the proximal tubule would cause the concentration of chloride in the tubule lumen to rise. This would reduce the concentration gradient across the tubule wall so that back-diffusion of chloride from the interstitial space into the lumen would be less. Therefore, without a change in active reabsorption, a higher delivery of chloride and sodium into the loop of Henle would be associated with an increased net reabsorption of chloride, and therefore of sodium.

It is clear that the glomerulus and the nephron up to the collecting duct have a considerable buffering capacity which minimizes changes in the delivery of sodium into the collecting duct – thus making it easier for the collecting duct to adjust the amount of sodium that emerges in the urine. As might be expected the pattern of sodium reabsorption in the collecting duct is totally different from those parts of the nephron that precede it. In the collecting duct it is probable that under normal circumstances there is no parallelism between the amount of sodium delivered into it and the amount reabsorbed. In contrast the collecting duct usually handles sodium in a manner which can be independent of the amount of sodium that is delivered into it[41,42]. For instance the natriuresis of chronic sodium loading is not accompanied by any change in proximal tubule sodium reabsorption; and a natriuresis can be produced acutely with small amounts of intravenous saline without any detectable change in proximal tubule reabsorption[17,43]. Presumably in both these instances there is little change in sodium delivery to the collecting duct. Alternatively it is well established that large infusions of saline, hyperoncotic albumin, or whole blood may be given in such a way that they produce the same fall in proximal tubule sodium reabsorption, and yet have very different effects on urinary sodium excretion[44-47]. The collecting duct's behaviour as regards sodium handling seems to be mainly determined by the need to maintain sodium and volume balance. The lack of relation between the amount of sodium delivered into the collecting duct and the amount that emerges in the urine is demonstrated in Table 1, the data for which have been obtained from Sonnenberg[47].

Table 1 Changes in sodium delivery into the collecting duct and urinary sodium excretion during blood volume exchange and expansion

		Na $\mu Eq/min/g$ KW	
		End distal delivery	Urinary excretion
Blood volume	DOCA + high sodium intake	1·68	0·70
exchange	Sodium deprived	5·31	0·02
Blood volume	DOCA + high sodium intake	6·92	11·98
expansion	Sodium deprived	8·17	2·70

Two groups of rats were studied; one of these had been given DOCA and a high sodium intake and the other had been deprived of sodium. After an exchange transfusion, a manoeuvre which serves as control for when blood volume is expanded, the amount of sodium delivered into the collecting duct (labelled 'end distal delivery') was considerably greater in the sodium-deprived rats, and yet in keeping with the need for sodium balance the urinary excretion of the sodium-deprived rats was less than that of the sodium-loaded rats. When the blood volume was expanded the end distal delivery of sodium rose substantially in both groups of rats. It was highest in the sodium-deprived rats, but again, the urinary excretion of sodium was highest in the sodium-loaded animals. These results also demonstrate another phenomenon which underlines the independence of the collecting duct's way of handling of sodium from the amount of sodium delivered into it: it is that the amount of sodium excreted in the urine can sometimes be greater than the amount of sodium delivered into the collecting duct. This is demonstrated in the sodium-loaded DOCA rats after blood volume expansion when the amount of sodium excreted in the urine (11·98 $\mu Eq/min$) is nearly twice that delivered into the collecting ducts (6·92 $\mu Eq/min$).

In the present state of knowledge it would appear that changes in glomerular filtration rate, or of sodium reabsorption in the proximal tubule or in the loop of Henle, are usually irrelevant to the changes that occur in urinary sodium excretion. The exceptions are gross salt-loading or depletion. In order to understand, therefore, what controls urinary sodium excretion it is necessary to find out what controls sodium-handling in the collecting duct. Unfortunately this is the site which is most difficult to get at, and has been least investigated.

There are certain intrarenally produced substances such as dopamine, bradykinin, prostaglandin and angiotensin, all of which are known to alter urinary sodium excretion[48,49]. Some of them may do so by their actions on the collecting duct. Nevertheless it must be pointed out that the release of these substances is subservient to extrarenal influences.

When investigating the control of urinary sodium excretion in response to volume changes it is more relevant to find out what influences the collecting duct from outside the kidney. Aldosterone is probably not very important as its anti-natriuretic effect is so easily circumvented by a slight increment in sodium balance[50,51]. On the other hand angiotensin in physiological concentrations is probably the most potent anti-natriuretic agent known[52]. To counterbalance these, at least two unidentified substances with natriuretic properties have been demonstrated in urine[53]. Aldosterone certainly[54], and the natriuretic hormones possibly, act on the collecting duct. It is not known whether angiotensin or the natriuretic hormone acts on the collecting duct directly or by causing vascular changes which in turn cause changes in hydrostatic pressure. Acute changes in arterial pressure certainly affect sodium reabsorption, and it has been shown that this is due to a change in sodium handling in the collecting duct[55]. Persistent changes in arterial pressure, however, unless they are very great, do not seem to affect urinary sodium excretion, and the renal nerves have also only been shown to produce short-term changes in urinary sodium excretion associated with alterations in sodium reabsorption in the proximal tubule[56]. It is not known whether the renal nerves can influence the collecting duct's handling of sodium. No terminals have been found at this site.

When contemplating the perennial puzzle of how urinary sodium excretion is controlled in normal circumstances, and particularly in disease, one has the impression that many of the pieces are missing. It is not unlikely that some of these are circulating substances which control sodium transport, some of which act on the upper nephron thus permitting yet others to control what emerges from the lower nephron.

References

1. Semple, S. J. G. and de Wardener, H. E. (1959). The effect of increased renal venous pressure on circulatory 'autoregulation' of isolated dog kidneys. *Circ. Res.*, **7**, 643
2. de Wardener, H. E. and Miles, B. E. (1952). The effect of haemorrhage on the circulatory autoregulation of the dog's kidney perfused in situ. *Clin. Sci.*, **11**, 267
3. de Wardener, H. E., McSwiney, R. R. and Miles, B. E. (1951). Renal haemodynamics in primary polycythaemia. *Lancet*, **2**, 204
4. Schnermann, J. (1975). Regulation of single nephron filtration rate by feedback – facts and theories. *Clin. Nephrol.*, **3**, 75
5. Schnermann, J., Ploth, D. W. and Hermle, M. (1976). Activation of tubuloglomerular feedback by chloride transport. *Pflugers Arch.*, **362**, 229
6. Lewy, J. E. and Windhager, E. E. (1968). Peritubular control of proximal tubular fluid reabsorption in the rat kidney. *Am. J. Physiol.*, **214**, 943
7. Smith, H. W. (1951). *The Kidney. Structure and Function in Health and Disease*, p. 331. (New York: Oxford University Press)
8. Walker, A. M., Bott, P. A., Oliver, J. and McDowell, M. C. (1941). The collection and analysis of fluid from single nephrons of the mammalian kidney. *Am. J. Physiol.*, **134**, 580

9. Curran, P. F. and MacIntosh, J. R. (1962). A model system for biological water transport. *Nature (Lond.)*, **193**, 347

10. Diamond, J. M. and Tormey, J. M. (1966). Studies on the structural basis of water transport across epithelial membranes. *Fed. Proc.*, **25**, 1458

11. Tisher, C. C. and Cirksena, W. J. (1968). Sodium localisation by electron microscopy (E.M.) in single perfused renal tubules (abstract) *Proc. Amer. Meeting Amer. Soc. Nephrol., 2nd Washington*, p. 21

12. Dresser, T. P., Lynch, R. E., Schneider, E. G. and Knox, F. G. (1971). Effect of increases in blood pressure on pressure and reabsorption in the proximal tubule. *Am. J. Physiol.*, **220**, 444

13. Hayslett, J. P. (1973). Effect of changes in hydrostatic pressure in peri-tubular capillaries on the permeability of the proximal tubule. *J. Clin. Invest.*, **52**, 314

14. Koch, K. M., Aynedjian, H. S. and Bank, N. (1968). Effect of acute hypertension on sodium reabsorption by the proximal tubule. *J. Clin. Invest.*, **47**, 1696

15. Sato, K. (1973). Re-evaluation of some micropuncture techniques: some of the factors which affect the rate of fluid absorption by the proximal tubule. In M. Hohenegeer (ed.). *Biochemical Aspects of Kidney Function*, (Munich: Goldman)

16. Brenner, B. M., Troy, J. L. and Daugharty, T. M. (1971). On the mechanism of inhibition in fluid reabsorption by the renal proximal tubule of the volume expanded rat. *J. Clin. Invest.*, **50**, 1596

17. Giebisch, G., Klose, R. M. and Windhager, E. E. (1964). Micropuncture study of hypertonic sodium chloride loading in the rat. *Am. J. Physiol.*, **206**, 687

18. Spitzer, A. and Windhager, E. E. (1970). Effect of peritubular oncotic pressure changes on proximal tubular fluid reabsorption. *Am. J. Physiol.*, **218**, 1188

19. DiBona, G. F. (1977). Neurogenic regulation of renal tubular sodium reabsorption. *Am. J. Physiol.*, **233**(2) F73

20. Burg, M. B. and Orloff, J. (1968). Control of fluid absorption in the renal proximal tubule. *J. Clin. Invest.*, **47**, 2016

21. Morel, F. and Murayama, Y. (1970). Simultaneous measurement of unidirectional and net sodium fluxes in microperfused rat proximal tubules. *Pflugers Arch.*, **320**, 1

22. Morgan, T. and Berliner, R. W. (1969). *In vivo* perfusion of proximal tubules of the rat. Glomerulotubular balance. *Am. J. Physiol.*, **217**, 992

23. Radtke, H. W., Rumrich, G., Kloss, S. and Ullrich, K. J. (1971). Influence of luminal diameter and flow velocity on the isotonic fluid absorption and ^{36}Cl permeability of the proximal convolution of the rat kidney. *Pflugers Arch.*, **324**, 288

24. Wiederholt, M., Hierhelzer, K., Windhager, E. E. and Giebisch, F. (1967). Microperfusion study of fluid reabsorption in proximal tubules of rat kidneys. *Am. J. Physiol.*, **213**, 809

25. Brenner, B. M. and Troy, J. L. (1971). Post glomerular vascular protein concentration: evidence for a causal role in governing fluid reabsorption and glomerulotubular balance by the renal proximal tubule. *J. Clin. Invest.*, **50**, 336

26. Asterita, M. F. and Windhager, E. E. (1975). Estimate of relative thickness of peritubular intestinal space in *Necturus* kidney. *Am. J. Physiol.*, **228**, 1393

27. Boulbaep, E. L. (1972). Permeability changes of the proximal tubule of *Necturus* during saline loading. *Am. J. Physiol.*, **222**, 517

28. Grandchamp, A. and Boulpaep, E. L. (1974). Pressure control of sodium reabsorption and intercellular backflux across proximal kidney tubule. *J. Clin. Invest.*, **54**, 69

29. Ullrich, K. J. (1970). Recent advances in nephrology – physiological aspects. *IVth Int. Cong. Neph.*, **1**, 8 (Karger)

30. Conger, J. D., Bartoli, E. and Earley, L. E. (1976). A study 'in vivo' of peritubular oncotic pressure and proximal tubular reabsorption in the rat. *Clin. Sci. Mol. Med.*, **51**, 379

31. Holzgreve, H. and Schrier, R. W. (1975). Evaluation of peritubular capillary microperfusion method by morphological and functional studies. *Eur. J. Physiol.*, **356**, 59

32. Holzgreve, H. and Schrier, R. W. (1975). Variation of proximal tubular reabsorptive capacity by volume expansion and aortic construction during constancy of peritubular capillary protein concentration in rat kidney. *Eur. J. Physiol.*, **356**, 73

33. Bartoli, E., Conger, J. D. and Earley, L. E. (1973). Effect of intraluminal flow on proximal tubular reabsorption. *J. Clin. Invest.*, **52**, 843

34. Häbeler, D. A. and Shiigai, T. (1977). Flow dependent volume reabsorption in the proximal convolution of the rat kidney – the role of glomerular borne tubular fluid for the maintenance of glomerulotubular balance. Proceedings of the VI Workshop Conference, Hoechst: New aspects on renal function (Schloss, Reisenburg, July 1977). *Excerpta Medica* (in press)

35. Bojesen, E. (1954). The renal mechanism of 'dilution diuresis' and salt excretion in dogs. *Acta Physiol. Scand.*, **32**, 129

36. Leyssac, P. P. (1963). Dependence of glomerular filtration rate on proximal tubular reabsorption of salt. *Acta Physiol. Scand.*, **58**, 236

37. Rostgaard, J. and Thuneberg, L. (1972). Electron microscopical observations on the brush border of proximal tubule cells of mammalian kidney. *Z. Zellforsch.*, **132**, 473

38. Anagnostopoulos, T., Kinney, M. J. and Windhager, E. E. (1971). Salt and water reabsorption by short loops of Henle during renal vein constriction. *Am. J. Physiol.*, **220**, 1060

39. Morgan, T. and Berliner, R. W. (1969). A study by continuous microperfusion of water and electrolyte movements in the loop of Henle and distal tubule of the rat. *Nephron*, **6**, 388

40. Morgan, T. O. (1969). A study of the factors controlling sodium, potassium and water movement in the nephron using the technique of microperfusion. M.D. Thesis, Sydney University, Australia

41. Kuschinsky, W., Wahl, M., Wunderlich, P. and Thurau, K. (1970). Different correlations between plasma protein concentration and proximal fractional reabsorption in the rat during acute and chronic saline infusion. *Pflugers Arch.*, **321**, 102

42. Willis, L. R., Schneider, E. G., Lynch, R. E. and Knox, F. G. (1972). Effect of chronic alteration of sodium balance on reabsorption by proximal tubule of the dog. *Am. J. Physiol.*, **223**, 34

43. Davis, B. B., Walter, M. J. and Murdaugh, H. V. (1969). Renal response to graded saline challenge. *Am. J. Physiol.*, **217**, 1604

44. Howards, S. S., Davis, B. B., Knox, F. G., Wright, F. S. and Berliner, R. W. (1968). Depression of fractional sodium reabsorption by the proximal tubule of the dog without sodium diuresis. *J. Clin. Invest.*, **47**, 1561

45. Knox, F. G., Howards, S. S., Wright, F. S., David, B. B. and Berliner, R. W. (1968). Effect of dilution and expansion of blood volume expansion on proximal sodium reabsorption. *Am. J. Physiol.*, **215**, 1041

46. Knox, F. G., Schneider, E. G., Willis, L. R., Standhoy, J. W. and Ott, C. E. (1973). Effect of volume expansion on sodium excretion in the presence and

absence of increased delivery from superficial proximal tubules. *J. Clin. Invest.*, **52**, 1642

47. Sonnenberg, H. (1972). Renal response to blood volume expansion: distal tubular function and urinary excretion. *Am. J. Physiol.*, **223**, 916
48. Klahr, S. and Rodriguez, H. J. (1975). Natriuretic hormone. *Nephron*, **15**, 387
49. de Wardener, H. E. (1977). Natriuretic hormone. *Clin. Sci. Mol. Med.*, **53**, 1
50. Relman, A. S. and Schwartz, W. B. (1952). The effect of DOCA on electrolyte balance in normal man and it's relation to sodium chloride intake. *Yale J. Biol. Med.*, **24**, 540
51. August, J. T., Nelson, D. H. and Thom, G. W. (1958). Response of normal subject to large amounts of aldosterone. *J. Clin. Invest.*, **37**, 1549
52. Barraclough, M. A., Jones, N. F. and Marsden, C. D. (1967). Effect of angiotensin on renal function in the rat. *Am. J. Physiol.*, **212**, 1153
53. Clarkson, E. M., Raw, S. M. and de Wardener, H. E. (1976). Two natriuretic substances in extracts of urine from normal man when salt-depleted and salt-loaded. *Kidney Intern.*, **10**, 381
54. Uhlich, E., Baldamus, C. A. and Ullrich, K. J. (1969). Einfluss von aldosteron auf den natriumtransport in den sammelrohren der saugetierniere. *Pflugers Arch.*, **308**, 111
55. Kunau, R. T. and Lamiere, N. H. (1976). The effect of an acute increase in renal perfusion pressure on sodium transport in the rat kidney. *Circ. Res.*, **39**, 689
56. Bello-Reuss, E., Pastoriza-Munoz, E. and Colindres, R. E. (1977). Acute unilateral renal denervation in rats with extra-cellular volume expansion. *Am. J. Physiol.*, **232**, F26

13
Neurocirculatory control of sodium and water excretion

R. J. LINDEN

It is not possible to cover this topic adequately in the space of this presentation. Realizing this eventuality the organizers limited me, with qualifying phrases such as 'role of efferent renal nerves' and 'cardiac and venous receptors' and 'general concept of filling of the circulation'. Perhaps I can connect the three aspects together by giving examples of our researches in Leeds where a study of atrial receptors, situated at the veno-atrial junctions, allows the conclusions that these receptors are stimulated to increase their discharge by an increase in blood volume; the effects of stimulation by small balloons are responses which include a reflex increase in urine volume effected by both a change in activity in renal nerves and a blood-borne agent, as well as an increase in heart rate. There is an effect on sodium excretion. Before describing these experiments it is pertinent to look at the evidence for effects of changes in activity in renal nerves on the function of the kidney.

RENAL NERVES

The kidney is a richly innervated organ, the nerves emanating from a renal plexus on and around the surface of the extra-renal portion of the renal artery[1,2]. The innervation of the renal blood vessels is derived mainly from the plexus and is said to be solely sympathetic[2]. Astrom and Crafoord[3] recorded action potentials in renal efferent nerves and demonstrated rhythmic inhibition during systole identical to that in splanchnic nerves. They also showed that the rhythmic discharge could be affected by the carotid sinus; the discharge in the renal nerves increased and became continuous after blockade of carotid sinus nerves.

Elevation of intrarenal pressure by venous occlusion, obstruction of ureters, elevation of arterial perfusion pressure and mechanical pressure each caused an increase in activity in afferent nerves from the kidney[3,4]. No function has been ascribed to these afferent nerves.

In contrast many studies have shown that the renal efferent nerves have an effect on the functions of the kidney. Only examples of reports of investigation in this vast field can be given. Denervation diuresis has been recognized since 1859[5]. It was left to Berne[6], using anaesthetized and unanaesthetized dogs, to conclude that the higher urinary volume and sodium excretion observed in the denervated kidney in the anaesthetized animal was due to a prior vasoconstriction resulting from the anaesthetic. In the unanaesthetized dog the glomerular filtration rates of urinary sodium excretion were the same in the innervated and denervated kidneys. There has been dispute concerning the statement that the increase in sodium excretion resulting from the stimulation of renal nerves in anaesthetized animals is mediated by an increase in glomerular filtration rate alone; some evidence is reviewed in an excellent article on the control of sodium excretion by de Wardener[7]. It is now apparent that the renal nerves can affect other kidney functions as well as glomerular filtration rate (e.g. Bonjour et al.[8]). Pomeranz et al.[9] have produced reflex responses (from carotid sinuses) or direct responses (stimulating splanchnic nerves) and were able to obtain a reduction in blood flow in the outer cortex, an increase in blood flow in the medulla with no alteration in total renal blood flow. Thus there was a redistribution of blood flow; but de Wardener[7] thinks it possible that this does not represent changes in true blood flow. More recently DiBona[10] has reviewed the evidence showing, and he accepts, that there is nervous control of renal tubular sodium reabsorption.

Renin can be released on stimulation; by using an intensity of stimulation of renal nerves which did not reduce total renal blood flow or glomerular filtration rate, there was a response of a release of renin and a reduction in sodium excretion[11]; stimulation in a non-filtering kidney releases renin[12], the release of renin in response to stimulation of the renal plexus can be inhibited by propranolol[13], and the renin response to slow haemorrhage was altered by renal denervation[14]; all these effects were found in anaesthetized animals.

REFLEXES AFFECTING THE KIDNEY

It has been shown that these renal efferent nerves can be affected by afferent nerves from elsewhere in the body. Occlusion of the carotid arteries in anaesthetized animals so as to lower the pressure in the carotid sinuses and lessen the stimulus to baroreceptors, resulted in vasoconstriction in the kidney[15-17], and an increase in carotid sinus pressure decreased renal resistance[18]. These same authors[15-18] have shown that an increase in activity in afferent nerve fibres from the 'cardiopulmonary area' also affects the efferent renal nerves to decrease renal resistance. It is also pointed out that these two sets of afferent nerves interact, with the nerves from the 'cardiopulmonary area' having a larger effect on renal nerves, and preferentially over their effects in other parts of the body. Both sets of afferent nerves also affect renin release[18]. Stimulation of receptors in the ventricles depresses renin release[19]. A fuller discussion of the interaction of these groups of receptors may be found in a recent excellent review[20].

SUMMARY OF EFFECTS OF EFFERENT NERVES ON RENAL FUNCTION

All this evidence suggests that efferent nerves to the kidney can affect mechanisms in the kidney known to affect sodium excretion as enunciated by Nashat[21]:

1. glomerular filtration and hence the filtered load;
2. the intrarenal distribution of blood flow between groups of nephrons that retain or lose sodium;
3. the reabsorption capacity of the tubular cells brought about by:
   (a) neural mechanisms.
   (b) the presence of specific or non-specific hormones capable of altering tubular function.
   (c) the physical environment of the tubular cells.

But the prevailing opinion is that given by de Wardener[7] when he concludes 'it appears that renal function in a denervated kidney in a conscious animal is not distinguishable from that in a normal kidney'. Many reports hold the view that in the conscious animal and man the renal nerves have no function. An argument in favour of this view is that anaesthetic causes an increase in sympathetic 'tone' to the kidney and this allows reductions of this tone to have an effect. For example the most recent investigation with this viewpoint examines renal responses in conscious dogs under stresses of volume expansion and volume depletion (haemorrhage) and concludes that 'renal nerves do not have a significant role in the regulation of sodium excretion in conscious animals'[22].

However, searching in conscious animals which possess many and various mechanisms for the control of sodium excretion by removing one, the renal nerves, appears destined to be fruitless. Who would remove one of five thermostats from a waterbath and expect the temperature not still to be controlled? Instead it is better to look for examples of evidence which suggest the nerves do have an effect.

There is evidence in conscious animals that psychologically stressful situations lead to profound renal vasoconstriction, which is often abolished or reduced during habituation but may persist in spite of repetition[23,24] and the effect of carotid occlusion depends on the resting activity in renal nerves[24]. A series of investigations into patients with autonomic failure by Wilcox[25], suggests that their inadequate sodium homeostasis may in part be a result of the diminution of renal nerve activity. An augmented sympathetic tone to the kidneys is said to be a major determinant of salt retention in dogs with congestive heart failure[26], with vena caval constriction[27,28] and in patients with heart failure[29]. These examples are adequate to sustain an argument that renal nerves may have some function in normal sodium homeostasis. Certainly two reviewers[10,21] believe that the finding of nerves supplying the proximal and distal tubules and the demonstration, using fluorescence histochemical and electron-microscope techniques, of adrenergic nerve terminals in direct contact with tubule basement membranes, furnishes anatomical evidence to support a neural control of tubular reabsorption.

ATRIAL RECEPTORS AND URINE FLOW

With this objective of the control of blood volume, Gauer[30] commented on Starling's law of the heart and stressed the conceptual rigidity of the viewpoint that the regulation of cardiac output was through the regulation of venous return. Claiming that he was basing his conclusions on 'direct observation of the heart in the intact animal' he proposed the 'working hypothesis that in the circulation, volume and pressure as physiological parameters of different physical dimensions are regulated independently'. Such a hypothesis seems superficially attractive but in fact a fundamental failure of this argument is that pressure and volume are intimately connected through the elasticity of the vessels and compartments—thus arterial baroreceptors can well be regarded as 'volume' receptors. With no evidence, but a remarkable foresight, Gauer[30] ended his article relating ventricular size to blood volume and suggesting that 'adjustment of ventricular size could be initiated . . . from receptors in the heart itself, particularly the atria'.

Since then numerous investigators have reported investigations involving bleeding and infusions, and have related the ensuing changes in blood volume to changes in pressure, particularly in the atria and pulmonary vasculature; they have also contrasted the simultaneous changes in impulse discharge from receptors in the atria and arterial baroreceptors[31,32]. Because there have been large simultaneous changes in atrial pressure and receptor discharge in nerves from the atria during these manoeuvres it has been concluded that the atrial receptors are volume receptors and control blood volume. Obviously this conclusion is not valid from the evidence—it demonstrates only concomitant variation—no cause and effect relationship has as yet been shown. It is easy to agree with Goetz et al.[33] that there is as yet no evidence that atrial receptors are volume receptors. But part of a story which could lead eventually to such a conclusion has unfolded. Stimulation of atrial receptors affects the kidney and causes an increase in urine flow.

The first intimation that urine flow might be affected by stimulation of receptors within the chest came from Gauer and his group. Henry et al.[34] first showed that distension of a large balloon in the left atrium so as to block the mitral orifice and raise the pressure in the left atrium about $20\,cmH_2O$ resulted in an increase in urine flow.

However, a balloon distended so as to block the mitral orifice and raise the left atrial pressure by about $20\,cmH_2O$ does not stimulate atrial receptors only. There is a fall in cardiac output and systemic blood pressure and an accumulation of the blood in the pulmonary circulation behind the blocked mitral valve, causing a rise in pressure in all parts of the pulmonary circulation. Obviously there will be secondary effects in the systemic circulation. To obviate these difficulties we repeated the experiments of Henry et al.[34] but the distensions of the large balloon which blocked the mitral orifice were interspersed by experiments involving only the stimulation of atrial receptors brought about by distending the small balloons at the pulmonary vein–atrial junctions[35]. During stimulation of the atrial receptors alone by distensions of the small balloons there were no changes in mean atrial pressure or mean pressure in the pulmonary circulation. Distensions of the two separate balloon systems were carried out in random order in each dog and in the event all distensions of each of the two balloon systems resulted in an increase in urine flow. There is no reason to believe that the increases in urine flow obtained by the two methods are in any way qualitatively different. It is probable that the large balloons are stimulating more atrial receptors than the smaller ones resulting in a larger increase in urine flow. Further support for involving the atrial receptors in the response of an increase in urine flow was obtained by stimulating the right atrial receptors without altering the right atrial pressure and without obstructing venous return[36]; the resulting increase in urine flow was in all respects the same as that obtained by stimulating left atrial receptors.

Evidence[37] that this response involves atrial receptors comes from the blockade of branches of vagal nerves which are known to carry the afferent nerve fibres involved in the response of the reflex increases in heart rate. After control distensions in which the response of an increase in urine flow was obtained the atrial receptors were stimulated in eight dogs with the vagi cooled or sectioned, the left at the upper border of the aorta and the right vagus either at the lung root or in the neck. In all but one of the eight dogs the response of an increase in urine flow was abolished or greatly reduced (see Table 1 of Ledsome and Linden[35]). The results were in all respects similar to those obtained when investigating the heart rate reflex obtained by the stimulation of atrial receptors[38]. It was possible to conclude that the increase in urine flow was caused by a reflex from the atrial receptors and that the afferent limb was in the vagi. Since that series of experiments the application of the same cooling techniques in twenty more dogs has always resulted in abolition of the increase in urine flow confirming the original conclusion.

It has also been observed[39] that this reflex has an efferent nervous limb to the kidney. Nervous impulses in efferent sympathetic nerves to the heart (right ansa subclavia), to the kidney, to the spleen, and in the abdominal sympathetic trunk below the origin of the renal artery were recorded in anaesthetized dogs. The discharge was observed to change in response to stimulation of left atrial receptors only in the nerves to two areas: during stimulation of the atrial receptors the discharge in the nerves to the heart increased but that in the nerves to the kidney decreased. In all other nerves there was no change. It is probable that these nerves to the kidney cause changes in blood flow and thus contribute to the diuresis; some evidence for this statement has recently been provided by Mason and Ledsome[40]. However, the efferent nerves are not necessary for the increase in urine flow. The increase in urine flow has been obtained even in denervated kidneys and in isolated and perfused kidneys. Stimulation of atrial receptors still resulted in an increase in urine flow following complete blockade of efferent sympathetic nerves in anaesthetized dogs brought about by the injection of bretylium tosylate (10 mg/kg) and propranolol (1 mg/kg) which completely blocked reflex activity of sympathetic nerves. The reflex increase in urine flow was also obtained in the presence of atropine. There is no doubt that one limb of this diuretic reflex response involves a blood-borne agent.

Because of the time relations of the diuretic response to the obstruction of the mitral orifice, Gauer and Henry[41] expanded Gauer's (1955)[30] original hypothesis and postulated that activation of the atrial reflexes causes the diuresis by means of a reflex inhibition of the secretion of antidiuretic hormone from the posterior pituitary gland. This hypothesis was put forward even though it had been suggested earlier[42] that the antidiuretic hormone was not involved; in these experiments it had been shown that the diuresis could still be obtained in the presence of large amounts of infused vasopressin. Later Mason and Ledsome[42] observed that decreasing a large infusion rate of vasopressin to a smaller but still large infusion rate resulted in a diuresis similar to that observed by distension of the balloons of the left atrium. They followed this by further experiments[44] which involved graded infusions of vasopressin which modified the diuresis elicited by distension of the left atrium. Neither of these experiments demonstrated that the atrial receptors were involved in the release of antidiuretic hormone, but they allowed the conclusion that even with large concentrations of antidiuretic hormone in the blood a diuresis could still be obtained.

It is still popularly believed that stimulation of the atrial receptors causes a reflex inhibition of the secretion of antidiuretic hormone, and many papers have been cited as supporting this hypothesis (see Ledsome and Linden[35] for criticism). One of the difficulties in dissecting the information contained in previously published investigations is that the methods used have not been specific to atrial receptors. The following methods have been used: negative pressure breathing, immersion of subjects, centrifugation of subjects, dialysis, infusions, methods causing mitral obstruction and lastly distension of the balloons at the junction of the pulmonary veins and the left atrial receptors. The methods other than the last either alter the composition of the blood or cause mechanical changes in the circulatory system with secondary reflex effects, and hence it cannot be argued that only the left atrial receptors were stimulated.

We examined[45] effects of distending both the large balloon in the body of the left atrium (in the manner of Henry et al.[34]), and of stimulating the left atrial receptors with the small balloons, on the urine flow and on the level of antidiuretic activity in the plasma of the anaesthetized dog. First it was shown that our bioassay had sufficient sensitivity to detect changes in the concentration of the antidiuretic hormone of dogs anaesthetized with chloralose. We used the method of Gupta et al.[46] who described a method for the bioassay of the antidiuretic hormone in plasma which had a sensitivity far greater than any published report. This method permitted the direct injection of plasma into rats without any previous extraction procedure. In order to avoid any errors which may occur in the measurements of this activity from variations in the sensitivity of a rat to standard doses of vasopressin, it was necessary to inject all three samples of dog plasma from a single experiment (i.e. control sample before distension, test sample during distension and control sample after release of distension) into one rat. The unknown samples (of plasma) were injected alternately with fixed doses of vasopressin (20 μU). This procedure permitted an assessment of any variation in the sensitivity of the rat to vasopressin and in the absence of such variations it is possible to define differences in the antidiuretic activity of samples of plasma.

It was clearly shown that the diuresis caused by distension of the large balloon in the left atrium so as to block the mitral orifice, or by distension of the small balloon to stimulate only the atrial receptors, was not accompanied by a reduction in the antidiuretic activity of plasma (although in fact on each occasion of distension there was a diuresis). It was at this stage in the investigations that the conclusion was drawn that the blood-borne agent does not take the form of a diminution in concentration of antidiuretic activity of the plasma (e.g. the antidiuretic hormone) and, therefore, is a diuretic substance.

The conclusion that stimulation of the atrial receptors did not alter the concentration of antidiuretic hormone in the blood, and thus that the changes in antidiuretic hormone in blood were not responsible for the diuresis observed during stimulation of atrial receptors, was supported by further experiments[47,48]. In dogs anaesthetized with chloralose the large balloon was placed in the left atrial appendage and the ureters catheterized as before. But in these dogs the posterior pituitary gland was destroyed. The posterior pituitary gland was approached through a hole in the sphenoid bone through which an insulated metal probe was inserted 1 cm into the brain and a current of 400 mA was passed for 20 s; the probe was then withdrawn 2 mm and the same current passed; a current was passed at 2 mm intervals as the probe was withdrawn. At post mortem the pituitary was charred and was observed both macroscopically and microscopically not to contain the antidiuretic hormone. After ablation of the pituitary gland no antidiuretic activity was detectable in the plasma at any time during the experiments.

A diuresis was obtained in each dog during distension of the balloon in the left atrium; the reflex diureses obtained after pituitary ablation were in no way different from those obtained with the pituitary intact. It was therefore concluded that the diuresis obtained by stimulation of atrial receptors is not caused by reduction of antidiuretic hormone in the blood. This study[47,48] also showed that the diuresis which results from distension of the balloon in the left atrium was present after renal denervation and the administration of bretylium tosylate which blocks postganglionic sympathetic nerve fibres, thus providing further evidence in favour of a blood-borne agent mediating the diuresis, even when the posterior pituitary gland is ablated. Such evidence as this also allows the conclusion that the same mechanisms are responsible for the diuresis after the pituitary ablation as before.

It was therefore concluded that distension of the balloons in the left atrium results in a diuresis which is mediated by a blood-borne agent which does not originate from the pituitary gland. Since it had already been shown that the diuresis was not accompanied by a consistent reduction in antidiuretic activity in the plasma (see above) and that the water-loaded, ethanol-anaesthetized diuretic rat was unaffected by the plasma from the dog during stimulation of the atrial receptors, it was concluded that the blood-borne agent causing the increase in urine flow was unlikely to be an antidiuretic agent and was most likely to be a diuretic agent as yet of unknown origin.

Atrial receptors and afferent nerves

Two sets of afferent nerves emanate from the atria. The atrial receptors described above discharge into fast-conducting myelinated fibres and were thought to be involved in the heart rate–urine response reflex[49]. Recently, Thoren[50] has observed atrial receptors discharging into very slow-conducting non-myelinated fibres ('C' fibres). To distinguish which fibres mediated the urine response a series of experiments were completed in chloralose anaesthetized dogs in which the large balloons were distended to block the mitral orifice and cause the diuresis[51].

Responses of an increase in urine flow were obtained in seven dogs with the vagi at $36 \pm 1\,°C$ (first control), either 18 or $12\,°C$, and $36 \pm 1\,°C$ (second control). The response at 18 or $12\,°C$ was expressed as a percentage of the average of the control responses; the response at $18\,°C$ was 69.8% (mean; range 65.2–77.7; $n = 3$) of control and that at $12\,°C$ was 27.92% (mean; range 7.6–48.5; $n = 4$).

In eight dogs the effect of cooling the vagi on the increase in the activity of atrial receptors produced by the distension of a balloon in the left atrium was studied and calculated as above. In seven receptors (four dogs) which discharged into myelinated fibres (mean conduction velocity 17.6 m/s; range 6–27) the response at $18\,°C$ was 68.2% (mean; range 28–100) of control and that at $12\,°C$ was 25.4% (mean; range 5.5–42.3).

In four dogs, six receptors which discharged into non-myelinated fibres (conduction velocity <2 m/s) were examined. In five the responses were slightly reduced by cooling the vagi to $12\,°C$ (mean response 95.1% (range 77.7–100) of control) and in a sixth the response was reduced to 43% at $18\,°C$ and abolished at $17\,°C$.

Thus on cooling the vagi, only the effects on the responses of the receptors which discharged into myelinated fibres were similar to the effect on the urine response observed previously. The effect on the response in non-myelinated fibres was not related. From these findings it is concluded that the atrial receptors which discharge into myelinated fibres in the vagus are the most likely receptors to mediate the increase in urine flow.

Atrial receptors and renal efferent nerves

Experiments similar to those above recording action potentials in afferent nerves were completed but, instead, the discharge in efferent nerves to the kidney were examined whilst cooling both vagi in a graded manner[52].

As reported above distension of small balloons at the pulmonary vein–atrial junctions in anaesthetized dogs has been shown to cause a reflex reduction in activity in efferent renal nerves[39]. Distension of such balloons has also been shown to stimulate atrial receptors which discharge into myelinated and non-myelinated vagal fibres. Using graded cooling of the cervical vagi, the response in myelinated fibres to distension of the balloons was blocked at temperatures which were different from those at which the response in non-myelinated fibres was blocked; findings allowed the conclusion that myelinated fibres only were involved in a reflex increase in urine volume (see above). In this series of experiments small balloons were positioned in the left pulmonary vein–atrial junctions and the atrial appendage. Both cervical vagi were placed on cooling thermodes in pools of paraffin. Activity in efferent renal nerves was recorded along with the ECG and pressures in the femoral artery, left atrium and trachea. The reflex increase in heart rate was prevented by giving bretylium tosylate (10 mg/kg). The atrial receptors were stimulated and the activity in renal nerves observed with the vagi warm (32–37 °C), with the vagi cool (12 °C or 18 °C), and finally with the vagi warm again.

Twelve nerve preparations were examined in six dogs. Distension of the balloons with the vagi warm resulted in a decrease in impulse frequency of 28 % (mean; range 10–80). These responses were not significantly affected during cooling of the vagi to 18 °C, but were significantly reduced or abolished at 12 °C (mean 6 %; range 0–26, $p < 0.001$). This reduction in response was the same as that described in afferent myelinated fibres in the vagi during graded cooling, in contrast to the response in non-myelinated fibres[53].

In a second group of experiments, balloons were distended with the vagi at a temperature of 9 °C; at this temperature all responses in myelinated fibres are blocked and most responses in non-myelinated fibres are transmitted. In six dogs, fifty units were obtained; none showed a significant response.

From these results, it is concluded that during stimulation of atrial receptors, the vagal fibres which are involved in reflex reduction in activity in renal efferent nerves are myelinated, and that non-myelinated fibres are unlikely to be involved in this reflex.

Thus the atrial receptors at the pulmonary vein–atrial junctions discharging into myelinated fibres, are responsible for the increase in urine flow and decrease in renal nerve activity.

Atrial receptors and sodium excretion

Recently using large balloons to block the mitral orifice and small balloons to stimulate only the atrial receptors the urine responses have been evoked; again in chloralose-anaesthetized dogs. The dogs have been prepared with one kidney denervated and one remained innervated[54]. The urine was collected every 10 min from a cannula in each ureter.

Interim results suggest that with the large balloon (nineteen experiments) there was an increase in urine flow in the innervated kidney of 100 % ± 19.4 (SEM) and in the denervated of 87 % ± 18.8 (SEM); and the difference was statistically significant ($p < 0.01$). Sodium excretion increased by 74 % (±22.5) in the innervated and 43.8 % (±21.4) in the denervated kidney. Though the change in the denervated kidney was not in itself significant, the difference between the responses of the two kidneys was significantly different ($p < 0.01$). Thus the innervated kidney excreted more water and more sodium than the denervated kidney.

With the small balloons (twelve experiments) and thus less stimulus, the responses were smaller but similar – except now the denervated kidney increased its sodium excretion by 14 % ± 6.4 (SEM) and this increase was statistically significant ($p < 0.05$). This value was also less than that from the innervated kidney which confirms the above conclusion – more sodium was excreted by the innervated kidney. At the moment we do not know whether to regard the small amount of sodium excreted by the denervated kidney, in response to the blood-borne, possibly diuretic, substance as biologically important or not. Experiments are being conducted to solve this problem.

Concluding note

Stimulation of atrial receptors involves two responses: an increase in heart rate resulting from the changes only in efferent sympathetic nerves (and no positive inotropic response) and an increase in urine flow caused by a blood-borne diuretic substance and involving changes in activity in efferent sympathetic nerves to the kidney with no known function, but possibly involving renal blood flow. The functional significance of this reflex has been postulated[37] as possibly being involved in the control of heart volumes in that an increase in atrial receptor discharge increases heart rate and thus decreases heart volumes and causes an increase in urine flow which would cause a decrease in extracellular liquid, blood volume, and thus heart volume. Such a hypothesis would envisage the atrial receptors as being the first link in the negative feedback on heart volumes.

This hypothesis does not completely deny the working hypothesis of Gauer and Henry[41] in which they insist that the atrial receptors are involved in the control of blood volume, but it must be remembered that there are no cause and effect relationships existing which could provide the evidence that blood volume is regulated by atrial receptors. It is difficult not to hold the view that extracellular fluid is not regulated by a single mechanism but by many mechanisms; the atrial receptor reflex may be only one part of a complex group of mechanisms and its importance is certainly not known. However, the fact that atrial receptors do not influence the concentration of anti-diuretic hormone in the blood as claimed by Gauer and Henry[41], Goetz et al.[33] and Pelletier and Shepherd[55], but possibly cause an increase in a 'diuretic substance' (see above) does not alter the argument for or against the atrial receptors being a possible control mechanism related to blood volume. There is also some evidence that this mechanism may be deranged in heart failure. It has been shown[56] that the atrial receptors discharge less in dogs with chronic heart failure than in normal dogs, even though the atrial pressures are much higher in dogs with the known increase in extracellular liquid in heart failure. A change in receptor discharge may be one of the causes of the known increase in extracellular liquid in heart failure.

SUMMARY

Afferent nerves from the kidney exist but have no known function. Increase in discharge in efferent nerves to the kidney of anaesthetized animals causes changes in sodium excretion by several mechanisms. That these effects have not been demonstrable in conscious animals by removing the nerves and comparing the function of a denervated and an innervated kidney, is not evidence of nil effect of nerves in conscious animals. There is evidence in dogs and man, particularly in diseased states, that the presence of nerves allows retention of sodium and the absence allows excessive loss. Evidence has also been presented that, in anaesthetized animals, reflexes are obtainable which affect sodium excretion: atrial receptors, when stimulated, cause an increased excretion of sodium, mediated by efferent nerves to the kidney.

References

1. Mitchell, G. A. G. (1950). The renal nerves. *Br. J. Urol.*, **22**, 269
2. Christensen, K., Lewis, E. and Kuntz, A. (1951). Innervation of the renal blood vessels in the cat. *J. Comp. Neurol.*, **95**, 373
3. Astrom, A. and Crafoord, J. (1968). Afferent and efferent activity in the renal nerves of cats. *Acta Physiol. Scand.*, **74**, 69
4. Kady, N. N. and Nashat, F. S. (1975). The effects of raising the intrarenal pressure on the blood flow to the innervated and denerved kidneys of anaesthetized dogs. *J. Physiol.*, **247**, 8P
5. Bernard, C. (1859). *Lecons sur les Proprieties. Physiologiques et les Alterations Pathologiques des Liquides de l'Organisms.* (Paris: Bailliere)
6. Berne, R. M. (1952). Hemodynamics and sodium excretion of denervated kidney in anaesthetized and unanaesthetized dog. *Am. J. Physiol.*, **171**, 148
7. de Wardener, H. E. (1973). The control of sodium excretion. In J. Orloff and R. W. Berliner (eds.). *Handbook of Physiology*, Section 8, pp. 677–720. 'Renal Physiology'. (Washington, DC: Amer. Physiol. Soc.)
8. Bonjour, J. P., Churchill, P. C. and Malvin, R. L. (1969). Change of tubular reabsorption of sodium and water after renal denervation in the dog. *J. Physiol.*, **204**, 571
9. Pomeranz, B. H., Birtch, A. G. and Barger, A. C. (1968). Neural control of intrarenal blood flow. *Am. J. Physiol.*, **215**, 1067
10. DiBona, G. F. (1977). Neurogenic regulation of renal tubular sodium reabsorption. *Am. J. Physiol.*, **233**, F73
11. La Grange, R. G., Sloop, C. H. and Schmid, H. E. (1973). Selective stimulation of renal nerves in the anaesthetized dog. *Circ. Res.*, **33**, 704
12. Johnson, J. A., Davis, J. O. and Witty, R. T. (1971). Effects of catecholamines and renal nerve stimulation on renin release in the non-filtering kidney. *Circ. Res.*, **24**, 646
13. Johns, E. J., Lewis, B. A. and Singer, B. (1976). Angiotensin release and the sodium retaining effect of renal nerve activity in the cat. *J. Physiol.*, **257**, 49P
14. Tanigawa, H., Dua, S. L. and Assaykeen, T. A. (1974). Effect of renal and adrenal denervation on the renin response to slow haemorrhage in dogs. *Clin. Exper. Pharmacol. Physiol.*, **1**, 325
15. Oberg, B. and White, S. (1970a). Circulating effects of interruption and stimulation of cardiac vagal efferents. *Acta Physiol. Scand.*, **80**, 383
16. Oberg, B. and White, S. (1970b). The role of vagal cardiac nerves and arterial baroreceptors in the circulatory adjustments to hemorrhage in the cat. *Acta Physiol. Scand.*, **80**, 395
17. Mancia, G., Shepherd, J. T. and Donald, D. E. (1975). Role of cardiac, pulmonary and carotid mechanoreceptors in the control of hind-limb and renal circulation in dogs. *Circ. Res.*, **37**, 200
18. Little, R., Wennergren, G. and Oberg, B. (1975). Aspects of the central integration of arterial baroreceptor and cardiac ventricular receptor reflexes in the cat. *Acta Physiol. Scand.*, **93**, 85
19. Thames, H. D. (1977). Reflex suppression of renin release by ventricular receptors with vagal afferents. *Am. J. Physiol.*, **233**, H181

20. Donald, D. E. and Shepherd, J. T. (1978). Reflexes from the heart and lungs: physiological curiosities or important regulatory mechanisms. *Cardiovasc. Res.* (in press)
21. Nashat, F. S. (1974). Topics in renal physiology, p. 221 and p. 224. In R. J. Linden (ed.). *Recent Advances in Physiology.* (London: Churchill)
22. Lifschitz, M. D. (1978). Lack of a role for the renal nerves in renal sodium reabsorption in conscious dogs. *Clin. Sci. Mol. Med.,* **54,** 567
23. Seal, J. B. and Zbrozyra, A. W. (1978). Renal vasoconstriction and its habituation in the course of repeated auditory stimulation and naturally elicited defence reactions in dogs. *J. Physiol.* (in press)
24. Gross, R. and Kirkheim, H. (1978). Effects of bilateral common carotid occlusion on sympathetic activity and renal function in conscious dogs. *J. Physiol.* (in press)
25. Wilcox, C. S., Aminoff, M. J. and Slater, J. D. H. (1977). Sodium hoseostasis in patients with autonomic failure. *Clin. Sci. Mol. Med.,* **53,** 321
26. Barger, A. C., Muldowney, F. P. and Liebowitz, M. R. (1959). Role of the kidney in the pathogenesis of congestive heart failure. *Circulation,* **20,** 273
27. Gill, J. R., Carr, A. A., Fleischmann, K. E., Casper, A. G. T. and Bartter, F. C. (1967). Effect of Pentolium on sodium excretion in dogs with constriction of the vena cava. *Am. J. Physiol.,* **212,** 191
28. Azer, M., Cannon, R. and Kaloyanides, G. J. (1972). Effect of renal denervation on the antinatriuresis of caval constriction. *Am. J. Physiol.,* **222,** 611
29. Brod, J. (1972). Pathogenesis of cardiac oedema. *Br. Med. J.,* **1,** 222
30. Gauer, O. H. (1955). Volume changes of the left ventricle during blood pooling and exercise in the intact animal. *Physiol. Rev.,* **35,** 143
31. Gupta, P. D., Henry, J. P., Sinclair, R. and Von Baumgarten, R. (1966). Responses of atrial and aortic baroreceptors to nonhypotensive hemorrhage and to transfusion. *Am. J. Physiol.,* **211,** 1429
32. Henry, J. P., Gupta, P. D., Meehan, J. P., Sinclair, R. and Share, L. (1968). The role of afferents from the low pressure system in the release of antidiuretic hormone during nonhypotensive haemorrhage. *Can. J. Physiol. Pharmacol.,* **46,** 287
33. Goetz, K. L., Bond, G. C. and Blowham, D. D. (1975). Atrial receptors and renal function. *Physiol. Rev.,* **55,** 157
34. Henry, J. P., Gauer, O. H. and Reeves, J. L. (1956). Evidence of the atrial location of receptors influencing urine flow. *Circ. Res.,* **4,** 85
35. Ledsome, J. R. and Linden, R. J. (1968). The role of the left atrial receptors in the diuretic response to left atrial distension. *J. Physiol.,* **198,** 487
36. Kappagoda, C. T., Linden, R. J. and Snow, H. M. (1973). Effect of stimulating right atrial receptors on urine flow in the dog. *J. Physiol. (Lond).,* **235,** 493
37. Linden, R. J. (1975). Reflexes from the heart. In E. Sonnenblick (ed.). *Progress in Cardiovascular Diseases.* (New York: Stratton)
38. Ledsome, J. R. and Linden, R. J. (1964). A reflex increase in heart rate from distension of the pulmonary vein–atrial junctions. *J. Physiol. (Lond).,* **170,** 456
39. Karim, F., Kidd, C., Malpus, C. M. and Penna, P. E. (1972). The effects of stimulation of the left atrial receptors on sympathetic efferent nerve fibres. *J. Physiol.,* **227,** 243
40. Mason, J. M. and Ledsome, J. R. (1974). Effects of obstruction of the mitral orifice or distension of the pulmonary vein–atrial junctions on renal and hind-limb vascular resistance in the dog. *Circ. Res.,* **35,** 24
41. Gauer, O. H. and Henry, J. P. (1963). Circulatory basis of fluid volume control. *Physiol. Rev.,* **43,** 423
42. Ledsome, J. R., Linden, R. J. and O'Connor, W. J. (1961). The mechanisms

by which distension of the left atrium produces diuresis in anaesthetized dogs. *J. Physiol.*, **159**, 87

43. Mason, J. M. and Ledsome, J. R. (1971). The effect of changes in the rate of infusion of vasopressin in the anaesthetized dog. *Can. J. Physiol. Pharmacol.*, **49**, 933

44. Ledsome, J. R. and Mason, J. M. (1972). The effects of vasopressin on the diuretic response to left atrial distension. *J. Physiol.*, **221**, 427

45. Kappagoda, C. T., Linden, R. J., Snow, H. M. and Whitaker, E. M. (1974). Left atrial receptors and the antidiuretic hormone. *J. Physiol.*, **237**, 663

46. Gupta, K. K., Chaudhury, R. R. and Chuttani, P. N. (1967). Plasma anti-diuretic hormone concentrations in normal subjects and in persons with oedema of cardiac and renal origin and in normal pregnancy. *Indian J. Med. Res.*, **55**, 643

47. Kappagoda, C. T., Linden, R. J., Snow, H. M. and Whitaker, E. M. (1973). Left atrial receptors and diuresis in the dog. *J. Physiol.*, **237**, 48

48. Kappagoda, C. T., Linden, R. J., Snow, H. M. and Whitaker, E. M. (1975). Effects of destruction of the posterior pituitary on the diuresis from left atrial receptors. *J. Physiol.*, **244**, 757

49. Linden, R. J. (1973). Function of cardiac receptors. *Circulation*, **48**, 463

50. Thoren, P. (1976). Atrial receptors with non-medullated vagal afferents in the cat. Discharge frequency and pattern in relation to atrial pressure. *Circ. Res.*, **38**, 357

51. Kappagoda, C. T., Linden, R. J. and Sivananthan, N. (1978). Atrial receptors and urine flow. *J. Physiol.* (in press)

52. Kappagoda, C. T., Linden, R. J., Mary, D. A. S. G. and Weatherill, D. (1978). Atrial receptors which effect a reflex decrease in renal sympathetic activity. *J. Physiol.* (in press)

53. Kappagoda, C. T., Linden, R. J. and Sivananthan, N. (1977). The receptors which mediate a reflex increase in heart rate. *J. Physiol.*, **266**, 89P

54. Kappagoda, C. T., Linden, R. J. and Sreeharan, N. (to be published)

55. Pelletier, C. L. and Shepherd, J. T. (1973). Circulatory reflexes from mechanoreceptors in the cardio-aortic area. *Circ. Res.*, **33**, 131

56. Greenberg, T. T., Richmond, W. H., Stocking, R. A., Gupta, J. P. and Henry, J. P. (1973). Impaired atrial receptor responses in dogs with heart failure due to tricuspid insufficiency and aortic stenosis. *Circ. Res.*, **32**, 424

14
Capillary and extracapillary factors influencing the distribution of salt and water

M. A. FLOYER

Of the research on the circulation during the past 25 years, the heart has claimed the greatest attention, with the arteries a good second. Research on capillaries has been more scanty, and research on the interstitial space even less. But if we question the purpose of the circulation, the answer is that it should maintain a flow of blood, at ideal rate and pressure, through the capillaries. Likewise, the purpose of the capillaries is to maintain optimal conditions of composition, volume, and pressure in the areas immediately surrounding the cells, namely the interstitial space. Perhaps, therefore, study of the interstitial space may lead to further understanding of the working of the circulation. Our lack of concern for this backwater of the circulation is perhaps illustrated by the fact that about 80 years ago Starling[1] suggested that four forces control equilibrium fluid between the capillaries and the interstitial space. Of these, only one (plasma oncotic pressure) had been measured with any accuracy until a short time ago. Although never verified experimentally, Starling's hypothesis has been taught as a 'law' to many generations of students. In this paper I would like to review some of the work done on the interstitial space, and to suggest ways in which this may affect our understanding of the circulation in health and disease.

In the oedema of heart failure, it is presumed that capillary pressure increases with increasing venous pressure and that this results in imbalance of the Starling forces, allowing large amounts of fluid to enter the interstitial space. But mean capillary pressure must be affected by the degree of vaso-constriction resulting from low cardiac output, as well as by the raised venous pressure. This may be one reason for the absence of oedema in acute heart failure until salt and water retention has increased plasma volume. It is also possible that there is some change in the nature of the interstitial space affecting the amount of fluid it can contain, or the state in which it held it. When there is 'overload' or increased pressure in a body compartment there are two possible explanations: either there is too much fluid in the space, or else the size of the space, or the pressure/volume relationship within it, has changed.

We have been studying the pressure/volume relationships within the interstitial space for the last few years. We were led to this problem by an interest in the mechanism of arterial hypertension. The 'volume' hypothesis put forward by Ledingham and Guyton[2,3] suggests that a small persistent overload of fluid may be a factor in the maintenance of raised blood pressure in many instances. However, raised plasma volume or extracellular volume cannot be demonstrated in many forms of hypertension. The alternative explanation is that there is a changed pressure/volume relationship of the blood vessels or of the interstitial space, thus increasing central venous pressure and interstitial fluid pressure even though blood volume and interstitial fluid volume remain normal. Before discussing the results of experiments performed to test this idea, it is necessary to describe some of the techniques used in studying the interstitial space.

STRUCTURE OF THE INTERSTITIAL SPACE

The interstitial space consists of interlacing collagen fibres between which are large glycoaminoglycan molecules, especially hyaluronic acid. These are large molecules $(1-8 \times 10^8)$[4,5] and consist of a random coil made up of sugar units with a negative charge for each 400 mW unit. At the concentration in the tissues (probably about 1%) there is a large degree (about 80%) of overlap of the glycoaminoglycan molecules[4,6]. Studies of Brownian movement suggest that there is no free fluid in the interstitial space and that all fluid is contained in the gel of collagen and glycoaminoglycan molecules[7].

INTERSTITIAL FLUID VOLUME

This is measured by giving a substance which is thought to penetrate the capillary wall thoroughly but does not enter cells. Many substances are used, each giving a different volume. However, all methods show that the interstitial fluid volume is large, being several times that of the plasma.

INTERSTITIAL 'FLUID' PRESSURE

Interstitial pressure has been measured by several methods. Early attempts putting a needle into the tissues showed that a reliable pressure can only be measured if a small amount of fluid is introduced first; positive pressures of several mmHg are then recorded[7-9]. If pressure is measured continually after the introduction of a small amount of fluid through the needle, reliable readings are obtained for about 30 min, during which the pressure falls from 2–3 mmHg above atmospheric to about 0; after this further reliable readings cannot be obtained. Presumably reabsorption of fluid causes the solid tissues to block the end of the needle, preventing the necessary free flow of fluid between tissues and manometer. However, studies by Guyton and his colleagues[10], confirmed recently in this laboratory[2,11], have shown that if a needle is placed in the interstitial tissue and left for several hours connected to a sensitive manometer with low volume displacement, subatmospheric pressure reading can be obtained.

Guyton measured interstitial pressure by implanting a perforated capsule in the tissues[10,12]. Initially he used table tennis balls with multiple holes which were placed under the skin of dogs. After the capsule has been in place for a few weeks, pressure is measured by inserting a needle through the skin and one of the holes, and is about 7 mmHg below atmospheric. We have confirmed this observation in rats and in man using polythene hollow cylinders with multiple holes about 1 mm diameter[8,13]. Soon after implantation these capsules are filled with fluid with a protein concentration similar to that of plasma, but 4–6 weeks later the protein concentration has fallen to about one-third of that in the plasma with a raised albumin/globulin ratio. Pressure, initially above atmospheric, falls to 5–7 mmHg below atmospheric as the protein concentration falls.

Another way of measuring interstitial pressure is the wick method, described by Scholander and colleagues[14]. A wick is made by pulling long-fibre cotton wool into the end of a cannula 2–3 mm internal diameter, the apparatus resembling a small paint-brush with a hollow handle. The cannula is filled with saline and the wick is wetted; it is then inserted under the skin through a trocar or a small incision and is pushed a little way from the site of entry. The cannula is connected to a manometer. Following insertion, the pressure falls and reaches a steady level of 2–4 mmHg below atmospheric after 15–30 min. Pressures measured in this way are consistently higher (less negative) than by the capsule. Insertion of a wick results only in a small scar which heals rapidly, and the method can be used for clinical studies[15].

THE NATURE OF THE SUBATMOSPHERIC INTERSTITIAL PRESSURE

It is necessary to know what is the cause of the subatmospheric pressure which is measured by the capsule and wick (and by the needle if left in for long enough). If there is no free fluid in the tissues it is difficult to know how a fluid pressure can be measured. Snashall et al.[15] suggested that the capsule and wick hold free fluid in contact with the interstitial gel, and that the subatmospheric pressure measured is due to the osmotic pressure of the gel. When an unsaturated gel is in contact with free water, two forces determine the equilibrium of fluid distribution between gel and sol phases. The boundary layer of gel molecules, prevented from diffusing into the water by the gel structure, acts as a semi-permeable membrane. Water is attracted into the gel by the osmotic effect of the gel molecules and of the positively charged ions held in the gel by the negative charges on its chains. Entry of water causes the gel to swell, setting up elastic forces which tend to force water out. When the osmotic and elastic forces are equal no more fluid will enter the gel and it is said to be saturated. Snashall et al.[15] suggested that the interstitial gel is normally in an unsaturated state and that the subatmospheric pressure measured in the tissues is the force necessary to prevent free fluid from entering the gel. The wick and capsule allow free fluid to be held in the tissues in contact with the interstitial gel and to reach equilibrium with it. The gel must exert a similar force on fluid filtered from the capillaries and this must represent one of the Starling forces.

PRESSURE/VOLUME RELATIONSHIPS IN THE INTERSTITIAL SPACE

Guyton and his colleagues[16] have shown that the compliance of the interstitial space varies with the degree of hydration. If the tissues are dehydrated, there is a sharp fall in interstitial pressure following the removal of a relatively small amount of fluid. If the tissues are over-hydrated, pressure rises fairly rapidly until atmospheric pressure is reached, when there is a sudden marked rise in compliance; at this point large volumes of fluid can enter the interstitial space with little rise in pressure. At this point oedema begins to form. It is presumed that when the interstitial pressure reaches atmospheric, the osmotic and elastic forces in the gel are equal. No more fluid will enter the gel, and free fluid accumulates in the tissues, the pressure rising little until the fascial planes or skin are stretched.

Further evidence that free fluid appears in the tissues only when the gel is saturated was obtained by Guyton and colleagues[17]. They measured the resistance to bulk fluid flow of the subcutaneous tissue in animals with different degrees of hydration. Under normal conditions the resistance to flow was very high, but when, with increasing hydration, the interstitial pressure rose to atmospheric, resistance to flow suddenly decreased by a factor of 100 000.

OTHER FACTORS WHICH MAY AFFECT INTERSTITIAL SPACE COMPLIANCE

We have been studying the interstitial space compliance in rats and in human subjects in order to test the hypothesis that interstitial space compliance is reduced in hypertension. In 1966 we found that interstitial space compliance is reduced in rats with experimental hypertension following partial renal artery constriction.

Interstitial space compliance is measured by giving an animal or human subject an infusion of saline, measuring interstitial pressure before and after the effusion, and estimating the amount of fluid which has entered the interstitial space. If a saline infusion of about half the plasma volume is given to a rat in 2 min, central venous pressure rises sharply and then falls in about 10 min to a steady level a little above the base-line. Tissue pressure, measured by capsule, rises slowly during and after the infusion and reaches a new steady level after 10 min. It is presumed that this indicates the passage of some of the infused fluid from circulation to interstitial space. If no fluid enters or leaves cells, the increase in the interstitial fluid is the volume of the infused saline less the volume by which the plasma is expanded and the amount which appears in the urine. Plasma volume increase is either estimated by direct measurement before the infusion and again after equilibrium has been reached, or is calculated from the change in packed cell volume.

Lucas and Floyer[18] investigated interstitial space compliance following bilateral nephrectomy in rats. They measured interstitial space compliance as described above a given time after the removal of one kidney. Following this the animals were divided into two groups. In the controls, the remaining ureter was anastomosed with the inferior vena cava, giving an animal which becomes uraemic and acidotic but in which a perfused kidney is present. Compliance was measured in the same way at the same time after this operation; there was no change in the interstitial space compliance. In the experimental group the second kidney was removed; the blood urea, pH, and electrolyte concentration were exactly the same as in the control group. However, measurement of interstitial space compliance in these animals without a kidney showed that interstitial space compliance had fallen fourfold.

Lucas and Floyer also showed that following bilateral nephrectomy the plasma volume/interstitial fluid volume ratio rises. They suggested that the hypertension which occurs after bilateral nephrectomy (renoprival hypertension) is caused both by salt and water retention and by reduced interstitial space compliance resulting in increased interstitial pressure and forcing more interstitial fluid into the plasma. They also[18,19] speculated that there might be a renal hormone, secreted when the kidney is well-perfused, which acts on interstitial tissue and raises compliance; this effect would be abolished following bilateral nephrectomy or when the kidney is poorly perfused, as after partial renal artery constriction. They suggested that this might be a physiological mechanism which would be especially important in animals which drink infrequently. If interstitial tissue compliance is high when an animal has drunk a large volume of water, it will be possible to store much water in the tissues without raising the interstitial pressure sufficiently to force the interstitial fluid into the circulation whence it will be excreted. Raised compliance will also delay tissue pressure from reaching the point at which oedema will occur. However, when the animal becomes dehydrated, compliance must fall in order that sufficient fluid is returned from the interstitial space into the plasma in order to maintain plasma volume. A hormone secreted by the well-perfused kidney which raised interstitial space compliance would benefit such animals and would fit the experimental results described above.

Recently, Brain et al.[20] have measured both interstitial and vascular compliance in human subjects by measuring central venous and interstitial pressure (using a wick) before and after saline infusions. In subjects with essential hypertension, there is a 2–4-fold decrease in both interstitial and vascular compliance compared with normal subjects. It was suggested that reduction of the interstitial space compliance might reduce the ability to store saline in the tissues, and might be responsible for the increased natriuresis and diuresis which occurs in hypertension.

If the suggestion that the kidney controls interstitial space compliance is confirmed, we may speculate further on the role which this mechanism plays in the oedema of heart failure. In heart failure the kidneys are vasoconstricted; this would be expected to reduce secretion of such a hormone. This might result in a more rapid rise of interstitial pressure towards atmospheric and might hasten the point at which oedema occurs. This would not be of much importance in the systemic circulation, but might be of great significance in the pulmonary circulation, in which a change in interstitial space compliance might precipitate pulmonary oedema.

We know very little in this field and much more work remains to be done on the interstitial space; it must be regarded not as a mere backwater but as an important functional part of the circulation.

References

1. Starling, E. H. (1896). On the absorption of fluid from the connective tissue space. *J. Physiol.*, **19**, 312
2. Ledingham, J. M. (1971). Blood pressure regulation in renal failure. *J. Roy. Coll. Phys. Lond.*, **5**, 103
3. Guyton, A. C., Coleman, T. G., Bower, J. D. and Granger, H. J. (1970). Circulatory control in hypertension. *Circ. Res.*, **26** and **27** (Suppl. II), 135
4. Laurent, T. C. (1970). Structure of hyaluronic acid. In E. A. Balazs (ed.). *Chemistry and Molecular Biology of the Intercellular Matrix*, vol. 2, pp. 703-732. (New York and London: Academic Press)
5. Ogston, A. G. (1966). On water binding. *Federation Proceedings*. Federation of American Societies for Experimental Biology, **25**, 986
6. Ogston, A. G. (1970). Biological functions of the glycoaminoglycans. In E. A. Balazs (ed.). *Chemistry and Molecular Biology of the Intercellular Matrix*, vol. 3, pp. 1231-1240. (New York and London: Academic Press)
7. McMaster, P. D. (1946). The pressure and interstitial resistance prevailing in the normal and edematous skin of animals and man. *J. Exp. Med.*, **84**, 473
8. Burch, G. E. and Sodeman, W. A. (1937). The estimation of subcutaneous tissue pressure by a direct method. *J. Clin. Invest.*, **16**, 845
9. Meyer, F. and Holland, G. (1932). Die Messung des Drukes in Geweben. *Arch. Exp. Path. Pharmakol.*, **168**, 580
10. Guyton, A. C., Armstrong, G. C. and Crowell, J. W. (1960). Negative pressure in the interstitial spaces. *Physiol.*, **3**, 70
11. Lee-Kelland, S. and Floyer, M. A. (Unpublished observations)
12. Guyton, A. C. (1963). A concept of negative interstitial pressure based on pressure in implanted perforated capsules. *Circ. Res.*, **12**, 399
13. Floyer, M. A. (1966). The mechanism underlying the response of the hypertensive subject to a saline load. In F. Milliez and L. Tcherdakoff (eds.). *L'Hypertension arterielle*, pp. 440-452. (Paris: L'Expansion Scientifique Française)
14. Scholander, P. F., Hargens, A. R. and Miller, S. C. (1968). Negative pressure in the interstitial fluids of animals. *Science*, **161**, 321
15. Snashall, P. D., Lucas, J., Guz, A. and Floyer, M. A. (1971). Measurement of interstitial 'fluid' pressure by means of a cotton wick in man and animals: an analysis of the origin of the pressure. *Clin. Sci.*, **41**, 35
16. Guyton, A. C. (1965). Interstitial fluid pressure. II. Pressure volume curves of the interstitial space. *Circ. Res.*, **16**, 452
17. Guyton, A. C., Scheel, K. and Murphree, D. (1966). Interstitial fluid pressure. III. Its effect on resistance to tissue fluid mobility. *Circ. Res.*, **19**, 412
18. Lucas, J. and Floyer, M. A. (1973). Renal control of changes in the compliance of the interstitial space. A factor in the aetiology of renoprival hypertension. *Clin. Sci.*, **44**, 379

19. Lucas, J. and Floyer, M. A. (1974). Changes in body fluid distribution and interstitial tissue compliance during the development and reversal of experimental renal hypertension in the rat. *Clin. Sci. Mol. Med.*, **47**, 1
20. Brain, A. J. S., Lucas, J. and Floyer, M. A. (1977). Evidence for a reduction in interstitial space compliance following plasma volume expansion in human essential hypertension: a factor controlling the distribution of a saline load. *Clin. Sci. Mol. Med.*, **52**, 21

15
Heart failure – pathophysiological considerations

E. BRAUNWALD

Heart failure is the pathophysiological state in which an abnormality of *cardiac* function is responsible for the failure of the heart to pump blood at the rate commensurate with the requirements of the metabolizing tissues. Heart failure is frequently, but not always, caused by a defect in myocardial contraction, and under these circumstances it may be termed *myocardial failure*. However, heart failure can occur in the face of normal myocardial function, as in acute valvular regurgitation. Heart failure must be distinguished from non-cardiac *circulatory* failure, of which hypovolaemic shock is an example.

When a defect in myocardial contraction occurs and/or an excessive haemodynamic burden is placed on the ventricle, the heart is dependent on three principal compensatory mechanisms for maintenance of its function as a pump:

1. the Frank–Starling mechanism, in which an increased preload, operating through lengthening of sarcomeres and optimal overlap between thick and thin myofilaments, acts to sustain cardiac performance;
2. myocardial hypertrophy with or without cardiac dilatation, in which the mass of contractile tissue is augmented;
3. increased release of catecholamines by adrenergic cardiac nerves and the adrenal medulla, which act on myocardial beta-receptors and augment myocardial contractility.

Initially, these three compensatory mechanisms may be adequate to restore relatively normal pumping performance of the heart, although intrinsic myocardial contractility may be substantially reduced or the haemodynamic burden on the heart is elevated. However, the potential of each of these compensatory mechanisms is limited, and the clinical syndrome of heart failure occurs when, despite the maximal utilization of these mechanisms, the pumping performance is inadequate.

The cardiac output is normal or depressed in the basal state in patients with the common forms of heart failure secondary to coronary artery disease, hypertension, primary myocardial disease, valvular disease, and pericardial disease (so-called low-output heart failure). When it is normal it fails to rise appropriately during exercise or declines precipitously when afterload is augmented. Cardiac output is usually elevated in patients with heart failure and conditions in which there is reduced afterload and/or hypermetabolism, such as hyperthyroidism, anaemia, beri beri, and Paget's disease (so-called high-output heart failure). The mechanisms responsible for the development of heart failure in patients whose cardiac outputs are initially high are complex and depend on the specific underlying disease process and its effect on the myocardium. In most of these conditions the heart is called upon to pump an abnormally large volume of blood in order to deliver an adequate quantity of oxygen to the metabolizing tissues. This increased volume load exerts an effect on the myocardium resembling that produced by an arteriovenous fistula or a regurgitant valvular lesion.

The inadequate delivery of oxygen to the metabolizing tissues, characteristic of heart failure regardless of the level of cardiac output, is reflected in an abnormally widened arterio-mixed venous oxygen difference. In mild cases, this abnormality may not be present in the basal state and may become evident only during the stress of increased activity. Oxygen extraction, as reflected in the arteriovenous oxygen difference, may be normal or even low in the presence of high output failure with multiple arteriovenous shunts. However, the arteriovenous oxygen difference would be higher were it measured at the venous end of the systemic capillary bed proximal to the admixture of the shunted blood.

A number of peripheral mechanisms are brought into play to conserve the limited cardiac output in heart failure. Among these are the redistribution of left ventricular output; vasoconstriction, mediated largely by the adrenergic nervous system, is primarily responsible for this redistribution of peripheral blood flow which develops or becomes more marked when an additional burden (such as exercise, fever, or anaemia) is imposed on the circulation in the presence of impaired myocardial function, and cardiac output cannot rise normally. As heart failure advances, there is a redistribution of left ventricular output, even in the basal state. This redistribution maintains the delivery of oxygen to vital organs such as the heart and brain, while blood flow to less critical areas such as the skin is reduced.

A progressive decline in the affinity of haemoglobin for oxygen due to an increase in 2,3-diphosphoglycerate (DPG) also occurs in heart failure. This shift in the oxygen–haemoglobin dissociation curve to the right represents an additional compensatory mechanism to facilitate oxygen transport; increased DPG, the tissue acidosis which produces a similar shift in the oxygen–haemoglobin dissociation curve and the slow circulation time characteristic of heart failure all act synergistically to maintain the delivery of oxygen to the metabolizing tissues in the face of a reduced cardiac output.

CONTRACTILITY OF HYPERTROPHIED AND FAILING MYOCARDIUM

There is general agreement that when an excessive load is imposed on a ventricle, the development of myocardial hypertrophy provides a fundamental compensatory mechanism that permits it to sustain this burden. There has been substantial interest in the analysis of the behaviour of isolated muscle removed from animals in which the heart had been subjected to a controlled major stress. A convenient experimental model is the cat with pulmonary artery constriction. Papillary muscles are removed from the right ventricles in which either hypertrophy or overt failure had developed and the excised muscles are then studied *in vitro*. Right ventricular hypertrophy and failure both reduce the maximum velocity of unloaded shortening (V_{max}) below the values observed in muscles obtained from normal cats; the changes are more marked in muscles obtained from animals in which heart failure had been present than in those with hypertrophy alone (Figure 1). Heart failure clearly depresses the maximum isometric tension, but hypertrophy without failure produces only a borderline depression of this variable[1].

Electron microscopic studies of myocardium removed from overloaded,

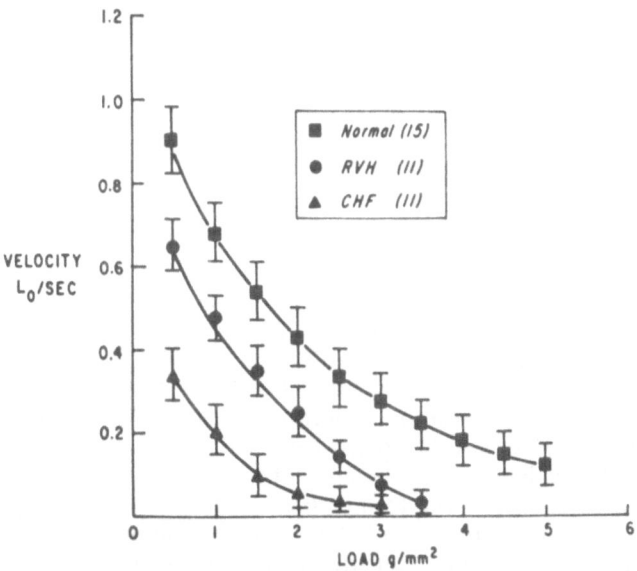

Figure 1 The force–velocity relations of the three groups of cat papillary muscles. Average values with $\pm$SEM are given for each point. Velocity has been corrected to muscle lengths per second (L_0/s). Numbers in parentheses are numbers of animals. (Reproduced with permission from *Circ. Res.*, **21**, 341 (1967))

dilated hearts fixed at the elevated falling pressures existing in life have revealed sarcomere lengths which averaged 2.2 μm, i.e., no longer than those at the apex of the length–active tension curve of normal cardiac muscle[2]. These observations suggest that the depressed contractility of failing heart muscle is *not* due to the disengagement of actin and myosin filaments. Thus, the depression of contractility of failing heart muscle appears to be related to an *intrinsic* defect of the muscle rather than to its operation at an abnormal position on a basically normal length–tension curve; also, these findings are *not* consistent with the hypothesis that the depressed contractility of failing heart muscle is due to its operation on the descending limb of the Frank–Starling curve.

The findings summarized above are, in general, consonant with those of a number of investigations on cardiac muscle isolated from animals with experimentally produced pressure overload, from left ventricular papillary muscles obtained from Syrian hamsters with hereditary cardiomyopathy, as well as from papillary muscles removed from the left ventricles of patients with heart failure due to chronic valvular disease[3]. The contractile performance of the intact right ventricles of cats with pulmonary artery constriction also reveal a marked depression which parallels that observed in the isolated papillary muscles removed from these ventricles. When compared with the normal, the active tension developed by the right ventricle at equivalent end-diastolic fibre lengths is markedly reduced in cats with heart failure[4] (Figure 2).

It may be concluded that the depression of the cardiac contractile state observed in the hypertrophied and failing ventricle represents an *intrinsic* property of the muscle. This depression is evident *in vitro*, when the muscle's physical and chemical milieu are controlled, and it is therefore not dependent on any altered humoral or other environmental factors existing *in vivo*. While the contractile state is uniformly depressed in the intact ventricle and in isolated muscles of cats with heart failure, the cardiac index and stroke volume are often maintained in the resting state, albeit at elevated ventricular end-diastolic volumes and pressures. It appears then that when the ventricle is chronically stressed by an increase in the impedance to emptying, the initial response is an increase in the total muscle mass. Initially, and if the pressure overload is not too extreme, this adaptation can allow the ventricle to generate an abnormally high systolic pressure and to empty normally, i.e., without depression of contractility.

Later, as the intrinsic contractile state of each unit of myocardium becomes depressed, increased muscle mass, operating in conjunction with increased sympathetic stimulation and perhaps the Frank–Starling mechanism, maintains overall circulatory compensation. The depression of contractility is manifest, in the mildest form, by a reduction only in the intrinsic velocity of shortening (V_{max}) of each myocardial fibre, but with little, if any, reduction in the development of maximal isometric force (P_0). As the intrinsic contractile state of each unit of myocardium becomes further depressed, a more extensive reduction in V_{max} occurs, and this is now accompanied by a reduction in P_0. At this point, cardiac output is maintained by an increase in muscle mass and cardiac dilatation. As contractility declines further, the ventricle becomes

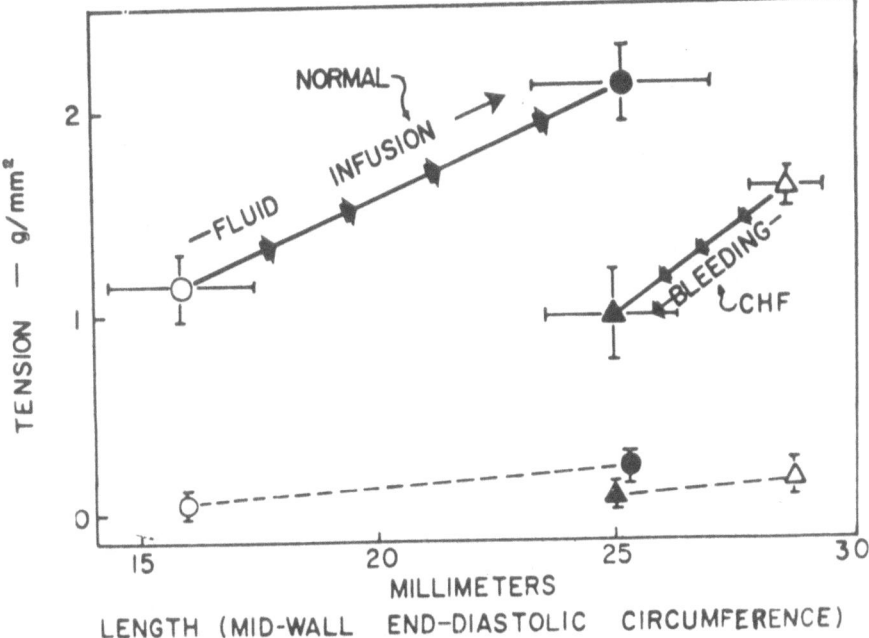

Figure 2 Intact ventricle length–tension relationships. Acute manipulation of end-diastolic volume to obtain ventricular Frank–Starling curves. Lines represent segments of active and resting length–tension curves (Frank–Starling relationship) of five normal (circles) and five failing ventricles (triangles). Solid lines represent active tension, while dashed lines refer to resting or diastolic tension. Open symbols refer to values obtained at spontaneously occurring end-diastolic volume, while solid symbols refer to values obtained after volume infusion in normal cats and bleeding of cats with heart failure. Average values ±SEM are shown. Active and resting tension are expressed as grams per square millimetre (g/mm²) on ordinate and normalized end-diastolic circumference, or muscle length, is in millimetres on abscissa. (Reproduced with permission from *Am. J. Physiol.*, **223**, 1150 (1972))

unable to empty normally. It operates on the ascending limb of a depressed, function curve[4,5] and the augmented ventricular end-diastolic volume must be regarded as aiding the maintenance of cardiac output, except in the terminal stages of heart failure. The elevation of ventricular end-diastolic volume and pressure, in accordance with the Frank–Starling mechanism, raises ventricular performance by stretching the sarcomeres to optimal levels, but at the same time causes pulmonary or systemic venous congestion and promotes the formation of pulmonary or peripheral oedema. While an improvement in function in response to positive inotropic stimuli, such as digitalis or sympathomimetic amines, can occur in failing muscle, the degree of augmentation falls and, at a late stage, the contractility of even the stimulated heart declines.

The character of the stress responsible for inciting the hypertrophy also appears to play a critical role in determining whether or not it is detrimental to myocardial contractility. When a volume overload is produced by the creation of an aortocaval fistula, resulting in progressive left ventricular dilatation and moderate left ventricular hypertrophy without clinical evidence of heart failure, the length–active tension relations of the dilated, hypertrophied ventricle remain essentially normal[6]; within 1 week of the creation of the fistula the left ventricular end-diastolic pressure rises and then remains constant, while the left ventricular end-diastolic diameter continues to increase progressively. During chronic adjustment to the volume load, the end-diastolic volume increases at any given end-diastolic pressure, but myocardial function, as reflected in the velocity of circumferential fibre shortening, usually remains normal. Also, in papillary muscles removed from animals with a volume overload resulting from experimentally produced atrial septal defect, contractility is entirely normal, without the changes in the force–velocity or length–tension curves noted in muscles obtained from animals with pressure-induced hypertrophy. However, in the presence of a very large shunt and clinical evidence of congestive heart failure, myocardial contractility does become markedly reduced[3].

In the presence of volume overload, the development of eccentric ventricular hypertrophy, which presumably is associated primarily with an increase in the number of sarcomeres laid down in series, allows the chronically dilated heart to deliver an increased stroke volume at a normal level of contractility and a normal extent of shortening of each individual sarcomere. Some increase in wall thickness and the change to a more spherical ventricular shape tend to maintain wall stress relatively constant and sarcomere length remains maximal. Thus, the ventricle compensates for a volume overload both with a change in ventricular geometry and an increase in the number of sarcomeres, resulting in an augmentation of stroke volume. In the compensated state the combination of ventricular dilatation and hypertrophy associated with chronic volume overloading allows enhancement of overall cardiac performance, with normal performance of each unit of an enlarged ventricle operating at an optimal sarcomere length.

MYOCARDIAL ENERGY PRODUCTION

Considerable effort has been directed toward elucidating the fundamental mechanism responsible for the relative decrease in the useful external work delivered by the myocardium in the common forms of low-output heart failure. Recent observations on the relation between left ventricular performance and myocardial oxygen consumption have shown that when contractility becomes depressed acutely, myocardial oxygen consumption also declines. Patients with chronic impairment of left ventricular performance and reduction of the velocity of myocardial fibre shortening also exhibit reduction of coronary blood flow and myocardial oxygen consumption per unit of muscle[7].

To determine whether energy supplies are adequate in cardiac hypertrophy and failure, the contents of high-energy phosphate were compared in the papillary muscles of normal cats, cats with hypertrophy without failure and cats with overt right ventricular failure induced by pulmonary artery constriction. The concentrations both of adenosine triphosphate (ATP) and of creatinine phosphate (CP) were normal in the papillary muscles removed from failing hearts and non-failing, hypertrophied hearts studied *in vitro*[8]. Since, as already pointed out (Figure 1), the mechanical performance of these isolated muscles was impaired[1], this depression of contractility could not be attributed to a reduction of total myocardial high-energy stores. In addition, there appear to be no reductions of ATP and CP concentrations in papillary muscles removed from failing human hearts. Thus, it would appear that energy production and the total reserve of high-energy phosphate compounds are not *primarily* responsible for the reduced contractility of the hypertrophied or failing heart, regardless of any changes in mitochondrial function. However, the possibility has certainly not been excluded that ATP is depleted in a small compartment vital for muscular contraction.

MYOCARDIAL ENERGY UTILIZATION

The activity of myofibrillar ATPase has been reported to be reduced in the hearts of patients who had died of heart failure and in dogs with naturally occurring heart failure[3]. Furthermore, there is evidence that reductions in the activities of both myofibrillar and actomyosin ATPase occur in heart failure induced by pulmonary artery constriction in cats and by constriction of the ascending aorta in guinea pigs. These depressions of enzymatic activity could occur if an altered low-molecular weight subunit of the myosin molecule, i.e., the portion of the molecule responsible for the ATPase activity, were produced in the overloaded heart and if it reduced contractility by lowering the rate of interaction between actin and myosin filaments[3]. The synthesis of a myosin with an abnormally low intrinsic ATPase activity could explain many of the functional changes in failing heart muscle, such as depression of the force–velocity curve.

EXCITATION–CONTRACTION COUPLING

Studies in a number of *in vitro* systems have indicated that there is impairment of the delivery of Ca^{++} for activation of the contractile process in heart failure. A variety of cellular structures, including the sarcolemma, the sarcoplasmic reticulum (SR) and the mitochondria affect the myoplasmic concentration of Ca^{++}. It has been proposed that structural damage to these organelles or changes in the intracellular concentrations of other cations, adenine nucleotides or free fatty acids may interfere with mechanisms regulating the myoplasmic concentration of Ca^{++} and thus participate in the production of heart failure. The uptake of Ca^{++} by these structures is dependent on a Ca^{++}-activated ATPase and depression of the activity of this enzyme, or defects in Ca^{++} accumulation sites could play a role in the development of myocardial failure, in that a reduction in Ca^{++} pumping could be responsible for a reduction of Ca^{++} bound to the SR and eventually for less Ca^{++} available for the contractile process.

The reduction in contractility of papillary muscle obtained from cats with constriction of the pulmonary artery is accompanied by a reduction in the muscle's resting membrane potential, maximum rate of rise, and overshoot, as well as in the duration of the action potential[3]. While the precise mechanism responsible for these changes in electrical properties is unknown, they may be related to elevations of the intracellular $[Na^+]$ and depression of intracellular $[K^+]$ and could be associated with diminished entry of Ca^{++} into myocardial cells, which in turn could impair myocardial contraction. The ATPase isolated from the SR obtained from the right ventricles of dogs with heart failure has been found to be depressed[9] and in failing calf hearts the rate of Ca^{++} uptake by the SR and the activity of microsomal Ca-activated ATPase obtained are reduced to about 50% of normal[5]. A disturbance in the uptake of Ca^{++} by the SR could interfere with cardiac performance, since inadequate reduction of the intracellular $[Ca^{++}]$ at the end of systole could result in delayed or incomplete relaxation. In studies employing murexide, a dye which rapidly binds Ca^{++} in solution, it has been demonstrated that the rate of Ca^{++} uptake by the SR obtained from failing heart muscle in humans, rabbits, and hamsters, is slowed and that the total binding of Ca^{++} is reduced[3].

Experimental heart failure in the rabbit produced by aortic regurgitation in which there is depression of myocardial contractile performance *in vitro*, appears to be associated with a significant alteration in the intracellular distribution of Ca^{++}. While total intracellular $[Ca^{++}]$ is normal, mitochondrial $[Ca^{++}]$ has been found to be greatly increased. The rate of uptake and of binding of Ca^{++} to the SR are reduced. With greater quantities of Ca^{++} accumulated in the mitochondria, contractility might then be reduced by limiting the quantity of Ca^{++} available to initiate contraction; moreover, if enough Ca^{++} enters the mitochondria, uncoupling of oxidative phosphorylation can occur. Interestingly, uptake of Ca^{++} by the SR has been reported to be significantly reduced in rabbits with aortic regurgitation sacrificed *before* objective signs of heart failure had developed. This finding, very early in the course of failure, suggests that this reduction of Ca^{++} uptake is responsible for, rather than a consequence of, the impairment of contractility[10].

The hamster with hereditary cardiomyopathy offers the opportunity for study of the function of the SR in a naturally occurring form of myocardial failure. There is a depression of the rate of Ca^{++} binding by the SR, and this depression becomes more severe as the heart failure progresses[11]; abnormalities of phospholipid and cholesterol composition which have been described in the SR of the cardiomyopathic hamster might explain these changes. Also, both the rate and extent of energy-linked Ca^{++} binding by mitochondria have been reported to be greatly reduced in these failing hearts[11]. Abnormalities in the accumulation of Ca^{++} by the SR have been demonstrated in other forms of heart failure as well[3], including the spontaneously failing dog heart–lung preparation, ischaemic failing heart muscle, the substrate-depleted failing rat heart, the heart with isoproterenol-induced necrosis, the failing heart with potassium deficiency and cardiac muscle removed from patients with cardiomyopathy who were recipients of cardiac transplants. However, while disturbances of Ca^{++} transport frequently accompany heart failure, the nature of the abnormality of Ca^{++} transport differs in various forms of heart failure.

FUNCTION OF THE AUTONOMIC NERVOUS SYSTEM

In view of the importance of the adrenergic nervous system in the normal regulation of the circulation, considerable attention has been directed to the activity of this system in heart failure. A crude index of adrenergic nervous activity, at rest and during exercise, is provided by the concentration of noradrenaline (NA) in arterial blood. No change, or else only very small increases, were noted during exercise in normal subjects, whereas much larger elevations occurred in patients with heart failure, presumably reflecting the greater activity of their adrenergic nervous systems during exercise.

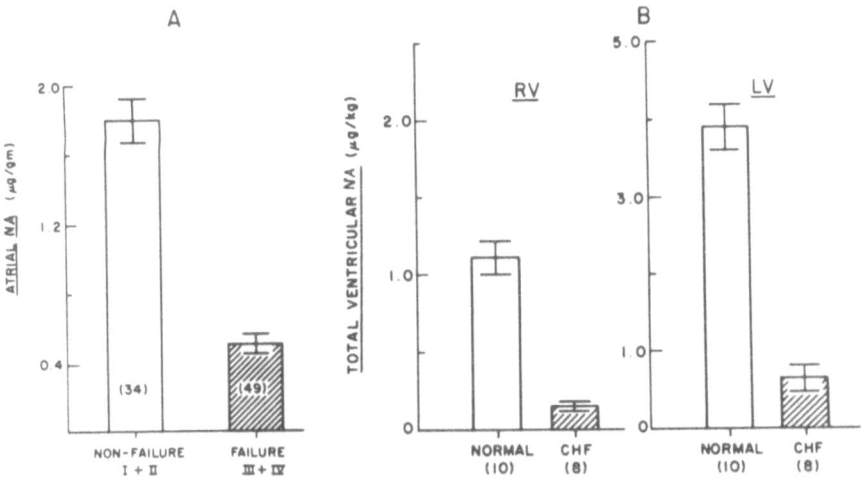

Figure 3 Effects of heart failure on the cardiac stores of noradrenaline: (A) Concentration of NA in atrial appendage biopsies taken during cardiac operations from 34 patients without heart failure (Classes I and II) and 49 patients with heart failure (Classes III and IV). Average values and their standard errors are shown. (B) Total ventricular NA content in normal dogs and in dogs with pulmonary stenosis, tricuspid insufficiency, and congestive heart failure (CHF). Average values are given with their standard errors. RV — right ventricle, LV — left ventricle. (Reproduced with permission from Little, Brown and Company, 1976; *Mechanisms of Contraction of the Normal and Failing Heart*, 2nd ed.)

Measurement of 24 h urinary NA excretion revealed marked elevations in patients with heart failure, indicating that the activity of the adrenergic nervous system, and presumably secretion of catecholamines by the adrenal medulla, are also augmented at rest in these patients; abnormality of adrenergic nervous activity is also reflected in the very low concentrations of NA in the atrial tissue of these patients, sometimes to lower than 10% of normal (Figure 3). The NA concentrations have also been shown to be markedly depressed in papillary muscles removed from the left ventricles of patients with severe left ventricular failure who underwent mitral valve replacement[12].

Since the changes in cardiac NA concentration occurring in some patients with heart failure appeared to be severe enough to impair adrenergic function, an attempt was made to define the mechanism by which this depletion occurred. In dogs with right ventricular failure produced by creation of pulmonary stenosis and tricuspid insufficiency, the reduction of cardiac NA concentration was *not* shown to be the result of a simple dilution of sympathetic nerve endings in a hypertrophied muscle mass, since the total ventricular NA contents were lower, both in the hypertrophied right and the non-hypertrophied left ventricles (Figure 3).

After the production of heart failure in the guinea pig by constriction of the aorta, the left ventricular NA concentration immediately fell to values approximately 30% of normal. The infusion of a large dose of NA raised cardiac NA stores much less in guinea pigs with heart failure than in normal animals. This impaired capacity to retain administered NA might be due either to a reduction in the total number of neurons in the myocardium or to a diminution of the number of intraneuronal binding sites. The rate of NA synthesis, estimated by measurement of the turnover of radioactive-labelled amine in the guinea pig heart, and the synthesis of NA, is diminished roughly in proportion to the change in pool size[3].

The cardiomyopathic Syrian hamster also exhibits cardiac NA depletion terminally[13]. This is accompanied by a marked increase in NA turnover rate to a level which approaches the maximum achievable under stress, leaving little, if any, reserve. These findings are compatible with the concept that heart failure is accompanied by a progressive increase in tone in the adrenergic cardiac nerves which leads to a concomitant reduction in cardiac NA stores. Marked reductions in the activity of tyrosine hydroxylase accompany the cardiac NA depletion in dogs with experimental heart failure, while no alterations in enzyme activity occur in the hearts of animals in which NA depletion has been produced with reserpine[3]. These findings suggest that the reduction in the activity of this enzyme is responsible for the depletion of cardiac NA in heart failure. An absence of fluorescence in the terminal varicosities of adrenergic fibres in close association with cardiac muscle cells in the NA depleted, failing heart has been noted. Recovery from heart failure is associated with virtual restoration both of the NA concentration and of the histochemical appearance of adrenergic nerve distribution, suggesting that a reversible abnormality, presumably of neurotransmitter synthesis, occurs in the terminal portion of the cardiac adrenergic innervation in heart failure.

NA exerts a strongly positive inotropic effect, even in the failing heart; and the adrenergic nervous system may be considered to provide important potential support to the failing myocardium. However, with supramaximal stimulation of the cardiac adrenergic nerves, the increments of heart rate and contractile force that occur in animals with heart failure and cardiac NA depletion are abolished or are much smaller than in normal dogs[3] (Figure 4). Thus, it is likely that when heart failure is accompanied by depletion of cardiac NA stores, the quantity of NA released by the adrenergic nerve endings in the heart is deficient in relation to the impulse traffic along these nerves. However, the contractile state is normal in isolated right ventricular papillary muscles obtained from cats with cardiac NA depletion produced surgically or pharmacologically. Therefore, it may be concluded that the stores of NA in the heart are *not* fundamental for maintenance of the heart's intrinsic contractile state. However, since the reduction of stores of cardiac NA in heart failure is associated with a diminished release of the neuro-transmitter, this depletion of NA may be responsible for loss of the much-needed adrenergic support and reflex control of the failing heart, and in this manner it could intensify the severity of heart failure.

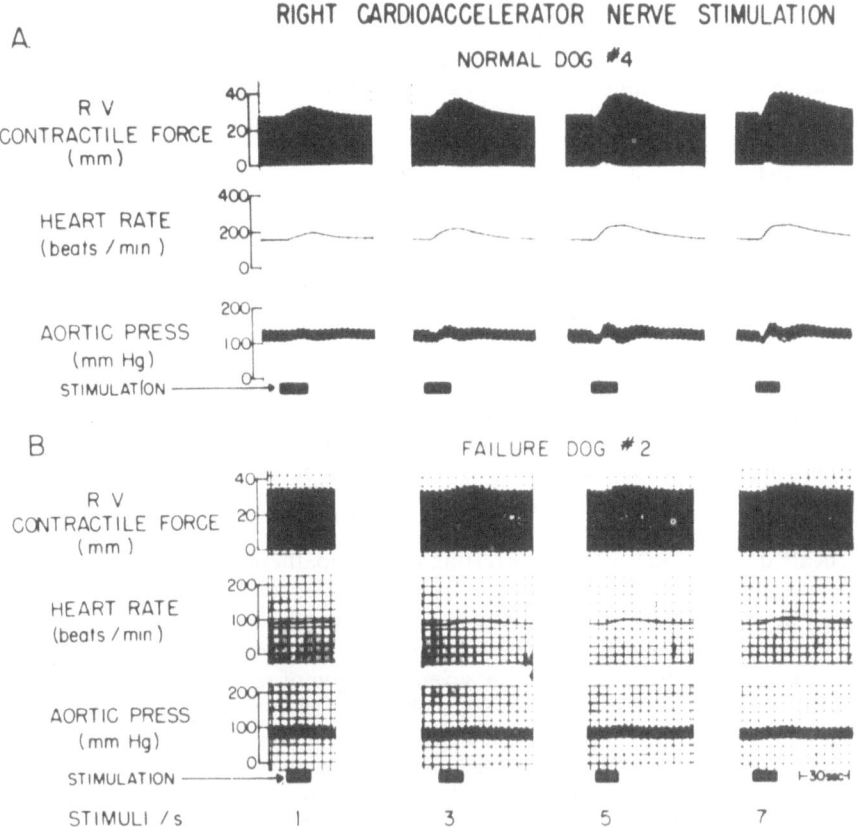

Figure 4 Records showing the effect of right cardioaccelerator stimulation in (A) a normal dog, and (B) a dog with congestive failure. (Reproduced with permission from *Circ. Res.*, **14**, 51 (1966))

Evidence indicating that the NA-depleted, failing heart is increasingly dependent on circulating catecholamines for the maintenance of basal haemodynamic function, has been obtained from experiments in calves with experimentally produced heart failure and cardiac NA depletion[14]. In the later stages of heart failure, when levels of circulating catecholamines are elevated and the cardiac NA stores are depleted, the contractility of the myocardium is supported by adrenergic stimulation derived from extra-cardiac sources. In patients with heart failure, interference with the adrenergic nervous system by propranolol or guanethidine, in doses that do not lower arterial pressure, frequently cause sodium and water retention as well as intensification of heart failure.

The possibility of defective adrenergic control of heart rate in patients with heart failure has been studied by observing the reflex chronotropic responses both to upright tilt and nitroglycerin-induced hypotension[15]. An attenuation of the normal increase in heart rate, both before and after atropine, confirms that a defect exists in the adrenergic component of baroreceptor-mediated reflex heart rate control in patients with cardiac dysfunction; the severity of this defect is, in general, proportional to the impairment of cardiac reserve. Similar observations have been made in dogs with experimental heart failure. A reduction in responsiveness of the beta-receptors as a cause of impaired sympathetic influence could be excluded by noting a normal response of heart rate to isoproterenol, suggesting that the adrenergically mediated heart rate response results from NA depletion rather than from a defect in the beta-adrenergic receptor mechanism in the sino-atrial node. In addition, the heart rate at maximal exercise is reduced in patients with cardiac dysfunction, suggesting that the ability of the adrenergic nervous system to speed the heart is impaired in these subjects. Thus, cardiac dysfunction appears to be associated with a marked impairment of autonomically mediated changes in heart rate.

Heart failure is associated with marked disturbances of parasympathetic function as well. The degree of parasympathetic restraint on the automaticity of the sino-atrial node is markedly reduced in patients with heart disease; after pharmacological blockade of the adrenergic system with propranolol, heart rate is similar in normal subjects and in patients with heart disease. However, when resting parasympathetic tone is then inhibited with atropine in these adrenergically blocked subjects, the degree of cardiac acceleration is markedly reduced in patients with heart failure as compared to normal subjects. Patients with heart disease also exhibit a marked reduction in heart rate slowing for any given elevation of systemic arterial pressure compared to normal subjects. Since this slowing can normally be virtually abolished by parasympathetic blockade, these findings suggest an abnormality of heart rate control by the parasympathetic nervous system in patients with heart failure[16]. The sensitivity of the baroreceptor reflex to transient hypertension has also been shown to be significantly reduced in dogs with hypertrophy alone and reduced further in dogs with heart failure.

Although the precise mechanism responsible for the demonstrated impairment of parasympathetic function in heart failure is not clear, this disturbance may be of considerable functional importance, since the ability to alter heart rate constitutes an extremely important mechanism by which the cardiac output is adjusted; indeed, under normal circumstances changes in heart rate account in large measure for changes in cardiac output. Patients with heart failure exhibit an inability to elevate stroke volume normally during exercise, and when this limitation of stroke volume occurs together with defective control of heart rate as a consequence of abnormalities of both the sympathetic and parasympathetic limbs of the autonomic nervous system, the inability of these patients to raise cardiac output appropriately is readily appreciated.

EXTRACELLULAR FLUID ACCUMULATION

Oedema formation, i.e., a clinically apparent increase in the interstitial fluid volume, is a cardinal manifestation of untreated chronic heart failure; indeed, this fluid accumulation is responsible for the adjective 'congestive' applied to heart failure. The *effective arterial blood volume*, an as yet poorly defined parameter of the filling of the arterial tree, is reduced in heart failure and other states leading to abnormal accumulation of extracellular fluid, and a series of physiological responses which are designed to restore this volume to normal are set into motion (Figure 5). A key element of these responses is

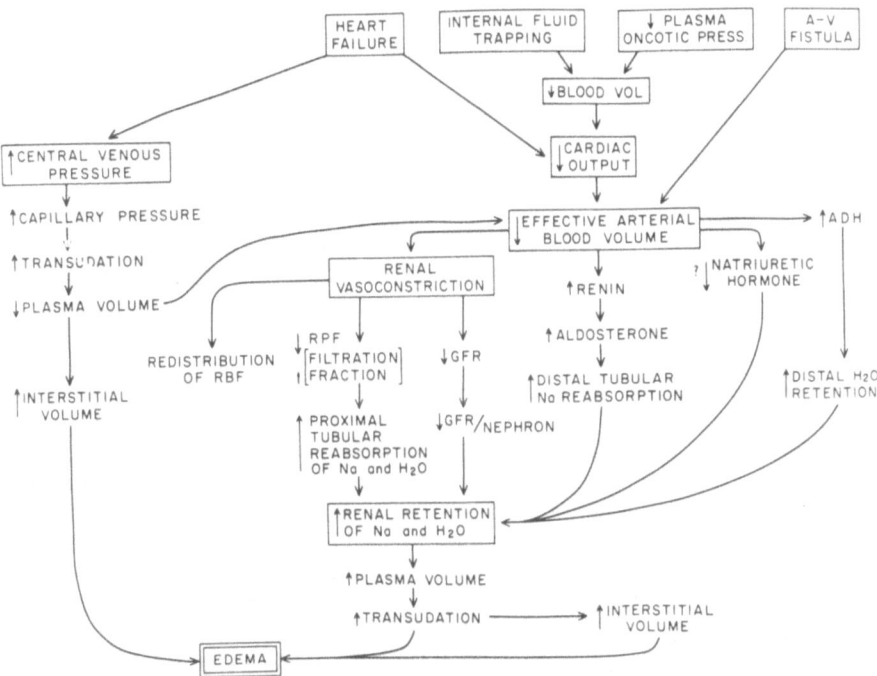

Figure 5 Sequence of events leading to the formation and retention of salt and water and the development of oedema. (Reproduced with permission from *Harrison's Principles of Internal Medicine.* (New York: McGraw-Hill, 1977))

the retention of an increment of salt and water, and in many instances this repairs the deficit of the effective arterial blood volume; often this occurs without the development of overt oedema. If, however, the retention of salt and water is insufficient to restore and maintain the effective arterial blood volume, the stimuli are not dissipated, the retention of salt and water continues, and oedema ultimately develops.

In heart failure, it is postulated that the defective systolic emptying of the chambers of the heart promotes an accumulation of blood in the heart and venous circulation at the expense of the arterial volume, and the afore-mentioned sequence of events is initiated. In many instances of mild heart failure a small increment of extracellular fluid volume may be achieved which repairs the deficit of effective arterial volume and establishes a new steady state because through the operation of Starling's Law of the Heart, an increase in the volume of blood within the chambers of the heart promotes a more force-ful contraction and thereby increases the stroke volume. However, if the cardiac disorder is more severe, fluid continues to be retained, even though this retention cannot repair the deficit of effective arterial blood volume. In addition to the sequence shown on the right-hand side of Figure 5, incom-plete ventricular emptying leads to an elevation of ventricular end-diastolic pressure. If the impairment of cardiac function involves the right ventricle primarily, then incomplete ventricular emptying leads to an elevation of right ventricular end-diastolic volume and pressure; as a consequence pressures in the systemic veins and capillaries also rise, thereby augmenting transudation of fluid into the interstitial space and enhancing the likelihood of peripheral oedema. If the impairment of cardiac function involves the left ventricle, the pulmonary venous and capillary pressures rise, leading in some instances to pulmonary oedema which may impair gas exchange and induce hypoxia, which may embarrass cardiac function still further. Also, pulmonary artery pressure rises, which in turn interferes with the systolic emptying of the right ventricle, leading to an elevation of right ventricular end-diastolic and central and systemic venous pressures, enhancing the likelihood of oedema formation.

The reduction of cardiac output is associated not only with a reduction of the effective arterial blood volume but of renal blood flow as well and the filtration fraction, i.e., the ratio of glomerular filtration rate to renal plasma flow, rises. In severe heart failure the blood flow to the outer renal cortex, in particular, is significantly reduced with less depression in the more central regions of the kidney, and glomerular filtration rate falls. This constriction of renal cortical vessels appears to play an important role in the retention of salt and water and the formation of oedema in heart failure. Indirect evidence suggests that at different stages of heart failure, activation of the adrenergic nervous system and of the renin–angiotensin systems is responsible for renal vasoconstriction. Activation of the former can be counteracted by the administration of alpha-adrenergic blocking agents which leads to a natri-uresis, a finding which indicates that the elevated renal vascular resistance in heart failure is mediated, at least in part, by adrenergic stimuli.

The intrarenal production of angiotensin-II may also contribute to renal vasoconstriction and to the salt and water retention in heart failure. Angiotensin-II also passes through the circulation and stimulates the pro-duction of aldosterone by the zona glomerulosa region of the adrenal cortex. In patients with heart failure, not only is aldosterone secretion elevated, but, as a consequence of a depression of hepatic blood flow, particularly during exercise, the metabolism of aldosterone is inhibited, i.e., the biological half-life of aldosterone is prolonged. The plasma level of the hormone is increased, a factor which contributes to oedema formation.

HEART FAILURE IN ANOXIA AND ISCHAEMIA

The depression of myocardial contractility which occurs in acute myocardial anoxia or ischaemia is associated with an abbreviation of the plateau of the action potential, suggesting an abnormality in the Ca^{++} current and therefore in the movement of Ca^{++} into the cell. The latter, in turn, may reduce the quantity of Ca^{++} released by the sarcoplasmic reticulum and thereby impairs contractility, as already discussed. Furthermore, the reduction of intracellular pH, as occurs in anoxia and particularly in ischaemia, augments the affinity of the SR for Ca^{++}, and thereby perhaps reduces its ability to release Ca^{++}. Indeed, studies on isolated SR have in fact shown that there is an impairment in the release of Ca^{++} early in the course of ischaemia, at a time that other membrane-associated functions are still normal. With more prolonged ischaemia there is also marked binding of Ca^{++} by the SR at a time when both mitochondrial and sarcolemmal Na, K-ATPase activities are severely impaired. It has been proposed that even when a normal quantity of Ca^{++} is made available for activating the contractile mechanism, the development of intracellular acidosis can impair contractility by displacing this ion from its binding side on troponin, thus reducing contractility[17].

More than 40 years ago, Tennant and Wiggers demonstrated that after ligation of a coronary artery, the contraction of cardiac muscle ceases and the affected area appears cyanotic, dilated and bulging. While patients with coronary artery disease usually do not show impaired left ventricular function in the absence of angina and of a previous myocardial infarction, transient episodes of myocardial ischaemia produce transient episodes of left ventricular failure. Myocardial ischaemia generally eliminates the normal contractile performance in a localized area of myocardium, resulting in an asynergic contraction. During brief periods of myocardial ischaemia, manifest clinically as angina pectoris, ventricular wall motion becomes abnormal and with the subsidence of ischaemia these mechanical changes revert to normal.

Regional loss of myocardial contractile activity, whether sustained or transient, may depress overall left ventricular function, producing reductions of stroke volume and stroke work, cardiac output and ejection fraction and elevations of end-diastolic volume and pressure. Clinical evidence of heart failure occurs when regional asynergy is so severe and extensive that the uninvolved myocardium cannot compensate adequately. Haemodynamic evidence of left ventricular failure develops when contraction ceases or becomes seriously impaired in 20–25% of the left ventricle; with loss of 40% or more of left ventricular myocardium, severe pump failure and the clinical picture of cardiogenic shock usually occur. The clinical evidence of impaired left ventricular function in most patients with acute myocardial infarction ranges from the barely detectable to the most severe forms of pump failure; the severity of heart failure is directly related to the extent of acute myocardial damage, whether the latter has occurred in a previously normal heart or is superimposed on previously damaged myocardium. Pulmonary râles, one of the principal clinical manifestations of heart failure, are secondary to a compensatory mechanism, i.e., cardiac dilatation, and possibly to increased stiffness of the left ventricle as well.

The abnormality in circulatory regulation that is present in ischaemic heart disease is shown in Figure 6. The process begins with an obstruction in the coronary vascular bed that results in regional myocardial ischaemia. If it is widespread, myocardial ischaemia depresses overall left ventricular function so that left ventricular stroke volume falls. A marked depression of left ventricular stroke volume ultimately lowers aortic pressure and reduces coronary perfusion pressure. This situation may intensify myocardial ischaemia and thereby initiate a vicious circle. The reduction of left ventricular

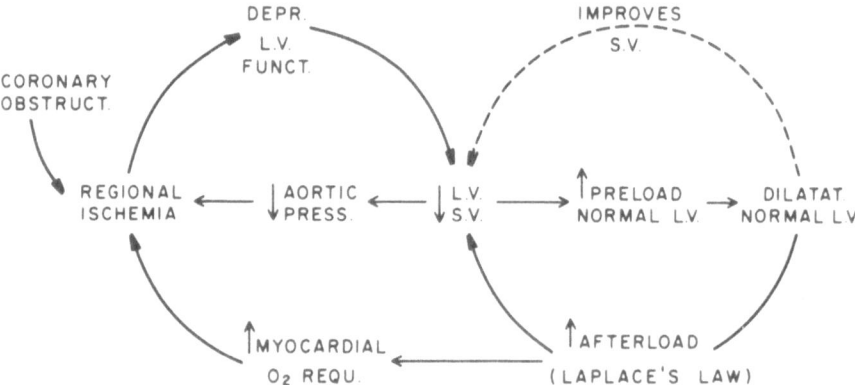

Figure 6 Schema showing changes in circulatory regulation in ischaemic heart disease. DEPR. L.V. FUNCT.—dilatation; O_2 REQU.—oxygen requirements. Solid lines indicate that the effect is produced or intensified; broken lines indicate that it is diminished. (Reproduced with permission from *N. Engl. J. Med.*, **290**, 1124 and 1420 (1974))

stroke volume also leads to an increased preload, that is, it dilates the well-perfused, normally functioning portion of the left ventricle. Although this compensatory mechanism tends to restore stroke volume, the dilatation of the left ventricle also elevates ventricular afterload, because at any given arterial pressure the dilated ventricle must develop greater tension. The increased afterload not only depresses left ventricular stroke volume but elevates myocardial oxygen consumption which in turn exaggerates regional myocardial ischaemia. The outcome of the coronary obstruction, then, depends on the balance attained between these processes. When regional myocardial ischaemia is limited and the function of the remainder of the left ventricle is normal, the compensatory mechanisms will sustain overall left ventricular function. If a large portion of the left ventricle becomes ischaemic, as occurs in massive coronary occlusion, overall left ventricular function becomes so depressed that the circulation cannot be sustained despite the dilatation of the remaining viable portion of the ventricle.

CONCLUSIONS

It may be useful to consider normal and impaired myocardial function, whatever the aetiology and pathogenesis, within the framework of the familiar Frank–Starling mechanism[3]. The normal relation between ventricular end-diastolic volume and performance is shown in Figure 7, curve 1. Normally, assumption of the upright posture tends to reduce venous return, and as a consequence, at any given level of exercise, the cardiac output is lower in the upright than in the recumbent position. On the other hand, the hyperventilation of exercise, the pumping action of the exercising muscles and the venoconstriction that occur all tend to augment ventricular filling. Simultaneously, the increase in adrenergic nerve impulses to the myocardium, and in the concentration of circulating catecholamines, and the tachycardia

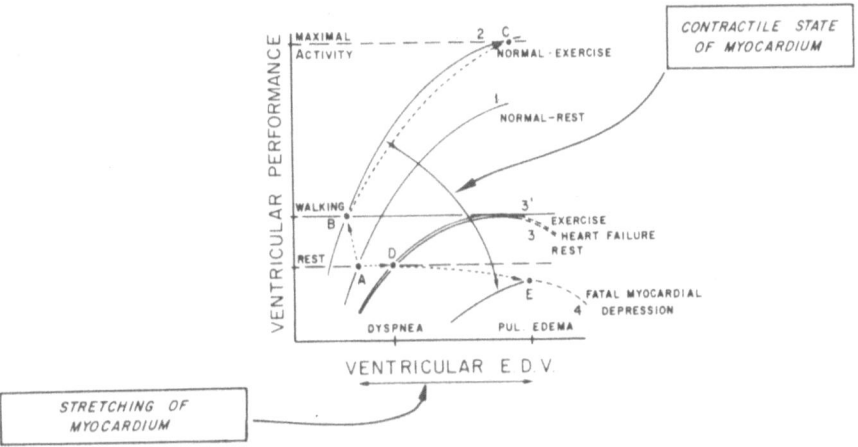

Figure 7 Diagram showing the interrelations between influences on ventricular end-diastolic volume (EDV) through stretching of the myocardium and the contractile state of the myocardium. Levels of ventricular EDV associated with filling pressures that result in dyspnoea and pulmonary oedema are shown on the abscissa. Levels of ventricular performance required when the subject is at rest, while walking and during maximal activity are designated on the ordinate. The dotted lines are the descending limbs of the ventricular-performance curves, which are rarely seen during life but show the level of ventricular performance if end-diastolic volume could be elevated to very high levels. (Reproduced with permission from *Mechanisms of Contractions of the Normal and Failing Heart*, 1st ed. (Boston: Little, Brown and Company, 1968))

that occur during exercise all result in an augmentation of the contractile state of the myocardium and an elevation of stroke volume, with either no change or even a decrease of end-diastolic pressure and volume. This state is represented by a shift from points A to B in Figure 7. Vasodilatation occurs in the exercising muscles, thus reducing peripheral vascular resistance and aortic impedance. This ultimately allows the achievement of a greatly elevated cardiac output during exercise, at an arterial pressure not greatly different from that occurring in the resting state. During intense exercise, cardiac output can rise to a maximal level only if use is made of the Frank–Starling mechanism, as reflected in increases in the left ventricular end-diastolic volume and pressure (Figure 7, point C).

In heart failure, the fundamental abnormality resides in depressions of the myocardial force–velocity relation and of the length–active tension curve, reflecting reductions in the contractile state of the myocardium. In many cases, such as those represented by Curve 3, Figure 7, cardiac output and external ventricular performance at rest are within normal limits, but are maintained at these levels only because the end-diastolic fibre length and ventricular end-diastolic volume are above normal – i.e., through the operation of the Frank–Starling mechanism. The elevations of left ventricular end-diastolic volume and pressure are associated with greater than normal levels of the pulmonary capillary pressure, contributing to the dyspnoea experienced by patients with heart failure (Figure 7, point D).

Since, as already noted, heart failure is frequently accompanied by depletion of cardiac noradrenaline stores and a reduction of the inotropic response to impulses in the cardiac adrenergic nerves, ventricular performance curves cannot be elevated to normal levels by the adrenergic nervous system, and the normal improvement of contractility that takes place during exercise is attenuated or even prevented (Figure 7, curves 3 to 3'). The factors that tend to augment ventricular filling during exercise in the normal subject push the failing myocardium even farther along its flattened length–active tension curve, and although left ventricular performance may be augmented somewhat, this occurs only as a consequence of an inordinate elevation of ventricular end-diastolic volume and pressure, and therefore of the pulmonary capillary pressure. The elevation of the latter intensifies dyspnoea and therefore has an important role in limiting the intensity of exercise that the patient can perform. According to this concept left ventricular failure becomes fatal when the myocardial length–active tension curve becomes depressed (Figure 7, curve 4) to the point at which either cardiac performance fails to satisfy the requirements of the peripheral tissues even at rest or the left ventricular end-diastolic and pulmonary capillary pressures are elevated to levels that result in pulmonary oedema, or both (Figure 7, point E).

SUMMARY

Heart failure is the pathophysiological state in which abnormality of cardiac function is responsible for the failure of the heart to pump blood at a rate commensurate with the requirements of the metabolizing tissues. Heart failure, and to a lesser extent, ventricular hypertrophy, both reduce the maximum velocity of unloaded shortening. When the ventricle is chronically stressed by an increase in afterload, the initial response is an increase in its total muscle mass. Initially, and if the pressure overload is not extreme, this adaptation can allow maintenance of a high systolic pressure without depression of contractility in the intact heart. Later, as the intrinsic contractile state of each unit of myocardium becomes depressed, increased muscle mass, operating in conjunction with increased sympathetic stimulation and the Frank–Starling mechanism, maintains overall circulatory compensation. The depression of contractility is manifest, in the mildest form, by a reduction in the intrinsic velocity of shortening (V_{max}) of each myocardial fibre, but with little, if any, decrease in the development of maximal isometric force. As the intrinsic contractile state of each unit of myocardium becomes further depressed, a more extensive reduction in V_{max} occurs, and this is now accompanied by a decrease in maximal isometric force. At this point, circulatory compensation is provided by an increase in muscle mass and cardiac dilatation. As contractility declines further, overt congestive heart failure occurs.

Both the ATP and CP concentrations are normal in muscles removed from failing hearts studied *in vitro*. Since the mechanical performance of these isolated muscles is impaired, this depression of contractility could not be attributed to a reduction of total myocardial high-energy stores. Thus, the energy production and the total reserve of high-energy phosphate compounds do not appear to be primarily responsible for the reduced contractility of the failing heart. However, the activity of myofibrillar and actomyosin ATPase has been reported to be reduced in the hearts of patients and experimental animals with heart failure. Studies in a number of *in vitro* systems also indicate that there is impairment of the delivery of Ca^{++} for activation of the contractile process in heart failure.

Heart failure is accompanied by depletion of cardiac noradrenaline stores; consequently, the quantity of noradrenaline released by the adrenergic nerve endings in the heart is deficient in relation to the impulse traffic along these nerves. Although the stores of noradrenaline in the heart are not fundamental for maintenance of the intrinsic contractile state of cardiac muscle, since the reduction of stores of cardiac noradrenaline in heart failure is associated with a diminished release of the neurotransmitter, this depletion may be responsible for loss of the much-needed adrenergic support of the failing heart, and in this manner it intensifies the severity of heart failure.

References

1. Spann, J. F., Jr., Buccino, R. A., Sonnenblick, E. H. and Braunwald, E. (1967). Contractile state of cardiac muscle obtained from cats with experimentally produced ventricular hypertrophy and heart failure. *Circ. Res.*, **21**, 341
2. Ross, J., Jr., Sonnenblick, E. H., Taylor, R. R. and Covell, J. W. (1971). Diastolic geometry and sarcomere length in the chronically dilated canine left ventricle. *Circ. Res.*, **28**, 49
3. Braunwald, E., Ross, J., Jr. and Sonnenblick, E. H. (1976). *Mechanisms of Contraction of the Normal and Failing Heart*, 2nd ed., 417 pp. (Boston: Little, Brown and Co)
4. Spann, J. F., Jr., Covell, J. W., Eckberg, D. L., Sonnenblick, E. H., Ross, J., Jr. and Braunwald, E. (1972). Contractile performance of the hypertrophied and chronically failing cat ventricle. *Am. J. Physiol.*, **223**, 1150
5. Ross, J., Jr. and Braunwald, E. (1974). Studies on Starling's law of the heart. IX. The effects of impeding venous return on performance of the normal and failing human left ventricle. *Circulation*, **30**, 719
6. McCullagh, W. H., Covell, J. W. and Ross, J., Jr. (1972). Left ventricular dilatation and diastolic compliance changes during chronic volume overloading. *Circulation*, **45**, 943
7. Henry, P. D., Eckberg, D., Gault, J. H. and Ross, J., Jr. (1973). Depressed inotropic state and reduced myocardial oxygen consumption in the human heart. *Am. J. Cardiol.*, **31**, 300
8. Pool, P. E., Spann, J. F., Jr., Buccino, R. A., Sonnenblick, E. H. and Braunwald, E. (1967). Myocardial high energy phosphate stores in cardiac hypertrophy and heart failure. *Circ. Res.*, **21**, 365
9. Mead, R. J., Peterson, M. B. and Welty, J. D. (1971). Sarcolemmal and sarcoplasmic reticular ATPase activities in the failing canine heart. *Circ. Res.*, **29**, 14

10. Ito, Y., Suko, J. and Chidsey, C. A. (1974). Intracellular calcium and myocardial contractility. V. Calcium uptake of sarcoplasmic reticulum fractions in hypertrophied and failing rabbit hearts. *J. Mol. Cell. Cardiol.*, **6**, 237
11. Sulakhe, P. V. and Dhalla, N. S. (1971). Excitation–contraction coupling in heart. VII. Calcium accumulation in subcellular particles in congestive heart failure. *J. Clin. Invest.*, **50**, 1019
12. Braunwald, E. and Chidsey, C. A. (1965). The adrenergic nervous system in the control of the normal and failing heart. *Proc. Roy. Soc. Med.*, **58**, 1062
13. Sole, M. J., Chi-Man, L. O., Laird, C. W., Sonnenblick, E. H. and Wurtman, R. J. (1975). Norepinephrine turnover in the heart and spleen of the cardiomyopathic Syrian hamster. *Circ. Res.*, **37**, 855
14. Vogel, J. H. K. and Chidsey, C. A. (1969). Cardiac adrenergic activity in experimental heart failure assessed by beta receptor blockade. *Am. J. Cardiol.*, **24**, 198
15. Goldstein, R. E., Beiser, G. D., Stampfer, M. and Epstein, S. E. (1978). Impairment of autonomically mediated heart rate control in patients with cardiac dysfunction. *Circ. Res.*, **36**, 571
16. Eckberg, D. L., Drabinsky, M. and Braunwald, E. (1971). Defective cardiac parasympathetic control in patients with heart disease. *N. Engl. J. Med.*, **285**, 877
17. Katz, A. M. (1976). Congestive heart failure. Role of altered myocardial cellular control. *N. Engl. J. Med.*, **293**, 1184

Part V
The Foxglove 1978

16
Some aspects of the clinical pharmacology of digoxin

D. G. GRAHAME-SMITH

'Vagueness is the rebellion of truth against intellect.'

BERTRAND RUSSELL

There is still a touch of vagueness about almost every scientific aspect of the basic and clinical pharmacology of cardiac glycosides. Things are not much better when the very practical field of digitalis therapy is considered, though in medical practice the problem is frequently solved by substituting dogma for vagueness! Two examples will serve to illustrate the general imprecision with which digoxin is used.

THE 1972 DIGOXIN BIOVAILABILITY PROBLEM[1]

In 1972 Burroughs Wellcome announced that their digoxin brand, 'Lanoxin', tablets had increased in biovailability. The change was such that there was almost a doubling in therapeutic potency. The story and implications are interesting.

'Lanoxin' tablets had been manufactured at the Wellcome Chemical Works in Dartford, Kent, from 1930 and the quality of tablet produced had been pharmaceutically consistent. In 1969 a change in the manufacturing process took place resulting in tablets, which although they satisfied regulatory pharmaceutical standards at the time, showed variable and lower dissolution rates. The manufacturing process in use many years before the change in 1969 was reinstituted in May 1972. Let us say that from 1930 to 1969 'Lanoxin' tablets had a bioavailability of 1; the change in 1969–72 led to a bioavailability of 0.5; in 1972 the change back restored the bioavailability to 1. All this knowledge stemmed from comparative studies involving *in vitro* tablet dissolution rates, plasma level/time curves and urinary excretion data after 'Lanoxin' administration, and retrospective plasma level data. The latter showed that on the same maintenance doses of 'Lanoxin' the steady

235

state plasma levels during the period 1969–72, were half those before and since[2]. Experience in the USA also showed widely varying digoxin variability amongst various brands of digoxin tablets. It is a matter of history now that this problem was fairly quickly sorted out, and led to revised standards for the pharmaceutical testing of digoxin tablets in Britain and the USA.

The point of this story is that the real problem was that during the period 1970–72 'Lanoxin' tablets had *half* the therapeutic potency they had during the previous 30 years and at the clinical level very few people noticed!

TEXTBOOKS: THEORY AND PRACTICE[3]

If one needs a better practical illustration of the imprecision with which digoxin is used then examine the disarray of recommendations amongst 25 medical textbooks and other reasonably authoritative sources on the indications and contraindications, dosage, cautions and so on for the use of digoxin. It seems inconceivable that for a drug with such a low toxic/therapeutic ratio, a known high clinical incidence of toxicity, and an action subject to so many variable influences, the information provided for prescribing can be so variable.

Although there is good consistency among the various sources in suggested intravenous doses there are wide differences in recommended oral doses, perhaps explained by the previously large variations in bioavailability. Only three sources suggest relating the loading dose to the patient's weight (a vet would never neglect this). Several sources still recommend digitalization until a satisfactory therapeutic response occurs or toxicity ensues; but because the symptoms of toxicity are notoriously difficult to assess, because toxic arrythmias may ensue before toxic symptoms occur and because, at least in the presence of cardiac failure with sinus rhythm, a satisfactory therapeutic response due to digitalis alone is very difficult to judge, such recommendations are not very helpful. In the majority of sources little guidance is given to determine the optimum daily dosage in individual cases, and frequently no mention is made of daily maintenance doses of less than 0.25 mg. There is incomplete discussion of the several non-cardiac factors known to alter the individual response to digoxin, factors such as renal insufficiency, extremes of age, electrolyte disturbances, and altered thyroid function.

One might expect textbooks to deal more carefully with correct therapeutic practice; instead some texts show a rather cavalier attitude to precision in drug therapy, an attitude which in general may be partly responsible for inefficient treatment and a burgeoning load of iatrogenic disease.

THE PRINCIPLES OF CLINICAL PHARMACOLOGY APPLIED TO DIGOXIN THERAPY

In the paper reviewing textbook recommendations[3], Aronson and I tried to distill from all sources, and from our own experience, recommendations which might apply to the majority of cases, based upon the consideration of the general clinical pharmacology of the drug. It is this general aspect of clinical pharmacology which can impose upon practical drug therapy the

PROCESSES OCCURRING ON DRUG ADMINISTRATION

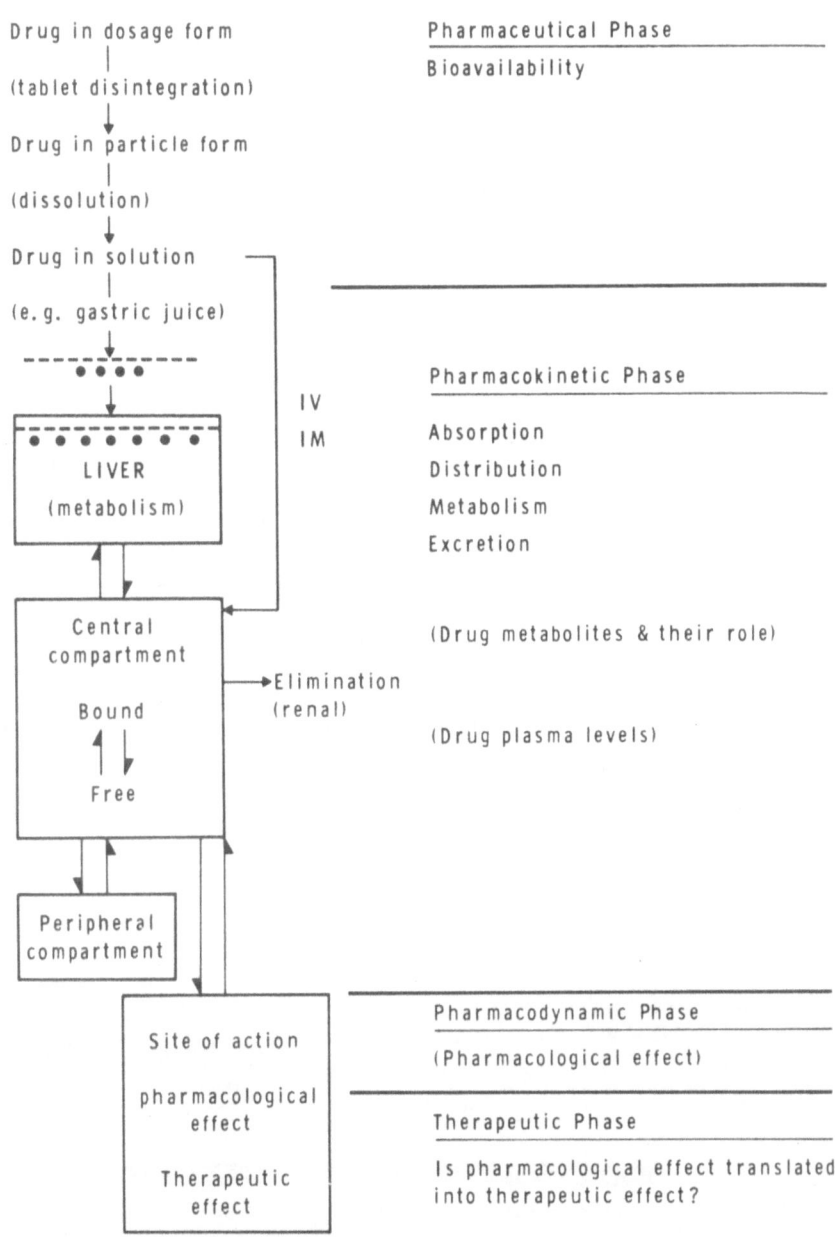

Figure 1 Principles of clinical pharmacology. The sequence of events in drug action.

same discipline as current medical science imposes upon the process of diagnosis.

The principles are shown in the sequence of events depicted in Figure 1. One factor not mentioned there is patient compliance with prescribed therapy. From the practical point of view this is one of the most important factors in determining the success of drug therapy. The general application and particular relevance of these principles to therapy with digoxin can be broken down into four phases.

1. Pharmaceutical phase (bioavailability)

The definition of bioavailability is an operational matter (see Figure 2). With an intravenous injection, 100% of a drug enters the circulation. By calculation of the area under the plasma level/time curve to time infinity ($AUC_{t0-\infty}$), 100% bioavailability can be studied. Equally bioavailability can be studied on the basis of urinary excretion. However it is done, 100% bioavailability can be defined by the study of the disposition of an intravenous dose of a drug.

The next step is to define the problem of absorption through the gut wall, and any first-pass effect through the liver, by dosage with an oral liquid preparation of the drug and assessment of plasma level/time ($AUC_{t0-\infty}$) and/or urinary excretion pattern.

Lastly there is the pharmaceutical problem of tablet dissolution within the gastrointestinal juices which is solved by tablet dosage and plasma level/time ($AUC_{t0-\infty}$), and/or urinary excretion studies.

In my view, bioavailability consists of A + B, but one may have to measure C anyway, to get A + B (see Figure 2). Such studies are a time-consuming business. Fortunately, and largely as a result of the 1972 bio-availability problem with digoxin, there is good evidence that the *in vitro*

BIOAVAILABILITY

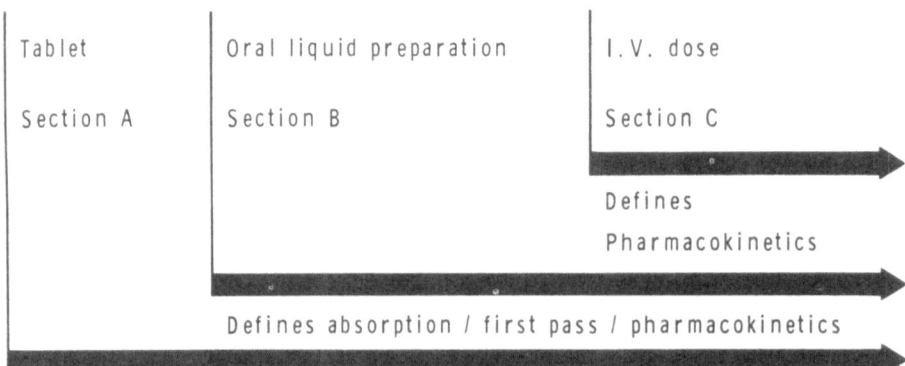

Figure 2   The stages of bioavailability testing.

dissolution characteristics of digoxin tablets reflects the *in vivo* bioavailability very well.

2. *Pharmacokinetic phase* (see ref. 3 for refs.)

(a) *Distribution*. In renal failure there is a lowered apparent volume of distribution of digoxin and the available data suggest that this may also be the case in hypothyroidism. Lowered apparent volume of distribution is another factor apart from decreased renal elimination of digoxin which may result in higher plasma levels than would occur following the same dose in the absence of renal failure, which is not taken account of in nomograms relating to creatinine clearance. Digoxin is widely distributed throughout the tissues of the body, being chiefly concentrated in the heart, kidneys, liver and skeletal muscle (including diaphragm). It is not, however, distributed into fat. Binding to plasma proteins does not play a very important part in the distribution of digoxin, though it does with digitoxin.

(b) *Metabolism*. Usually only a small amount of digoxin is converted to metabolites, both active and inactive, though individuals differ widely in the degree to which they metabolize the drug. There is no impairment of metabolism in congestive cardiac failure or hypothyroidism although there may be some increase in metabolism in renal failure. The matter of digoxin metabolism has not yet been settled completely and I find the discrepancy between studies confusing.

(c) *Excretion*. About 80% of an administered dose of digoxin is excreted in the urine unchanged in 7 days, mainly by glomerular filtration although a small amount is subject to both tubular secretion and reabsorption. The half-time of elimination $(T_{\frac{1}{2}})$ of digoxin from the plasma is about 1.6 days and in renal failure with complete anuria this value may increase up to 4.4 days when about 14% is eliminated daily by extra-renal (principally hepatic) mechanisms. In renal failure the fall in renal clearance of digoxin correlates linearly with the decline in creatinine clearance.

3. *Pharmacodynamic phase*

The 'bread and butter' clinical pharmacology discussed above in the pharmacokinetic phase provides information essential to the rational use of a drug, but it does not indicate the relationship of the plasma level/time curve to the pharmacodynamic effect. The pertinent question is, 'What function of the plasma level/time curve determines the pharmacodynamic effects?'

The pharmacodynamic phase is concerned with pharmacological effects. Some drug effects are reasonably well understood at the basic pharmacological level (e.g. muscle relaxants); with other drugs the mode of action underlying their pharmacological effects is more obscure (e.g. aspirin and in fact, digitalis). Some drug actions are superficially simple (for example, pharmacological antagonists such as β-adrenoceptor blocking agents and morphine antagonists). Other drugs have much more complex actions involving cascades of biochemical and pharmacological events, for example the action of ACTH on the adrenal cortex.

The effects of drugs in time is of importance. Some drugs are 'on–off', the degree of effect closely following the blood level, for example the β-blockade effect of propranolol. Some drugs are 'hit-and-run', the drug binding to receptors and continuing to act (i.e. not immediately reversible) despite a falling blood level. Examples of such 'hit-and-run' drugs might be hydrallazine and some monoamine oxidase inhibitors where the drug molecule binds to a receptor and dissociates rather slowly from it. Digoxin falls into this category. Another cause of the 'hit-and-run' phenomenon is when a drug sets in train a sequence of pharmacological effects which take time to run down, e.g. the anti-inflammatory effects of corticosteroids. With such drugs the relationship between blood levels and pharmacological effects may be very difficult to sort out and subject to great variation in the clinical situation.

In considering the pharmacodynamic effect of digoxin a considerable problem is posed by our lack of understanding of the precise mechanisms by which it acts. On the one hand there is the majority opinion that the positive inotropic effects of digoxin are due to inhibition of membrane-bound Na^+-K^+-ATPase, increasing either primarily or secondarily the intracellular pool of free Ca^{++} ion and facilitating excitation–contraction coupling[5]. I stand on this side at present. On the other hand, there is evidence that under certain circumstances cardiac glycosides stimulate Na^+-K^+-ATPase and therefore the Na^+-K^+ pump, and that somehow this is linked to the positive inotropic effect.

As I shall describe, if the red blood cell is anything like the heart (which it may not be), the inhibition theory is circumstantially more likely. Inhibition of Na^+-K^+-ATPase is generally agreed, though, to be the mechanism by which the electrophysiological and toxic effects are mediated.[8]

At the clinical level there are several factors known to alter patients' response to digoxin. The patient's electrolyte status may determine the degree of response to digoxin—thus, hypokalaemia potentiates the toxic effects of the drug in man, as may hypomagnesaemia. There is experimental evidence to suggest that hyponatraemia and hypercalcaemia may also increase the susceptibility to toxicity. The elderly may become toxic following doses of digoxin which would be well tolerated by younger patients, partly for pharmacokinetic reasons but perhaps also because of increased sensitivity.

Patients with hypothyroidism are more sensitive to digoxin, but whether this is due to increased plasma levels or to truly increased pharmacological sensitivity to the drug is not known.

4. *Therapeutic phase*

The pharmacological effect must be translated into a therapeutic effect, the definition of which is important. Slowing of the ventricular rate in atrial fibrillation has an obvious end-point. Heart failure in regular rhythm is more difficult. It is easy to imagine that however much of a positive inotropic effect is feasible with non-toxic doses of digitalis, the degree of such an effect might be insufficient to confer appreciable therapeutic benefit in some cases of severe cardiac failure. Even in mild heart failure there is controversy about the usefulness of digoxin, which will be referred to later.

HOW USEFUL IS THE PLASMA DIGOXIN LEVEL?

There is continuing discussion about, and some disillusionment with, the plasma concentrations of drugs as guides to therapy. When plasma levels of drugs or metabolites appear not to be useful guides to drug therapy then the reason lies in our incomplete understanding of the significance of the plasma level/time curve of the drug, or of the link, in time, between blood and tissue concentrations and pharmacological effect and therapeutic effect or the role of the metabolites, or the inappropriateness of the therapy. Another factor to take into account during chronic drug therapy is the occurrence of various tissue adaptations to the effect of the drug. Drug 'tolerance', receptor super-sensitivity subsequent to pharmacological blockade and changing drug metabolic pattern are all factors likely to cloud a simple relationship amongst plasma level/pharmacological effect/therapeutic effect. The complicated relationship between plasma levels and therapeutic effects may in certain instances be so obscure as to render it of little practical use.

Drugs with a high therapeutic index (high toxic/therapeutic dose ratio) and with an easily measurable clinical effect, for instance frusemide in oedema, present few problems in day-to-day therapeutics. The problems arise with drug therapies in which the clinical response is not easily defined, or in which the disease is variable, or in which the therapeutic effect is difficult to measure, as in rheumatoid arthritis, migraine, hay-fever, mental illness, for example, and with drugs which have a low therapeutic index. The treatment of heart failure in regular rhythm with digoxin exemplifies many of these difficulties which, it was hoped, the measurement of plasma digoxin levels might overcome.

The 'plasma level' of which everyone speaks is the plasma digoxin concentration at least 6 h after the last dose—so-called 'steady state' level—which certainly is not steady, but only falling slowly! What this level means pharmacodynamically is not known. The level is measured at this time because it is subject to less variability than is encountered during the phase of fast rise and fall. Whatever the level 'means' it has been measured now in millions of patients for two reasons:

1. most important, to help in the diagnosis of digoxin toxicity[9,10];
2. occasionally it is helpful in patients who are non-compliant or who are really taking too small doses and in whom, say, atrial fibrillation is not controlled.

There is general agreement that there is little point in measuring plasma digoxin levels to regulate the level for 'therapeutic' purposes, i.e. to get a really fine regulation of the level to produce a precise therapeutic effect. The therapeutic range is quite wide, certainly from 0.8 to 2.5 ng/ml in usual practice.

Recently we have assessed the usefulness of measuring plasma digoxin concentrations in the diagnosis of digoxin toxicity[10], mindful of the criticisms of Ingelfinger and Goldman[11] who concluded that the case had not been made that knowledge of plasma digoxin concentration was useful in the diagnosis of digitalis toxicity.

Eighty-three patients referred for plasma digoxin level estimations were studied. The mean plasma digoxin concentration in clinically toxic patients was higher than the mean concentration in non-toxic patients, but the overlap between the groups was extensive. This overlap could be accounted for partly by hypokalaemia in those toxic patients with plasma digoxin concentrations <3 ng/ml. We considered the various factors we studied and developed some practical guidelines for the use of plasma digoxin levels in the diagnosis of digoxin toxicity:

1. Patients with plasma digoxin concentration >3 ng/ml or plasma potassium concentration <3.5 mmol/l (whatever the digoxin concentration), should be considered toxic until proven otherwise;
2. patients with plasma digoxin concentration $\leqslant 3$ ng/ml without hypo-kalaemia should be considered to be probably toxic only if they are known to have at least *two* of the following features: $K^+ > 5$ mmol/l without obvious cause; creatinine >150 μmol/l; age >60 years; dose >6 μg/kg/day for at least a week.

These guidelines will allow accurate prediction of toxicity in patients who are toxic, at the expense of diagnosing toxicity in some who are not. Plasma digoxin concentration could not be predicted with more than 31% certainty by considering the magnitude of non-cardiac factors.

It still has to be shown whether an experienced physician, given all the information apart from the plasma digoxin level, improves the accuracy of his diagnosis of digoxin toxicity significantly by adding knowledge of the plasma digoxin concentration. I *think* it helps me, but I am not *sure* it does.

The pharmacodynamic approach

Because of the uncertainty about the precision of meaning of the plasma digoxin level we have been exploring the relationship between 'steady-state' plasma digoxin levels, a pharmacodynamic effect of digoxin and the therapeutic effects.

Drugs may have pharmacological effects in peripheral compartments (by which is meant biological compartments other than the therapeutic target organ), capable of measurement, which may reflect directly or indirectly the pharmacological effect through which the action of the drug is mediated. We have been particularly interested in the use of blood cells as indicators of pharmacological effect because these are easily available and show a range of functions potentially sensitive to drug effects.

There is essentially nothing new about this general approach. For many years the pharmacological effects of drugs have been measured rather than plasma levels, or even the clinical therapeutic effects. For instance, the prothrombin time is measured as an index of Warfarin effect, blood glucose is measured as an index of insulin effect, blood uric acid as an index of the effect of uricosuric agents and xanthine oxidase inhibitors, serum iron in iron therapy, reticulocyte responses with vitamin B_{12} therapy. There is un-doubtedly sufficient precedent to suggest that if the pharmacodynamic approach to monitoring drug therapy can be carried out technically the approach is likely to be a helpful one.

SOME ASPECTS OF THE CLINICAL PHARMACOLOGY OF DIGOXIN

The problem of monitoring digoxin therapy by measuring plasma digoxin concentrations at a given time after dose is a complex one because little is known about the precise relationships amongst the factors involved in the sequence of events determining the therapeutic outcome:

1. the time course of plasma concentrations after doses of digoxin;
2. concentrations and binding of digoxin at specific cardiac sites;
3. ensuing biochemical and pharmacological effects;
4. the therapeutic effect.

Our aim has been to explore techniques which would give an indication of pharmacological effects of digoxin, which might reflect a pharmacodynamic effect of digoxin on the heart, to relate these pharmacological effects to plasma digoxin concentrations and to see if these pharmacological effects bear any relationship to the therapeutic effect of digoxin. The first part of these studies had been described[12].

As mentioned previously glycosides inhibit Na^+-K^+-ATPase in many tissues including cardiac muscle. In red blood cells (RBC) inhibition of this enzyme is accompanied by a decreased uptake of K^+. To monitor K^+ uptake by RBC, ^{86}Rb may be used. If RBC Na^+-K^+-ATPase activity was inhibited in patients taking digoxin one would therefore expect the RBC of such patients to show inhibition of ^{86}Rb uptake.

Effect of digoxin therapy on patients' RBC ^{86}Rb uptake[12]
As patients were digitalized with digoxin, RBC ^{86}Rb uptake fell gradually to reach a nadir within 5 days. Within 3–11 days however RBC ^{86}Rb uptake

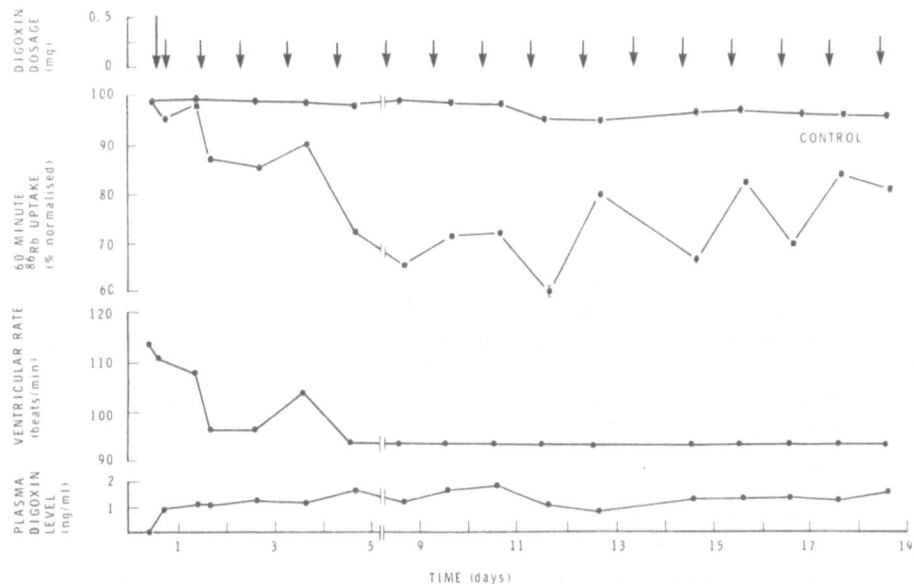

Figure 3 Response in ventricular rate, ^{86}Rb uptake and plasma digoxin level in a patient treated with digoxin.

began to fluctuate from day to day. The fall in RBC ^{86}Rb uptake during the first few days before fluctuations began was accompanied by a fall in the ventricular rate in patients in atrial fibrillation. The results on such a patient are shown in Figure 3.

Relationships amongst plasma digoxin concentrations, RBC ^{86}Rb uptake and the therapeutic response[12]
Fifteen patients were studied; in thirteen of these there was a definite fall in ^{86}Rb uptake of the patients' own RBC prior to the onset of fluctuations. In the two patients who had no fall in RBC ^{86}Rb uptake, one had no clinical response, treatment was stopped and sinus rhythm achieved with DC cardioversion. The other patient responded to therapy without a change in RBC ^{86}Rb uptake. The patients were divided into three groups for analysis:

Group I: those who remained in atrial fibrillation throughout.
Group Ia: those who were initially in atrial fibrillation but who reverted to sinus rhythm during treatment.
Group II: those with other supraventricular tachyarrhythmias.

Figure 4 shows the relationship between the percentage change in individual values of RBC ^{86}Rb uptake from the pretreatment values and the percentage change in ventricular rates at corresponding times. The values shown are those obtained before fluctuations began in RBC ^{86}Rb uptake and in the case of patients in Group Ia, before reversion to sinus rhythm. Figure 5 shows the relationship between plasma digoxin concentrations and the percentage changes in ventricular rates.

From these studies the following conclusions were drawn:

1. During digoxin therapy red cell ^{86}Rb uptake is initially inhibited, most probably indicating inhibition of RBC Na^+-K^+-ATPase.
2. The degree of inhibition of ^{86}Rb RBC uptake correlated well with the fall in ventricular rate in atrial fibrillation prior to fluctuations, a correlation which is better than that between the plasma digoxin level and fall in ventricular rate.
3. Comparison of Group I (atrial fibrillation throughout) and Group Ia (atrial fibrillation converting to sinus rhythm during therapy) suggests that in those patients who converted to sinus rhythm during therapy, the slowing of their ventricular rate whilst still in atrial fibrillation occurred with less inhibition of RBC ^{86}Rb uptake. For some reason lower plasma digoxin levels produce less inhibition of RBC ^{86}Rb uptake but more slowing of ventricular rate in Group Ia. It is tempting to speculate that this means that in this group of patients the heart is more sensitive to the effects of inhibition of Na^+-K^+-ATPase activity and therefore, the effects of digoxin.
4. The lack of correlation between changes in ventricular rate and RBC ^{86}Rb uptake in Group II (patients with supraventricular tachyarrhythmias other than atrial fibrillation) is not surprising. Cardiac glycosides do not really cause appreciable gradual slowing of the ventricular response in such arrhythmias, and one would not therefore expect a correlation with the gradual fall in ^{86}Rb uptake which occurred in these patients.

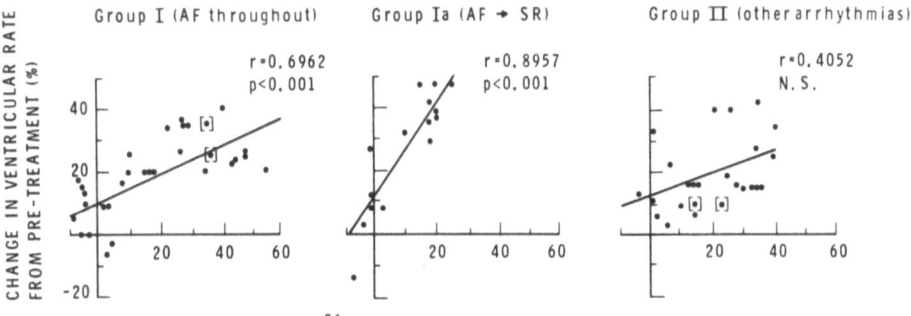

Figure 4 Relationship between change in ventricular rate and ^{86}Rb uptake in patients receiving digoxin. Group 1-patients who remained in atrial fibrillation throughout. Group 1a-patients who reverted from atrial fibrillation to sinus rhythm during treatment. Group 2-patients with other arrhythmias.

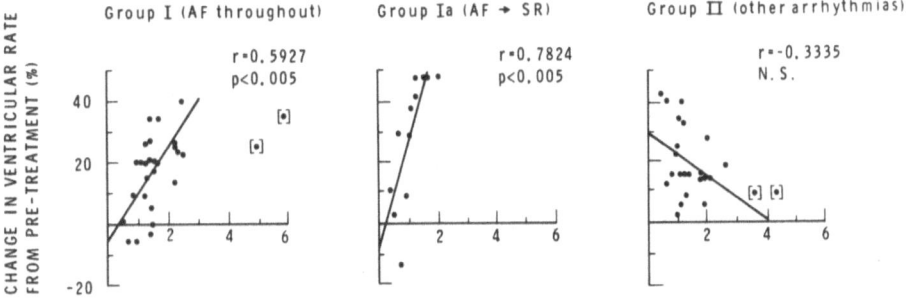

Figure 5 Relationship between change in ventricular rate and plasma digoxin concentration in the groups of patients defined in figure 4.

Multivariate analysis of the values for plasma digoxin, RBC ^{86}Rb uptake and the response of the ventricular rate in atrial fibrillation shows that combined measurement of plasma digoxin concentrations and RBC ^{86}Rb uptake gives a better index of response than either measurement alone. The correlations between plasma digoxin concentrations and RBC ^{86}Rb uptake (Group I, $r = 0.516$, $p < 0.01$; Group Ia, $r = 0.635$, $p < 0.05$; Group II, $r = 0.282$, not significant) show that the degree of ^{86}Rb uptake inhibition is related only in small part to plasma digoxin concentrations measured 6 h after the last dose.

The fluctuations in RBC ^{86}Rb uptake were a puzzle. Superficially it looked as if the RBC was trying to overcome the effects of digoxin.

Overall the studies were very encouraging as far as linking a peripheral, pharmacodynamic effect to a therapeutic effect upon the target organ. These studies have therefore been extended, utilizing further red cell functions as an index of the pharmacological activity of digoxin.

We reasoned that when a RBC is exposed to digoxin, digoxin will bind to the membrane Na^+-K^+-ATPase[13]. The assumption is that the enzyme would then be inhibited, that potassium influx would be inhibited, so that ^{86}Rb uptake would be inhibited. Inhibition of the enzyme would also be accompanied by inhibition of the efflux of sodium from the cell, so that the intracellular sodium concentration would rise[14,15]. We decided therefore to study all of these red cell functions in patients being digitalized for the control of the ventricular rate in atrial fibrillation and also in a separate group of patients, where digoxin was being used as treatment for heart failure in sinus rhythm.

As far as cardiac glycoside receptors on the RBC membrane are concerned the set of conditions we aimed to study were as follows: when a patient takes digoxin, the digoxin in the plasma will bind to specific cardiac glycoside receptors in the red cell membrane[13]. If the red blood cells are removed from the patient and exposed to 12-a-[^{3}H] digoxin under appropriate conditions, less binding of the [^{3}H] digoxin would take place than before he took digoxin. Therefore the fall in the amount of [^{3}H] digoxin binding when compared to the level prior to the patient receiving digoxin should give a guide to the number of receptors on the red cell occupied by the digoxin that he is receiving. We would assume that this is binding to Na$^+$-K$^+$-ATPase and that this would result in a fall in ^{86}Rb uptake of the RBC and a rise in red cell intracellular sodium concentration.

So the sequence of events measured in the second study was:

1. Plasma digoxin concentrations – *Pharmacokinetic phase*
2. Digoxin receptor occupation
3. RBC ^{86}Rb uptake inhibition *Pharmacodynamic phase*
4. RBC intracellular sodium concentrations
5. Ventricular rate in atrial fibrillation
   or
6. Systolic time interval (QS$_2$I) in heart *Therapeutic effect*
   failure in sinus rhythm[16]

The technique used to measure the number of digoxin sites on red cell membrane is briefly as follows: red cells are incubated with 12-a-[^{3}H] digoxin in a potassium-free Ringer solution. The [^{3}H] digoxin binds to red cell membrane and is resistant to washing off. After incubation the red cell is lysed, the membrane is washed and prepared by centrifugation and the [^{3}H] digoxin-bound assayed by liquid scintillation counting.

The binding of [^{3}H] digoxin is temperature-sensitive, saturable, inhibited by ouabain and K$^+$. In a group of ten normal individuals the maximum number of red cell membrane digoxin binding sites was 360 ± 68 molecules/cell (mean $\pm$ sd) and the dissociation constant $9.3 \pm 2.1 \times 10^{-9}$ M. The rate of dissociation is vastly slower than the rate of association.

Preincubation of red cells with non-radioactive digoxin followed by washing causing a decreased binding of [^{3}H] digoxin in subsequent incubation. This 'pre-binding' of digoxin, which might be considered equivalent to what happens *in vivo*, lowers the number of receptor sites available for subsequent binding of [^{3}H] digoxin, the other kinetics of binding remaining unchanged.

As a patient takes digoxin, the *in vitro* RBC [^{3}H] digoxin binding falls, indicating that receptor sites for digoxin on the red cell membrane have become occupied. Concomitantly RBC ^{86}Rb uptake falls. Intra-erythrocytic Na$^+$ concentration rises and the QS$_2$I decreases, indicating a positive inotropic effect in patients in heart failure in regular rhythm.

Table 1 shows the incidence amongst the patients studied of the various changes in the factors measured. Table 2 shows the concordance of biochemical and clinical responses in patients in heart failure in regular rhythm, and Table 3 the more detailed correlations between the biochemical variables, systolic time-intervals and plasma digoxin concentrations.

Table 1 Changes occurring on digoxin therapy

Clinical state	No. of patients	Fall in [^3H] digoxin binding	Fall in ^{86}Rb uptake	Rise in RBC {Na$^+$}	Measured clinical response (fall in ventricular rate* or fall in Qs$_2$I†)
Atrial fibrillation	4	2/3	3/4	4/4	4/4*
Heart failure in sinus rhythm	16	9/14	10/16	13/15	10/11†
(Changes coincident with clinical response)	—	(7/9)	(6/10)	(9/10)	—

Table 2 Concordance of biochemical and clinical responses; patients in heart failure in regular rhythm

	Biochemical response reflects clinical response	Biochemical response does not reflect clinical response
^{86}Rb uptake	11	7
[^{3}H] digoxin binding	8	2
Intracellular {Na$^+$}	12	0

It can be seen, particularly in Table 3, that digoxin binding correlated positively with QS$_2$I, the positive correlation arising in this situation because the more digoxin that is bound to the RBC ATPase the less can [^{3}H] digoxin bind; and the more digoxin that is bound, the shorter the QS$_2$I. ^{86}Rb uptake and intracellular sodium also both highly significantly correlated with the QS$_2$I. Plasma digoxin concentration correlated only weakly with [^{3}H] digoxin binding and ^{86}Rb uptake. There was no correlation of plasma digoxin concentrations and the change in QS$_2$I.

Therefore the indices of the pharmacodynamic effect of digoxin on the RBC during acute digitalization, correlate with the clinical response as measured by the QS$_2$I in heart failure in regular rhythm.

Table 3 Correlations between biochemical variables, systolic time intervals and plasma digoxin concentrations

^{86}Rb uptake	v	[^{3}H] digoxin binding	$r =$	$0.606, p < 0.001$
^{86}Rb uptake	v	Intracellular {Na$^+$}	$r =$	$-0.556, p < 0.001$
[^{3}H] digoxin binding	v	Intracellular {Na$^+$}	$r =$	$0.705, p < 0.001$
QS$_2$I	v	[^{3}H] digoxin binding	$r =$	$0.547, p < 0.001$
QS$_2$I	v	^{86}Rb uptake	$r =$	$0.547, p < 0.001$
QS$_2$I	v	Intracellular {Na$^+$}	$r =$	$0.578, p < 0.001$

[^{3}H] digoxin binding and ^{86}Rb uptake were the only variables to show significant appropriate correlations, which were weak, with the plasma digoxin concentrations in heart failure in regular rhythm.

These results concern the situation during acute digitalization, but in following some of those patients chronically we noted certain trends. These were that as digoxin therapy continued and despite maintenance of 'therapeutic' plasma concentrations, [^{3}H] digoxin binding began to increase to pretreatment levels, ^{86}Rb uptake rose toward pretreatment levels and intracellular {Na$^+$} concentration fell again to pretreatment levels. Concomitantly with these changes QS$_2$1 began to rise to predigitalization levels.

It looked as if the effect of digoxin was 'wearing off' biochemically, pharmacologically and clinically, despite therapeutic plasma levels.

We decided to study these trends in greater detail. We compared four groups of patients:

Group A – acute digoxin therapy (38). This group was studied 2–10 days after commencing treatment.

Group C – Control group (69). This consisted of the 38 patients comprising Group A but *before* they received any digoxin, and a further 31 hospital in-patients who at no time received digoxin.

Group D – (46). These patients had received digoxin for at least 2 months for treatment of cardiac failure in sinus rhythm (31) or for atrial dysrrhythmias (15).

Group T (13). These patients were considered toxic.

The important findings which emerged are summarized in Table 4, and point to the occurrence of a pharmacological tolerance of the RBC to digoxin

Table 4 Comparisons between RBC [^{3}H] digoxin binding, ^{86}Rb uptake and a cellular {Na$^+$} amongst control, acutely digitalized, chronically digitalized and toxic groups of patients

[^{3}H] digoxin binding	Intracellular {Na$^+$}	^{86}Rb uptake
A < C	A > C	A < C
D > A	D < A	D > A
C = D	C = D	C = D
T = A < C and D	T = A > C and D	T = A < C and D

C = Control; A = acute; D = Chronic; T = Toxic.

None of the differences between groups A and D are accounted for by differences in plasma digoxin concentrations.

during chronic therapy. During the acute phase of digoxin therapy, the number of digoxin receptors available for binding [³H] digoxin *in vitro* falls, concomitantly RBC ^{86}Rb uptake falls and intracellular {Na$^+$} rises, presumably because of Na$^+$-K$^+$-ATPase inhibition. As time goes on the number of receptors for digoxin on the red cell membrane appears to increase: presumably the total activity of RBC Na$^+$-K$^+$-ATPase increases toward predigitalization levels, and consequently ^{86}Rb uptake and intracellular {Na$^+$} levels normalize. All this occurs despite the maintenance of therapeutic plasma digoxin concentrations.

This is a most interesting phenomenon, suggesting that in some way the RBC membrane develops more receptors under the influence of digoxin. *Consider:*

Let x = the number of receptors normally in the RBC membrane;
Let y = the number of receptors occupied by digoxin during the acute phase of digoxin therapy;
$x - y$ = the number of receptors available for [³H] digoxin binding *in vitro*.

Therefore quantitatively in the acute stage the number of receptors available for binding has fallen from x to $x - y$.

To return binding to normal levels it is therefore necessary to postulate the 'growth' or 'turning-on' of y receptors so that $x - y + y$ receptors indicates the numbers of receptors in the chronic phase of therapy (which is x). We have yet to prove that digoxin still occupies y receptors in the red cell membrane during the chronic phase and that a further y receptors have been added, though our preliminary findings support this.

If indeed the latter is true, are these extra receptors (i.e. Na$^+$-K$^+$-ATPase) turned on by intracellular ion changes, or has the red cell membrane developed differently because of the effect of digoxin during its developmental phase?

If such changes take place in the heart then (presuming that inhibition of Na$^+$-K$^+$-ATPase is the mechanism by which cardiac glycosides exert their positive inotropic effect) one might expect the pharmacodynamic effect on the heart to diminish. The definitive evidence for this is still lacking. Our own investigations of patients followed chronically suggest that the digoxin effect on the QS$_2$I wears off, suggesting that any positive inotropic effect of digoxin wears off in a matter of weeks (see Figure 6).

These findings are relevant to the controversy as to whether the long-term use of digoxin is worthwhile in cardiac failure in regular rhythm, particularly with the availability of very effective oral diuretics.

What about the control of ventricular rate in atrial fibrillation? Traditionally it is accepted that digitalis is chronically effective in this condition. This must be proved while monitoring red cell functions. If red cell (and by implication heart) become apparently refractory to the Na$^+$-K$^+$-ATPase inhibitory effects of digitalis, and if ventricular rate really remains controlled, explanations for this paradox will be difficult.

If during chronic therapy more cardiac glycoside receptors become available and pharmacological effects therefore diminish, then one would expect the dose needed (and the plasma level needed) to produce digitalis intoxication to be greater than in the acute situation. I know of no evidence on this point. However when patients are toxic and in spite of having plasma digoxin concentrations higher than those found during acute and chronic digitalization, [³H] digoxin binding, ⁸⁶Rb uptake and intracellular {Na⁺} are *equivalent only* to the acute digitalization group (see Table 4). One would have expected evidence of an inhibition of the Na⁺-K⁺-ATPase activity greater than that seen in the *acute* digitalization group, but this is not so and remains to be explained.

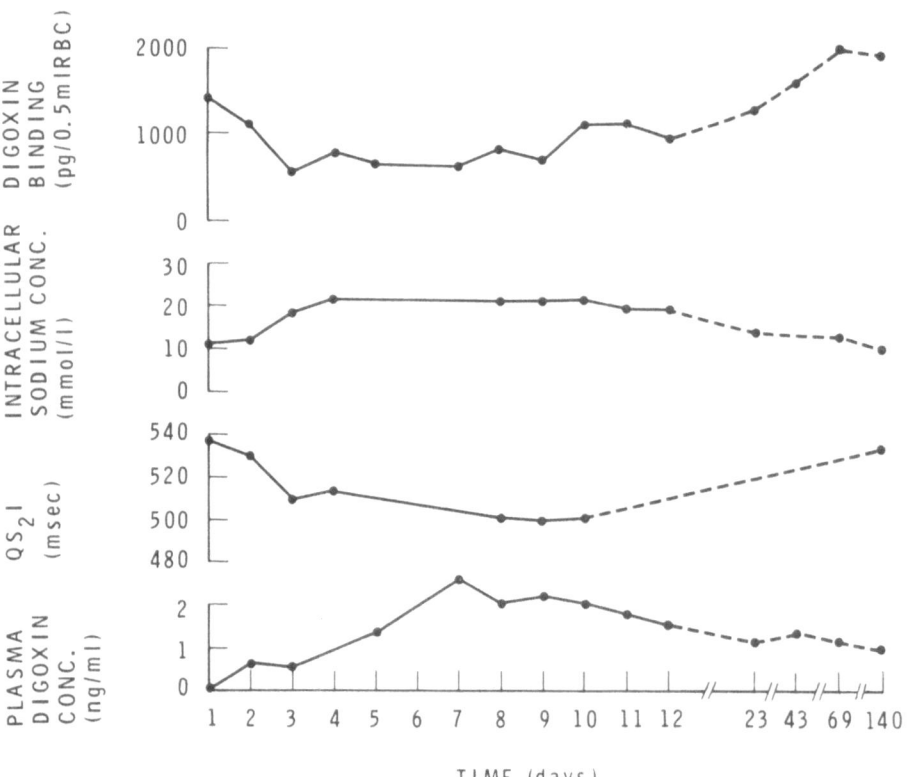

Figure 6. Digoxin binding, intracellular sodium concentration, QS₂1 and plasma digoxin level during chronic digoxin administration

These studies linking the pharmacokinetic, pharmacodynamic and therapeutic phases of digoxin therapy have brought to light some correlations which might prove of clinical relevance. In addition they have produced some unexpected findings which cast some doubt upon the efficacy of chronic digoxin therapy, and perhaps shed some light on the mechanisms of action, and the 'stability' of the cardiac glycoside receptor site population.

THERAPEUTIC GUIDELINES (see Ref. 3 for refs.)

It is unwise to be dogmatic and advise universal dosage requirements of any drug and particularly one with a low toxic:therapeutic ratio such as digoxin. However, one cannot criticise existing advice and duck the issues of how things should be done.

Route of administration

Because digoxin is rapidly absorbed the oral route is the route of choice. If, for some reason (vomiting, coma) the patient is unable to take an oral dose, or if extremely rapid digitalization is desired then slow intravenous infusion (over about 5 min) of the undiluted solution (e.g. digoxin injection, BP 0.25 mg/ml) is the best alternative. The intramuscular route should be avoided if possible—it is sometimes painful, has been shown to cause areas of necrosis at the site of injection in animals and may do so in man, and there is variable absorption of the drug from the site of injection.

Loading dose

A total loading dose of between 10 and 20 μg/kg body weight, followed by a suitable maintenance dose, generally results in plasma levels in the therapeutic range. Loading doses in patients with normal renal and thyroid function, normal electrolyte balance, and who are not elderly may be calculated on this basis. Such loading doses should be administered in three divided doses about 5 h apart: 12 μg/kg for a patient in sinus rhythm and 20 μg/kg for a patient in atrial fibrillation (resulting in total body digoxin levels of 8 and 13 μg/kg respectively) are appropriate, and carry 5% and 9% risks of toxicity.

Let us say one administers such a loading dose in three or four divided doses at 5 h intervals over a period of 10–15 h. The patient would be observed for early signs of toxicity before the administration of each dose and if no toxicity occurred the eventual full loading dose would be given. The maintenance dose would then be based on this, presumed correct, loading dose (see below).

When extremely rapid digitalization is thought necessary (as, for example, in a patient with fast atrial fibrillation and severe cardiac failure) the loading dose may be given as a single dose, the need for a rapid effect outweighing the increased risk of toxicity.

There is at present some controversy over the correct loading dose in renal failure. Overall it is safer to reduce the loading dose in renal failure by a half because of the hazard posed by reductions in the volume of distribution in renal failure which may lead to toxicity occurring when normal loading doses are given[17].

Maintenance dose

The maintenance dose should be based on the percentage of the loading dose eliminated daily, a value which depends on renal function. With a creatinine clearance (Cl_{cr}) of 100 ml/min about 34% of total body digoxin is eliminated daily; when Cl_{cr} falls to 0 ml/min only about 14% is cleared; between these two values the relationship is roughly linear and the percentage can easily be calculated from the formula:

$$\text{Percentage eliminated daily} = 14 + (Cl_{cr}/5)^{18}$$

Then:

$$\text{Daily maintenance dose} = \text{Loading dose} \times \text{percentage eliminated.}$$

Dialysis, whether peritoneal or haemodialysis, removes only about 2.3% of total body digoxin, and need not therefore be considered in deciding the correct maintenance dose.

Treatment without a loading dose

In some instances it may be difficult, or the physician may not desire, to administer the loading dose. In such cases the correct oral loading dose should be decided upon and the corresponding oral maintenance dose calculated as described above. This maintenance dose can then be given as a single daily dose; after about five half-times of elimination (7.5 days in a patient with normal renal function and 22 days in an anuric patient) a steady state will be reached. Such an approach, however, results in a loss of control over therapy if the correct calculations, as is so often the case, are difficult to make, and this may result in serious toxicity. Monitoring the patient's progress during rapid loading is the ideal, although not always attainable, means of therapy. A regression equation has been devised which may be of use in deciding the correct dose for daily treatment:

$$\text{Daily dose } (\mu g/\text{day}) = 3.56 \, Cl_{cr} + 93.0^{19}$$

It should be pointed out that one cannot rely totally on Cl_{cr} measurements in individual patients. Aside from the pitfalls in measuring Cl_{cr}, not all patients respond in a fashion which corresponds with the above outline, and each should be carefully observed and treated on his own merits. Nevertheless, the above approach provides a useful initial guide to therapy.

Special cases

(a) *Electrolyte imbalance.* There are scant data on the degree to which electrolyte abnormalities affect the response to digoxin but it has been estimated that a fall of plasma potassium to 3.0 mmol/l results in reduction in digoxin requirements of about one-third. Should hypokalaemia occur in a patient already taking digoxin it is best to stop therapy until the abnormality can be corrected or, if it is deemed necessary to continue, to reduce the dose by one-third. No figures are available for other electrolytes.

(b) *Old age and thyroid disease.* Unfortunately no data are available to enable the calculation of correct dosage regimens in these situations. Experience, however, seems to suggest that in the elderly and those with myxoedema the loading dose should be cut by up to a half; in the elderly, unless there is contrary evidence, renal function should be assumed to be diminished. In thyrotoxicosis doses require to be increased but no good guidance is available and the clinical condition must be carefully monitored. Equally important is the need to alter dosage schedules as thyroid disease is treated and requirements change, or as a patient becomes elderly while taking long-term therapy.

(c) *Cardioversion and cardiac operations.* It has been shown that plasma levels probably need to be lowered at least below 0.8 ng/ml (1.0 nmol/l) before cardiac operations if postoperative arrhythmias due to digoxin are to be avoided. No doubt a similar need exists where cardioversion is to be carried out, but no information is available. It is therefore best if digoxin therapy is stopped at least 3 days before operation or cardioversion if neither is urgent— plasma level measurement can help decide the timing more accurately in individual cases. When cardioversion is urgent the careful technique outlined by Hagemeijer and Van Houwe[20] may be useful in the absence of digoxin toxicity.

CONCLUSIONS

It is reckoned that about 300 000 patients a day take digoxin in the United Kingdom. Most hospital surveys have shown an incidence of toxicity varying from 10 to 25%. If we minimize the incidence of toxicity and put it at 2%, then 6000 people might be suffering from digoxin toxicity any day. Most toxicity is avoidable by the application of available knowledge. If further investigation supports the contention that digoxin is largely ineffective as a positive inotropic agent in heart failure in regular rhythm in the long term when compared with rest and modern diuretic therapy, then we should stop using it in this situation and an unnecessary hazard would be removed, but I do not believe the evidence is quite that conclusive yet. The next few years should sort this out.

If the mechanism by which digitalis produces its positive inotropic effect was known, and if this could be divorced from its electrophysiological toxic effects and symptomatic toxic effects, then the way might be open for the development of a more acceptable pump-promoting drug. So far this approach has not been very productive and perhaps advances in positive inotropic agents will take place outside the structural constraints of the cardiac glycoside molecule. However many things appear to be impossible until someone achieves them, so one should keep an open mind.

Acknowledgments

Most of the experimental work described in this paper was done by Dr J. K. Aronson (^{86}Rb uptake) and Dr A. R. Ford ([3H] digoxin binding) with excellent assistance from Mrs F. M. Wigley and Miss J. G. Carver. I am grateful to them for allowing me to describe the results and for discovering so many interesting things about what digoxin does to people.

References

1. Digoxin Bioavailability. (1974). Proceedings of a conference held at Leeds on 14 November 1973; ed. B. I. Hoffbrand, *Postgrad. Med. J.* **50** (Suppl. 6)

2. Shaw, T. R. D. (1974). Non-equivalence of digoxin tablets in the U.K. and its clinical implications. *Postgrad. Med. J.*, **50** (Suppl. 6), 24

3. Aronson, J. K. and Grahame-Smith, D. G. (1976). Digoxin therapy: textbooks, theory and practice. *Br. J. Clin. Pharmacol.* **3**, 631

4. Grahame-Smith, D. G. (1977). Monitoring drug therapy: the use of cellular biochemical and pharmacological techniques. *Neth. J. Med.*, **20**, 36

5. Lee, K. S. and Klaus, W. (1971). The subcellular basis for the mechanism of inotropic action of cardiac glycosides. *Pharm. Rev.*, **23**, 193

6. Ghysel-Burton, J. and Godfraind, T. (1975). Stimulation and inhibition by ouabain of the sodium pump in guinea-pig atria. *Brit. J. Pharmacol.* **55**, 249P

7. Cohen, I., Daut, J. and Noble, D. (1976). An analysis of the actions of low concentrations of ouabain on membrane currents in Purkinje fibres. *J. Physiol. (Lond.)*, **260**, 75

8. Smith, T. W. and Haber, E. (1973). *Digitalis*, **289**, 945, 1010, 1063, 1125

9. Beller, G. A., Smith, T. W., Abelmann, W. H. and Hood, W. B. (1971). Digitalis intoxication. A prospective clinical study with serum level correlations. *N. Engl. J. Med.*, **284**, 989

10. Aronson, J. K., Grahame-Smith, D. G. and Wigley, F. M. (1978). Monitoring digoxin therapy. The use of plasma digoxin concentration measurements in the diagnosis of digoxin toxicity. *Quart. J. Med.* NS, **47**, (April)

11. Ingelfinger, J. and Goldman, P. (1976). The serum digitalis concentration—does it diagnose digitalis toxicity? *N. Engl. J. Med.*, **294**, 867

12. Aronson, J. K., Grahame-Smith, D. G., Hallis, K. F., Hibble, A. and Wigley, F. M. (1977). Monitoring digoxin therapy: I. Plasma concentrations and an *in vitro* assay of tissue response. *Br. J. Clin. Pharmacol.*, **4**, 213

13. Erdman, E. and Hasse, W. (1975). Quantitative aspects of ouabain binding to human erythrocytic and cardiac membranes. *J. Physiol.*, **251**, 671

14. Schatzman, H. J. (1953). Herzglykoside als Hemmstoffe fur den aktiven Kalium und Natriumtransport durch die Erythrocyten-membran. *Helv. Physiol. Pharmacol. Acta*, **11**, 346

15. Astrup, J. (1974). Sodium and potassium in human red cells: variations among centrifuged cells. *Scand. J. Clin. Lab. Invest.*, **33**, 231

16. Weissler, A. M., Lewis, R. P. and Leighton, R. F. (1972). The systolic time intervals as a measure of left ventricular performance in man. In P. N. Yu and J. F. Goodwin (eds.). *Progress in Cardiology*, **1**, 159

17. Aronson, J. K. and Grahame-Smith, D. G. (1976). Altered distribution of digoxin in renal failure—a cause of digoxin toxicity? *Br. J. Clin. Pharmacol.*, **3**, 1045

18. Jelliffe, R. W. (1969). Therapeutic guidelines. Administration of digoxin. *Dis. Chest*, **56**, 56

19. Dobbs, S. M., Mawer, G. E., Rodgers, E. M., Woodcock, B. G. and Lucas, S. B. (1976). Can maintenance digoxin dose requirements be predicted? *Br. J. Clin. Pharmacol.*, **3**, 231

20. Hagemeijer, F. and Van Houwe, E. (1975). Titrated energy cardioversion of patients on digitalis. *Br. Heart J.*, **37**, 1303

17
The clinical value of digoxin in patients with heart failure and sinus rhythm

A. GUZ

Is the long-term use of digitalis glycosides worth while in patients with heart failure and sinus rhythm? I have very little doubt that most of my readers are divided into one of three groups; the majority who think it is crazy or perhaps even unethical to ask such a question towards the end of the 1970s; a very small minority who would say that they never use the drug except to block the AV node in atrial fibrillation and tachycardias; and finally a slightly larger minority who admit to being puzzled and bewildered by the literature and the evidence of their own clinical experience. I intend to review briefly some of the facts from a historical viewpoint, and to tell you about a small study that we have recently completed. This entire work has been done in collaboration with Dr David McHaffie from New Zealand.

Withering (1785)[1] identified an extract from *Digitalis purpurea* as the diuretic ingredient of the Shropshire woman's herbal brew, and in his study of 160 patients he showed that it could relieve dropsy in most of his cases. Although he knew that the drug 'influenced the pulse', the concept of heart failure was not recognized, and the primary cardiac action of the drug was not then known. The indications for its use were ill-defined and with more widespread prescription many patients, with little prospect of improvement, were exposed to serious risk from toxic side-effects. Withering knew of no other agent with comparable properties, and he succeeded where many others failed; by adopting a reliable dosage regime and using an experimental approach in each case. He was conscious of the questions that are still around today. How does digitalis work? What identifies patients who will benefit? How can the clinical response be measured? How may the risk of treatment be avoided?

Following its rejection as a dangerous drug of dubious efficacy at the end of the eighteenth century, and being sidetracked for much of the nineteenth century as a treatment for fevers[2], McKenzie[3] reintroduced digitalis into cardiovascular therapeutics because its atrioventricular nodal blocking properties slowed the ventricular response in atrial fibrillation. He showed that digitalis was particularly beneficial in patients with mitral stenosis and atrial fibrillation. With Lewis[4] he developed the concept that heart failure was caused by 'fatigue' of the ventricular muscle, and they proposed that relief in mitral stenosis resulted from cardiac slowing because this allowed the muscle to rest. This controversial aspect of the history of clinical cardiology has been reviewed by McMichael[5] who concluded that there was evidence from McKenzie's own work that a factor independent of heart rate control was contributing to clinical benefit. Nonetheless, McKenzie and Lewis considered atrial fibrillation as the specific indication for digitalis, and were convinced that few other cases benefited from it. In North America, some workers attempted to examine systematically the effects of digitalis in patients with a variety of cardiac conditions and rhythms. Comparisons of the action of digitalis in sinus rhythm and in atrial fibrillation were made by Christian[6], Luten[7] and Marvin[8]. These authors reported a total of over 130 patients and showed that digitalis was associated with improvement in about half the cases in which it was used. They proposed that patients with sinus rhythm benefited as much as those with atrial fibrillation. Gavey and Parkinson[9] reviewed the controversy, and from their own work concluded that for patients with non-rheumatic atrial fibrillation or sinus rhythm, there was a similar beneficial result from using digitalis. Patients with rheumatic atrial fibrillation, who showed the greatest reductions of heart rate, responded best of all.

With the advent of modern physiological studies, the place of digitalis as first choice in the treatment of heart failure became more firmly established. The glycosides were shown to have an acute action in increasing myocardial contractile force in isolated cardiac muscle, open-chest or intact anaesthetized animals, conscious resting animals, and anaesthetized or conscious resting man[10]. It has never been clear whether this inotropic effect improves ventricular pump performance at rest in the non-failing heart; in the failing heart the improvement has been more obvious. Surprisingly, studies of an acute effect during *exercise* have been few in number; no improvement in pump performance has been found in normal man[11,12]. Very recently Horwitz, Atkins and Saito[13] have been unable to demonstrate any inotropic action of ouabain given acutely to an exercising dog; the maximum running speed was in fact reduced.

Does the inotropic action persist in the long term? This crucial clinically relevant question does not seem to have been asked until recently. Mahler, Karliner and O'Rourke[14] could demonstrate a maintained improvement in several aspects of myocardial performance in the conscious dog given intramuscular digoxin for 8 days. Subsequently, Crawford, Karliner and O'Rourke[15] showed similar changes in normal man over a period of 10–14 days; these effects were small although significant. Dobbs, Kenyon and Dobbs[16] demonstrated a maintained shortening of left ventricular ejection time over a period of 1 month in patients with heart disease given digoxin. By contrast, Davidson and Gibson[17], in a careful study of this question in patients who had an aortic valve prosthesis, raised some doubts about whether the inotropic action of digoxin persists in the abnormal heart. A small inotropic effect could be detected 4–6 h after an oral dose of digoxin, but with continued dosage, no such effect could be demonstrated over the remaining 10 days of therapy, although the plasma levels of the drug were within the therapeutic range. Selzer[18] also found that the improvement in cardiac output diminished over time when digoxin was given to patients in left ventricular failure with sinus rhythm. Cohn et al.[19] confirmed these results and showed that in the majority of such patients there was partial or total loss of the initial benefit over a period of 4 h.

A different approach to the same problem has been the study of the effects of the withdrawal of digoxin administered in the long term to patients who have been in heart failure, but are in sinus rhythm. Starr and Luichi[20] doubted the maintenance of an inotropic action; they could not demonstrate any change in ballistocardiographic recordings following digitoxin withdrawal in a group of geriatric patients.

Such withdrawal has also been studied by documenting whether clinical deterioration occurs in such patients. Dall[21] found that maintenance digoxin could be stopped without detriment in 75% of a large group of elderly patients; unfortunately those subjects in sinus rhythm were not differentiated from those in atrial fibrillation. Fonrose et al.[22] thought that 'slight' signs of cardiac 'decompensation' occurred in 50% of another geriatric group of patients when digoxin was withdrawn. Dobbs et al.[16] in a double-biind trial substituted placebo for digoxin; 30% of 46 patients deteriorated on placebo, but this included four with atrial fibrillation. A common feature of deterioration in these studies was salt and water retention. Hull and Mackintosh[23] showed that digoxin withdrawal did not result in deterioration. In 17 out of 18 patients in sinus rhythm, provided that diuretic therapy was adjusted to control any salt and water retention.

We may conclude that there is doubt about any long-term inotropic action; this is entirely compatible with the results just described by Professor Grahame-Smith (pp. 235–254).

All these doubts and the prolonged controversy have led to an extraordinary 'state of the art'. The standard teaching remains that digitalis is indicated in *all* forms of heart failure whatever the cause and whatever the rhythm[24–26]. However, there is a lot of confusion and concern and this latter is heightened by the prevalence of 'digitoxicity' with long-term use[27]. An adverse reaction has been found in up to 19% of patients admitted to hospital who are using the drug, and there are reports of mortality in similar patients ranging from 7 to 50%. In spite of all this and the doubts expressed in a recent Editorial[28], the volume of prescriptions for digoxin in the UK has continued to rise steadily over the last 5 years. In this decade the digitalis glycosides have become the fourth most commonly prescribed drug in the United States[29].

What is the evidence that long-term stimulation (if indeed there is stimulation) of the diseased heart yields clinical improvement that could not be produced by alternative means? Diuretics now need a mention.

In Gavey and Parkinson's study[9] on digitalis, an examination was made of the response to diuretics in 16 patients with heart failure in sinus rhythm who had been refractory to cardiac glycosides. All had a diuresis, including some in whom oedema was not obvious. It is surprising that the demonstration that for some patients a diuretic was more effective than digitalis did not suggest the need for a comparison of the effects of the two drugs. Diuretics were regarded as little more than adjuvants to therapy because they did not influence 'myocardial insufficiency'.

Several observations suggested that the haemodynamic abnormalities in patients with heart failure could be improved without directly stimulating cardiac muscle. McMichael and Sharpey-Schafer[30] showed that mechanical lowering of right atrial pressure in such patients produced similar changes in central venous pressure and cardiac output to those produced by digitalis. These observations were extended when Pugh and Wyndham[31] provided evidence that the intravenous use of diuretics produced similar results. Later, Rader et al.[32] showed that diuretic therapy for heart failure could be used alone on a chronic basis; clinical improvement occurred in the majority of patients. There were changes in haemodynamic variables, but little correlation between such changes and the magnitude of the clinical response; this appeared to most closely parallel the relief of oedema produced by the diuretic. When these workers then added digoxin, increases in cardiac output were seen in some individuals with sinus rhythm, particularly where there had been no haemodynamic change with the mercurial diuretics, but there was no further diuresis or weight change in this sub-group and it was not possible to identify digoxin 'responders' on purely clinical criteria.

Modern diuretics such as frusemide and bumetanide are very potent agents for the relief of salt and water retention. These drugs will relieve oedema and symptoms in the majority of patients; the dose may be readily adjusted to the clinical response and the drugs have higher therapeutic/toxic ratios than does digoxin. It is, however, uncommon to find them being used alone, but rather in combination with long-term digoxin therapy.

It has become apparent that congestive heart failure is not simply a state of low cardiac output. It is instead a more complicated syndrome of impaired cardiac function characterized by salt and water retention. The signs and symptoms are predominantly those of intra- and extra-vascular space congestion and any treatment that relieves these features produces improvement in the patient irrespective of the haemodynamic change that ensues. If direct cardiac stimulation by digoxin is not required for relief of the signs and symptoms of heart failure in the majority of cases; if the long-term use of the drug is associated with serious risk of toxicity; and if there is doubt about long-term inotropism, then it is ethical and important to examine whether the drug provides benefits in the form of improved exercise capacity.

I would like to propose that the most important principle in such a study is to *separate* those responses expected from modern diuretics from the benefits obtained from augmenting myocardial contraction. The specific benefit of digoxin as a myocardial stimulant can only be examined *after* relief of salt and water retention by diuretics.

We have now done such a study on a very small number of patients in sinus rhythm with cardiac muscle disease. Patients with atrial fibrillation cannot be studied because not only may much of the benefit from digoxin at rest be due to the induced AV nodal block, but also this block is lessened on exercise.

All of these patients were in severe heart failure with large hearts; all had peripheral oedema and five out of the six had pulmonary oedema.

Before entry to the study, frusemide was given in order that body-weight be reduced to a steady 'dry' basal weight and this was maintained throughout the study. The dose of frusemide was increased in some cases to the point where serum creatinine levels were raised, but postural hypotension was avoided. This treatment was associated with striking improvement in all cases, but there remained variable degrees of exercise intolerance.

Steady-state exercise tests with increasing work loads were done in three pairs over the course of 3 months; diuretics were used throughout and if the body-weight changed by more than ± 1 kg between tests, the dose of diuretics was adjusted to correct the change. For half the patients digoxin was given only for the middle pair of tests and for the other half, digoxin was used only for the first and last pair of tests, but not for the middle pair. A minimum of 2 weeks was allowed for digitalization before tests and 4 weeks for the elimination of the drug from the body[33]. On each test day, any change in symptoms was noted, and this history was supplemented by the use of visual analogue scales to measure the sense of breathlessness and fatigue between tests[34]. Measurement of total body water, extracellular fluid volume and plasma volume were made once for every pair of tests to supplement the measurements of body-weight and clinical estimation of salt and water retention. We found we could control body-weight to within ± 1.5 kg of the starting weight, and these changes were reflected particularly by the extracellular fluid volume measurements.

The maximum level of exercise used was established by prior testing. It was usually the work load that produced 85% of the maximum heart rate predicted for age[35], or was a level 5 Watts below that which had previously stopped the test by producing chest pain, excess fatigue or breathlessness.

Five of the six patients completed all tests; the sixth was withdrawn from the study when he developed arrhythmias and angina following withdrawal of digoxin. None of these five patients showed any change in symptoms, no difference in workloads achieved, or any difference in heart rate, respiratory rate, ventilation, oxygen consumption, carbon dioxide production or respiratory quotient at each workload whether digoxin was added to, or removed from, the treatment regime.

All these patients retained salt and water and became oedematous if diuretics were withdrawn from the therapeutic regime, when the trial had finished.

This study had several limitations. It was not double-blind, and the digoxin dosage was not adjusted, beyond ensuring that serum digoxin levels were within the accepted therapeutic range. There was also no test of maximal exercise capacity. Nevertheless, in this group of patients where salt and water retention could be controlled with diuretics, digoxin did not improve the sense of well-being nor the capacity for exercise. The study showed that diuretics could be used as drugs of first choice for some patients with heart failure in sinus rhythm.

CONCLUSION

There is ample evidence that digoxin, when used in the short term, stimulates the heart, and may relieve the symptoms of cardiac failure in patients with normal rhythm. Its role in the treatment of the chronic heart failure syndrome with sinus rhythm remains uncertain. There are genuine doubts that the drug is effective with long-term administration and there is considerable risk of toxicity. A characteristic feature of congestive heart failure is that symptomatic benefit can be obtained by measures that relieve intra- and extravascular congestion. Since cardiac stimulation may not be required to achieve this, digoxin may not be essential treatment for such patients. It seems rational to suggest that the achievement of a 'dry' weight with diuretics should be the first objective in the treatment of congestive cardiac failure with sinus rhythm. Digoxin could *then* be administered and withdrawn as required, to ascertain whether the use of this drug further improved the clinical state.

There is a clear need for a 'double-blind' controlled trial on a large number of well-defined patients of the sort described above, to document whether long-term digoxin therapy is required when sinus rhythm prevails and when the patient is kept 'dry' with diuretics.

References

1. Withering, W. (1785). *An account of the foxglove, and some of its medical uses: with practical remarks on dropsy, and other diseases.* (Birmingham: M. Swinney)
2. Keele, K. D. (1966). Uses and abuses of medical history. *Br. Med. J.*, **2**, 1251
3. McKenzie, J. (1911). Digitalis. *Heart*, **2**, 273
4. Lewis, Sir Thomas (1942). *Diseases of the Heart*, 3rd edn. (London: Macmillan)
5. McMichael, J. (1975). *A Transition in Cardiology: The MacKenzie-Lewis Era.* Harveian Oration (London: Royal College of Physicians)
6. Christian, H. A. (1922). Digitalis effects in chronic cardiac cases with regular rhythm in contrast to auricular fibrillation. *Med. Clin. North Amer.*, **5**, 1173
7. Luten, D. (1924). Clinical studies with digitalis. I. Effects produced by the administration of massive dosage to patients with normal mechanism. *Arch. Int. Med.*, **33**, 251
8. Marvin, H. M. (1927). Digitalis and diuretics in heart failure with regular rhythm, with special reference to the importance of etiologic classification of heart disease. *J. Clin. Invest.*, **3**, 521
9. Gavey, C. J. and Parkinson, J. (1939). Digitalis in heart failure with normal rhythm. *Br. Heart J.*, **1**, 27
10. Smith, T. W. and Haber, E. (1973). Digitalis. *N. Engl. J. Med.*, **259**, 945, 1010, 1063, 1125
11. Williams, M. H., Zohman, L. R. and Ratner, A. C. (1958). Haemodynamic effects of cardiac glycosides on normal human subjects during rest and exercise. *J. Appl. Physiol.*, **13**, 417
12. Bruce, R. A., Lind, A. R., Franklin, D., Muir, A. L., McDonald, H. R., McNichol, G. W. and Donald, K. W. (1968). The effects of digoxin on fatiguing static and dynamic exercise in man. *Clin. Sci.*, **34**, 29
13. Horwitz, L. D., Atkins, J. M. and Saito, M. (1977). Effect of digitalis on left ventricular function in exercising dogs. *Circ. Res.*, **41**, 744
14. Mahler, F., Karliner, J. S. and O'Rourke, R. A. (1974). Effects of chronic digoxin administration on left ventricular performance in the normal conscious dog. *Circulation*, **50**, 720

15. Crawford, M. H., Karliner, J. S. and O'Rourke, R. A. (1976). Favourable effects of oral maintenance digoxin therapy on left ventricular performance in normal subjects: echocardiographic study. *Am. J. Cardiol.*, **38,** 843

16. Dobbs, S. M., Kenyon, W. L. and Dobbs, R. J. (1977). Maintenance digoxin after an episode of heart failure: placebo controlled trial in outpatients. *Br. Med. J.*, **1,** 749

17. Davidson, C. D. and Gibson, D. (1973). Clinical significance of positive inotropic action of digoxin in patients with left ventricular disease. *Br. Heart J.*, **35,** 970

18. Selzer, A. (1960). Comparative studies of acute and chronic effects of digitalis in cardiac failure. *Circulation*, **22,** 807

19. Cohn, K., Selzer, A., Kersh, E. S., Karpman, L. S. and Goldschlager, N. (1975). Variability of hemodynamic responses to acute digitalisation in chronic cardiac failure due to cardiomyopathy and coronary artery disease. *Am. J. Cardiol.*, **35,** 843

20. Starr, I. and Luichi, R. J. (1969). Blind study on the action of digitoxin on elderly women. *Am. Heart J.*, **78,** 740

21. Dall, J. L. C. (1970). Maintenance digoxin in elderly patients. *Br. Med. J.*, **2,** 705

22. Fonrose, H. A., Ahlbaum, N., Bugatch, E., Cohen, M., Genovese, C. and Kelly, J. (1974). The efficacy of digitalis withdrawal in an institutional aged population. *J. Am. Geriat. Soc.*, **22,** 208

23. Hull, S. M. and Mackintosh, A. (1977). Discontinuation of maintenance digoxin therapy in general practice. *Lancet*, **2,** 1054

24. *Price's Textbook of the Practice of Medicine* (1973). 11th edn. Ed. B. Scott. (London: Oxford University Press)

25. Beeson-McDermott. *Textbook of Medicine*, 14th edn., p. 891. (London: W. B. Saunders)

26. Goodman, L. S. and Gilman, A. (1975). *The Pharmacological Basis of Therapeutics*, 5th edn. p. 676. (New York: Macmillan)

27. Smith, T. W. (1975). Digitalis toxicity: epidemiology and clinical use of serum concentration measurements. *Am. J. Med.*, **58,** 470

28. Editorial (1976). Foxglove saga (continued). *Lancet*, **2,** 405

29. Schick, D. and Scheuer, J. (1974). Current concepts of therapy with digitalis glycosides. Part I. *Am. Heart J.*, **87,** 253

30. McMichael, J. and Sharpey-Schafer, E. P. (1944). The action of intravenous digoxin in man. *Quart. J. Med.*, **12,** 123

31. Pugh, L. G. C. and Wyndham, C. (1949). The circulatory effects of mercurial diuretics on congestive heart failure. *Clin. Sci.*, **6,** 41

32. Rader, B., Smith, W. W., Berger, A. R. and Eichna, L. W. (1964). Comparison of the haemodynamic effects of mercurial diuretics and digitalis in congestive heart failure. *Circulation*, **29,** 328

33. McHaffie, D. J., Purcell, H., Mitchell-Heggs, P. and Guz, A. (1978). The clinical value of digoxin in patients with heart failure and sinus rhythm. *Quart. J. Med.*, **188,** 401

34. Priestman, T. J. and Baum, M. (1976). Evaluation of quality of life in patients receiving treatment for advanced breast cancer. *Lancet*, **1,** 899

35. Astrand, P. and Rodahl, K. (1970). *Textbook of Work Physiology*. (Tokyo: McGraw-Hill, KogaKusha Ltd.)

Part VI
Harvey lecture

18
Essential cardiovascular regulation – the control linkages between bodily needs and circulatory function

A. C. GUYTON

It is a tribute to each of us that we represent the world of physiology and medicine in this dedication to Harvey and his work. But, more important, we ourselves are paying tribute to two attributes of Harvey's character that made him great: first, to his intelligence that gave him vision to understand the basic principles and logic of the circulation when other authorities of his times refused to open their minds; and, second, to the spirit that made him persist in telling his story of an almost heretic notion.

Today, the basics of the cardiovascular system seem to be elementary. Yet, if each of us should outline what he considers to be these basics, there would be serious disagreements, especially about cardiovascular regulation, the subject that I have chosen to discuss. Still, in the hope that I can bring together many of the diverse philosophies of cardiovascular regulation, I propose to begin with elementary aspects of regulation and to progress through more complex stages, hoping to weave a fabric of logic that might itself please Harvey. Fortunately, my task is made much easier by the fact that this audience is already well steeped in the fundamentals of circulatory function, and also by the fact that the collective impact of all the other papers that you have heard at this symposium represents perhaps the most thorough understanding of the circulation ever assembled, which in itself is our real tribute to Harvey.

BASIC PHILOSOPHY OF CARDIOVASCULAR REGULATION – THE TWO ESSENTIALS: ARTERIAL PRESSURE REGULATION AND LOCAL BLOOD FLOW REGULATION

From the great morass of literature that has been written about cardiovascular regulation, one would suspect that this subject would be too complex to find any basic dominating theme or philosophy. However, I would like to suggest that almost all aspects of cardiovascular regulation can be explained on the basis of two essential processes. The first of these is the establishment and maintenance of a stable and adequate pressure in the arteries; this provides a head of blood pressure at the vascular inlet of each tissue, providing the driving force to cause blood flow through each tissue as it is needed. The second is control of blood flow in each of the local tissues; in most instances this is related to the level of tissue metabolism, but in some instances to such factors as excretory load to be processed by the kidneys, heat delivery to the skin for body temperature control, or other similar factors. Obviously, the sum of all these regulations of local blood flows regulates the cardiac output at the same time.

Thus, the basic philosophy of circulatory control is indeed simple, though the many papers of this symposium have already attested to the fact that the practical means for expressing this control are not so simple.

Regulation of arterial pressure

Let us repeat again that the first essential for overall regulation of circulatory function is the maintenance of an adequate and relatively constant arterial pressure. The arterial pressure level must resist change despite many types of stresses, some of which are acute and some long-term. Haemorrhage, for instance, is a very acute stress; also, simply standing up is a severe stress to the circulation, or defaecating, or eating, or emotional stresses that alter the nervous drive to the circulation. On the other hand, some of the long-term stresses include dehydration, metabolic deficiencies, changes in altitude, and even the amount of salt that we eat over a lifetime. Therefore, it is no surprise that arterial pressure is regulated by multiple control mechanisms, each performing a specific role. Figure 1 demonstrates the function of several of these after a sudden abnormal step change in arterial pressure occurs at zero time[1]. Each curve depicts the quantitative 'feedback gain' – that is, the ability to correct the abnormal pressure – of a respective control mechanism at each interval of time after the initial stress. It is the sum of all these feedback effects that tends to return the arterial pressure towards its original control level. Note especially in this figure that the controls which operate within the first few seconds after the pressure change are almost entirely nervous reflex mechanisms. However, in general, the nervous controls become less effective with time, while others become far more potent. The most potent of all, one which develops very slowly, is the renal-body fluid pressure feedback control mechanism. Others that operate on an intermediate time frame include such factors as vascular stress-relaxation, shift of fluid between the circulation and the interstitium through the capillary membrane, and hormonal mechanisms such as the renin–angiotensin system and the aldosterone mechanism. Let us discuss first the acute nervous controls of arterial pressure.

NERVOUS CONTROL OF ARTERIAL PRESSURE

Arterial pressure control by the arterial baroreceptor system
Most conceptual aspects of the nervous control of the circulation are so

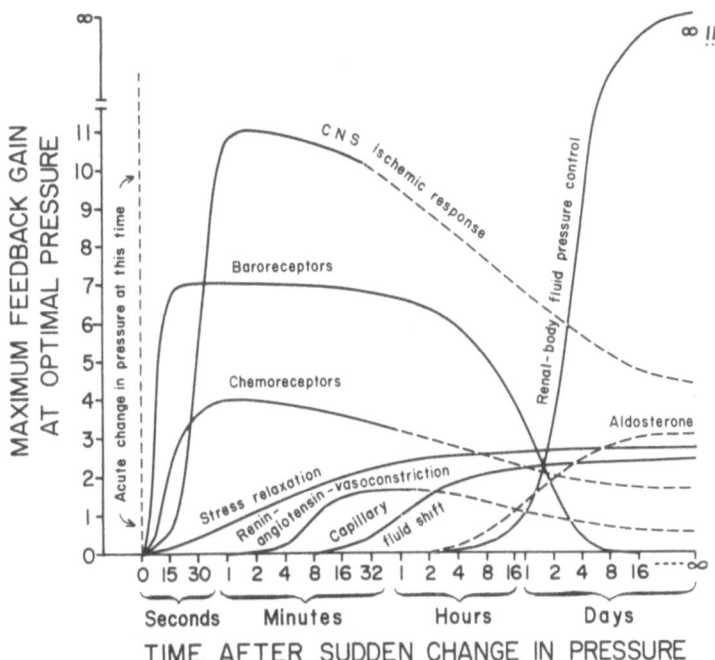

Figure 1 Feedback responses of the different pressure control mechanisms at different time intervals after some acute event changes the pressure from the normal value. (Preprinted from: Guyton *et al., Dynamics of Arterial Pressure Regulation.* W. B. Saunders Co.)

well known by this audience that they need little elaboration. On the other hand, it is often surprising how imprecisely we deal with the quantitative aspects of these control mechanisms. For instance, the carotid sinus and aortic high-pressure baroreceptor mechanism is frequently ascribed extreme capabilities both of acute pressure control and long-term pressure control, almost as if this mechanism were the only pressure controller in the body. Yet, strangely enough, complete removal of the carotid and aortic baroreceptors can be tolerated indefinitely. However, there is one major deficit in arterial pressure regulation. What is this deficit?

Figure 2 illustrates two 2 h tracings of the mean arterial pressure in a dog, first before baroreceptor denervation (upper panel) and, second, 3 weeks after denervation (lower panel)[2]. One can readily see from this figure the striking inability of the animal to maintain a constant level of arterial pressure in the absence of the baroreceptor system. Note that the pressure frequently remains for several minutes at a time at levels as high as 180 mmHg. But then it also frequently remains for several minutes at a time at pressures low as 45 mmHg. Thus, without the baroreceptor system the pressure may become excessively high or excessively low. Therefore, we can immediately state that the baroreceptor system provides an extremely important function to 'damp' the variations in arterial pressure.

On the other hand, do the baroreceptors play an important role in long-

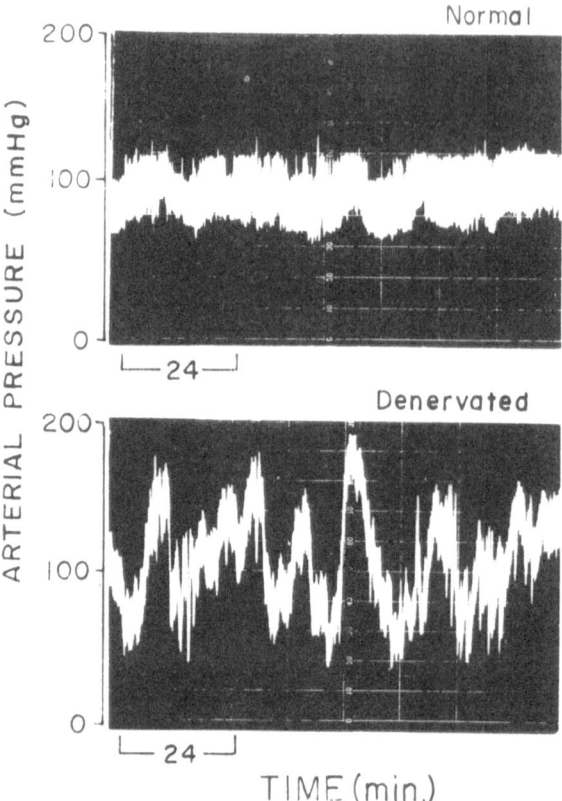

Figure 2 Two-hour recording of mean arterial pressure (mmHg) in a normal unanaesthetized dog (top record) and then again in the same dog several weeks after baroreceptor denervation (bottom record), illustrating marked variations in the mean arterial pressure in the absence of the baroreceptors. (Reprinted from Cowley *et al.*[2] by permission of the American Heart Association)

term arterial pressure control? For a period of 50 years, now, many physiologists have believed that this is true. Yet several authors have pointed out that, on the average, the decreases in arterial pressure below the normal control level, when averaged over a period of 24 h, compensate for the excesses in pressure that occur at other times of the day. The most complete study of this has been made by Cowley and his colleagues[2,3], over a period of years. They have now made multiple continuous recordings of arterial pressure for literally weeks at a time in a total of 65 denervated dogs. The recordings have been made while the animals were in the undisturbed state day and night, and the results have been analysed automatically by a computer. Figure 3 illustrates typical 24 h histograms for a single dog, as plotted by the computer, before denervation and several weeks after denervation[2]. One can readily see the broad spectrum of pressures after denervation in comparison with a much narrower spectrum before. Yet, the weighted average pressure level throughout the 24 h period was very little different whether

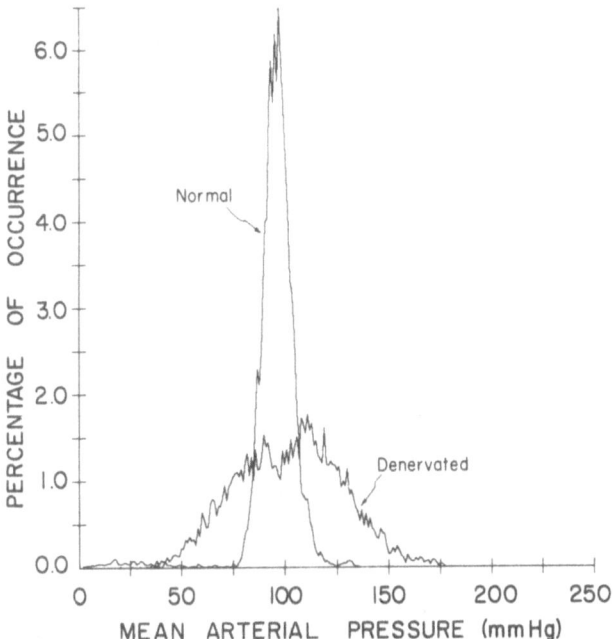

Figure 3 Histograms illustrating the frequency distribution of arterial pressure readings throughout 24 h recording intervals in a normal unanaesthetized dog and the same dog several weeks after denervation of its baroreceptors. (Reprinted from Cowley *et al.*[2] by permission of the American Heart Association)

the baroreceptors were intact or not. Indeed, in the total 65 dogs, the mean 24 h arterial pressures of the denervated dogs have averaged less than 1 mmHg different from those in normal dogs.

Thus, it appears that the baroreceptors have the single function of damping short-term pressure variations but not the capability of long-term arterial pressure control. This is exactly what would be predicted from the known property of the baroreceptors to reset to new pressure levels over a period of hours to several days[4-6].

Feedback gain of the sino-aortic baroreceptor pressure control mechanism. One can calculate the quantitative importance of the baroreceptors for damping minute by minute or hourly variations in pressure by comparing quantitatively the pressure variations in normal animals versus the variations in denervated animals. On the average in Cowley's studies, the variation was 2·6 times as great in the denervated as in the normal animals[2]. Using the following formula for calculation of the feedback gain of the control system,

$$G = \frac{\text{Variation after blocking the control system}}{\text{Variation with control system intact}} - 1$$

the gain of this control system is 1·6. For those who are not familiar with the meaning of feedback gain, this means that 1·6/2·6 of the variation that occurs without function of the baroreceptors is removed by the presence of

269

the baroreceptors, leaving only 1/2·6 of the variation still occurring. This level of sino-aortic feedback gain as calculated from Cowley's data is approximately equal to that found in a different way by Sagawa and his associates[7] and a little less than that found by Scher and his associates[8].

Control of arterial pressure by chemoreceptor and vasomotor centre ischaemic reflexes

Though the baroreceptor system has become widely recognized as an important pressure control system, relatively little has been written about the other nervous pressure control mechanisms, several of which are equally as important in their respective pressure-controlling roles as is the arterial baroreceptor system. For instance, both the peripheral chemoreceptors and the vasomotor centre become strongly stimulated when the pressure falls low enough to cause tissue ischaemia; and this stimulation causes reflex sympathetic excitation that helps to return the pressure towards normal. Heymans and Neil discussed long ago the importance of the chemoreceptor feedback system as a pressure regulator, especially when the arterial pressure falls below 70–80 mmHg[9]. Unfortunately, though, no one has yet fully documented the potency of this system for pressure control – that is, no one has measured the feedback gain. Anecdotal data suggest that at arterial pressures below 80 mmHg it might be as great as that of the arterial baroreceptor system. On the other hand, at the higher pressure levels, there seems to be sufficient evidence that the chemoreceptor system is not a significant pressure controller.

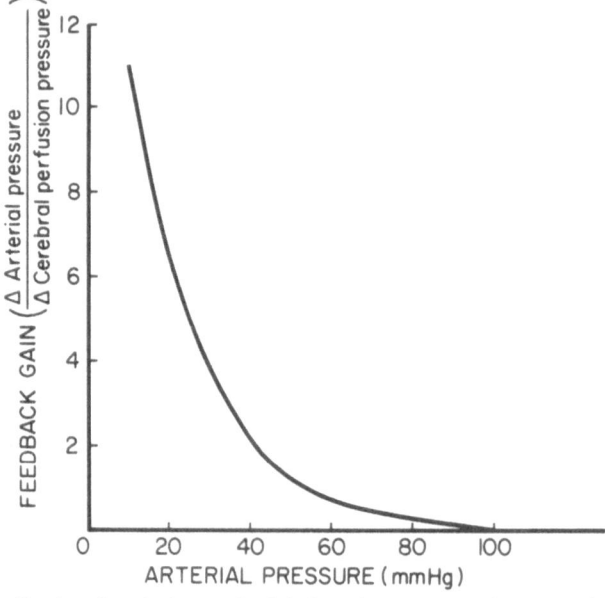

Figure 4 Feedback gain of the cerebral ischaemic response, demonstrating that this pressure-control mechanism is especially potent in preventing further decrease in arterial pressure when the pressure has already fallen to dangerously low pressures. (Drawn from data in Sagawa *et al.*[10])

By contrast, far more is known about both the pressure range and the potency of the vasomotor ischaemic mechanism for control of arterial pressure. Figure 4 illustrates a study by Sagawa *et al.* in which they determined the average feedback gain of the vasomotor ischaemic reflex at different arterial pressure levels[10]. Note that there is very little feedback gain of this reflex for control of arterial pressure at pressures above 60 mmHg. However, at lower pressures this mechanism becomes extremely potent as a pressure controller. Indeed, Sagawa measured feedback gains of 5–11 at mean arterial pressures of 10–25 mmHg. These are 3–7 times as great as the feedback gain of the baroreceptor system. Thus, the vasomotor ischaemic response is probably the most potent of all the nervous pressure feedback controllers; but it functions powerfully as a feedback controller only when the pressure falls to dangerously low levels. For this reason, it has often been described as the 'last-ditch stand' mechanism for maintenance of the arterial pressure, and it is certainly one of the major components causing the powerful agonal vasoconstriction observed throughout the circulation shortly before death from acute haemorrhage or trauma.

Low-pressure vascular stretch receptors and their 'feed-forward' control of arterial pressure

Recently, one of the most active areas of research in the field of nervous regulation of the circulation has been the study of the 'low-pressure' vascular stretch receptors and the circulatory reflexes that they cause. These low-pressure receptors are nervous stretch receptors located mainly in the walls of the atria but also in the great veins, the ventricles, and even the pulmonary vessels. One of the reflexes elicited by stretch of these receptors is the 'volume reflex' studied especially by Gauer and Henry[11] and by Linden and his colleagues[12]. But probably equally as important are the reflexes from the low-pressure receptors to the peripheral vasculature studied extensively by Shepherd and his colleagues[13]. The volume reflex causes increased excretion of urine when the low-pressure receptors are stimulated by stretch of the atria, thereby reducing the volume back towards normal. The low-pressure–peripheral vascular reflex causes peripheral vasodilatation when the low-pressure receptors are stretched, and this reflex helps to prevent a rise in pressure that otherwise might be caused by excess blood volume.

The question that is still not answered is the quantitative importance of the low-pressure receptor reflexes in the overall control functions of the circulation. However, I would like to suggest that these reflexes are probably very valuable in the daily life of the circulation. The reasons for believing this are the following: first, changes in blood volume are among the most stressful events for the circulatory system. After each meal, after each period of heavy sweating, or after any bout of heavy fluid intake, the blood volume shares in the changes of hydration of the body. Furthermore, there are ample studies to show that long-term changes in blood volume of as little as 2–5% can have very significant effects on the long-term level of arterial pressure, as we shall discuss later. Yet, it would be very disadvantageous if every temporary increase or decrease in the degree of body hydration caused these same tremendous changes in arterial pressure.

A second reason for believing in the importance of the low-pressure receptors for pressure control is that a very large volume of blood can be transfused into a normal animal in a period of a few minutes without severely changing the arterial pressure. For instance, the solid curve of Figure 5 illustrates the effect of a 5 min transfusion of blood into dogs at a volume equal to 30% of the dog's original blood volume[14]. The average increase in arterial pressure was only 15 mmHg. Yet, when this same experiment was repeated in dogs whose heads had been removed so that all the major circulatory nervous reflexes had been eliminated, the arterial pressure increased, as illustrated by the dashed curve, 120 mmHg, an 8-fold difference. Thus, it is clear that the nervous reflexes do play a tremendous role in moderating pressure changes in the face of blood volume stresses.

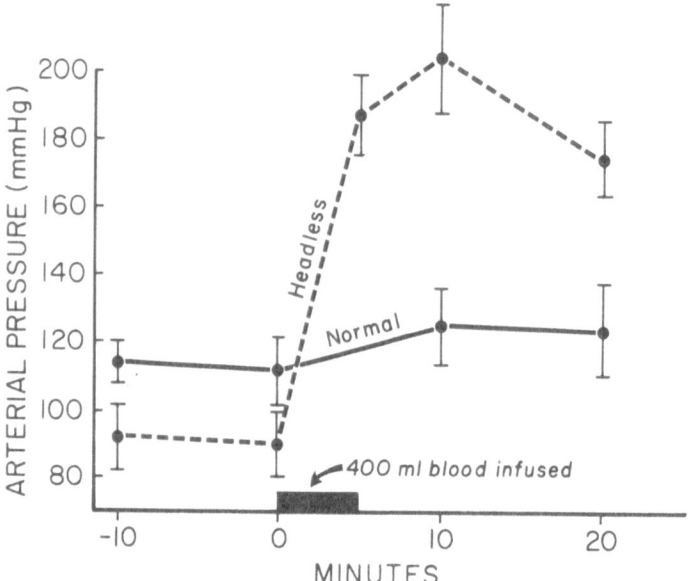

Figure 5 Effect on mean arterial pressure caused by infusion of 400 ml of blood into a group of normal anaesthetized dogs and a group of headless dogs without pressure-controlling reflexes. (Drawn from data in Dobbs, W. A., Ph.D. thesis, University of Mississippi School of Medicine, 1970)

Third, the sino-aortic baroreceptor system has a feedback gain of only 1·6. Yet, when one calculates the feedback gain that would be required of the sino-aortic system if it alone were moderating the pressure as much as illustrated in Figure 5, one derives a gain of 7, much greater than the 1·6 that has actually been measured for this system. Thus, it appears that a large share of the acute nervous control of arterial pressure in the face of blood volume changes is achieved in ways other than the sino-aortic baroreceptor reflexes. Since the chemoreceptor and vasomotor ischaemic reflexes operate primarily at low pressures, the only satisfactory candidate for this additional all-important pressure control seems to be the low-pressure receptors and their reflexes. However, these reflexes are not 'feedback' controllers of arterial pressure but, instead, 'feed-forward' controllers. Therefore, let us discuss what is meant by a *feed-forward controller* and explain some of its properties.

When the atria become excessively filled with blood, this automatically increases the cardiac output because of the Frank–Starling mechanism of the heart. Yet, if stretch of the low-pressure areas at the same time causes reflex peripheral vasodilatation of the arterioles, this can offset the tendency of the increased cardiac output to elevate the arterial pressure. That is, the reflex, feeds *forward* from the low-pressure area to the high-pressure area to head off a rise in pressure that would otherwise be caused by the elevated input pressure to the heart.

A *feed-forward* controller of arterial pressure has a special property not shared by a *feedback* controller which is the following: the feed-forward controller can exert all degrees of correction of an abnormal arterial pressure; it can correct the abnormal pressure a slight amount, it can correct the pressure entirely, or it can over-correct it. For instance, if a slight rise in atrial pressure should cause extremely intense peripheral circulatory vasodilatation, this might actually cause a fall in arterial pressure despite a simultaneous rise in cardiac output, this representing an over-correction.

On the other hand, the *feedback* controllers of pressure can never fully correct the abnormal pressure but can correct it only part of the way. The reason for this is a simple one: the reflex itself is elicited by an abnormal pressure, so that if ever the abnormality is fully corrected, no abnormality remains to keep driving the reflex. Therefore, the reflex fades away, and the abnormal pressure returns. Thus, in practice, the *feedback* controller of pressure always corrects the pressure by a given proportion. In the case of the sino-aortic baroreceptor system, this proportion seems to be approximately 60% correction but never the nearly 100% correction that normally occurs following acute volume stresses to the circulation. On the other hand, if our suspicions are correct about the feed-forward capabilities of the low-pressure receptor reflexes, it seems that their potency for correcting the arterial pressure is approximately that required to give only slightly less than full acute correction but not usually overcorrection when volume increases acutely.

Resetting (or adaptation) of the nervous mechanisms for pressure control
We have already pointed out that the baroreceptors do not seem to have a long-term effect in controlling pressure because they themselves eventually reset to whatever new level the animal's pressure approaches[4-6]. Without going into details, there is also much evidence that all or most of the other nervous mechanisms of pressure control reset in the same manner as the sino-aortic baroreceptor mechanism. Therefore, for the present, it appears that the nervous control mechanisms are capable of correcting abnormal pressure levels only for a few hours to a few days at most.

THE RENAL-BODY FLUID MECHANISM FOR PRESSURE CONTROL – THE BASIC LONG-TERM CONTROLLER

If the cardiovascular nervous reflexes are not the long-term controller of arterial pressure, then we must look for some more basic and more durable pressure controller. Historically, clinicians have long been aware of the relationship of salt and water to the control of pressure, but the fact that most hypertensive patients do not have elevated blood volumes or sodium concentrations has made it difficult to understand how a body fluid mechanism for pressure control could be of major importance. However, recent studies have demonstrated the tremendous importance of body fluid regulation as a means for long-term regulation of the arterial pressure, a mechanism that we shall discuss in the following sections of this paper.

The renal-pressure diuresis and natriuresis phenomenon as the basis of pressure control

From the earliest study of renal physiology, it was immediately learned that urine output of both water and salt is highly dependent on arterial pressure, falling to as little as zero at pressures of 40–50 mmHg and rising to many times normal when the arterial pressure is acutely elevated 50–100 mmHg above normal. This phenomenon has long been known as 'pressure diuresis' and 'pressure natriuresis'. Approximately 30 years ago it was quantitated by a number of different investigators, a quantitation that has stood the test of time in many laboratories in subsequent years[15-17]. Figure 6 illustrates approximately this relationship between arterial pressure and urinary output. Furthermore, both water output and sodium output follow essentially

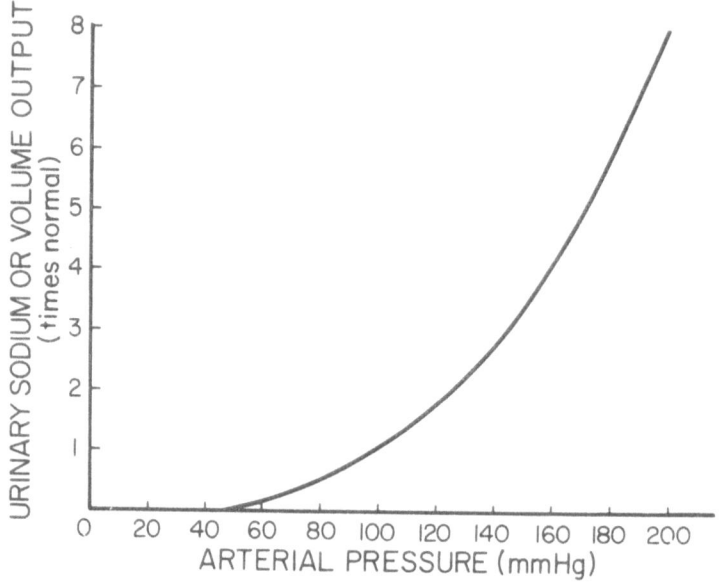

Figure 6 Effect of increasing arterial pressure on urinary sodium and urinary volume output. (Drawn from composite data in multiple papers in the literature[15-17])

the same curve. One can readily see from this curve that, if ever the arterial pressure rises too high, the urinary output of both water and sodium will increase markedly. This in turn removes salt and also dehydrates the person until the pressure falls back to the normal level.

Function of the fluid input–fluid output mechanism for pressure control in the intact animal

In the intact animal an increase in body fluid volume increases fluid output not only because of increased arterial pressure, but also because it activates several other mechanisms that indirectly enhance output. For instance, an increase of the fluid in the blood decreases the plasma colloid osmotic pressure, so that increased amounts of glomerular filtrate are formed and less tubular fluid is reabsorbed; thus more urine is formed. An increase in volume also decreases the rates of renin and aldosterone secretion, which allows the kidneys to excrete additional amounts of water and electrolytes. Because of these factors, as well as others not yet fully characterized, the relationship between arterial pressure and salt and fluid output in the intact animal when the body fluid volume is increased is considerably different from the curve shown in Figure 6 for the isolated kidney. This 'intact' relationship is shown in Figure 7 for salt output which illustrates a very steep curve relating pressure and output, roughly 20 times as steep as the pressure natriuresis curve of Figure 6[18]. The significance of this curve is as follows: in general, an increase in blood volume is eventually associated with an increase in pressure, while a decrease in blood volume will eventually decrease the pressure. Because of the very steep relationship between arterial pressure and the rate of excretion of salt (and water) as shown in Figure 7, even a very slight rise in pressure is associated with extremely rapid loss of extracellular fluid volume and return of the pressure back towards normal. Only a slight decrease in pressure is associated with marked retention of salt and water and, therefore, return of the pressure back towards normal.

The input–output pressure control diagram, and the equilibrium point. Now let us observe the 'intake' curve of Figure 7, which shows the level of salt intake at each respective arterial pressure. This intake is relatively constant in a normal person, though there is reason to believe that reduced arterial pressure will enhance salt intake if the person has full access to electrolytes when his pressure falls. If balance is to be achieved between salt intake and output, then there is only one point on the two curves where the system can continue to operate indefinitely; and this point is where the two curves cross each other, called the *equilibrium point*. One can see immediately that if the pressure rises to a level higher than that represented by the equilibrium point the output will necessarily be greater than the intake, and sooner or later the accumulated body salt as well as the blood volume will decrease, and the pressure will fall until it returns once again to the equilibrium point. Likewise, if the pressure falls below this equilibrium level, the intake will be greater than the output, and the salt and fluid will accumulate until either the arterial pressure rises high enough to reach the equilibrium point or until the person dies from fulminating oedema.

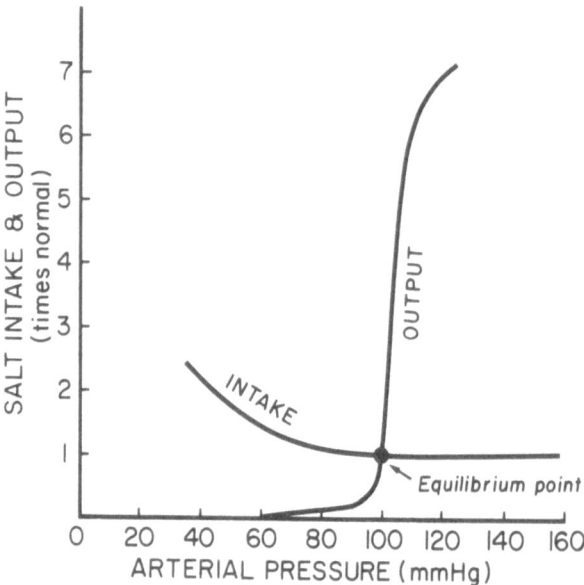

Figure 7 Normal relationship between arterial pressure on the one hand and both salt intake and output on the other hand, illustrating that the intake and output equilibrate at an arterial pressure of 100 mmHg. (The output curve was drawn from data in DeClue et al.[18])

It should be noted again that the relationship between arterial pressure and salt output (and water output as well) is a very steep one. This explains why the arterial pressure is normally controlled within a very narrow range despite tremendous changes in salt intake.

The infinite gain principle of the renal-body fluid pressure feedback control system. A special feature of the fluid intake–output mechanism for pressure control is that the output will never fall to equal input until the pressure decreases *all the way* back to the equilibrium point. Thus, if sufficient time is given for this mechanism to operate fully, it is able to correct the abnormal pressure absolutely and completely. In other words, this feedback control mechanism has *infinite feedback gain*[19-22]. When compared with the feedback gain of 1·6 that has been measured for the baroreceptor system, one can begin to understand the overriding importance of the renal-body fluid mechanism for pressure control.

However, still another feature of this mechanism should also be noted: its effect develops over a period of days and does not take place within seconds or even minutes as is true of the nervous controls. Therefore, it is easily understood why it is the nervous reflexes that provide most of the pressure control in acute situations even though this far more powerful body fluid mechanism becomes the dominant pressure controller over long periods of time.

The two determinants of the arterial pressure level. Another corollary of the above discussion and of the infinite gain principle illustrated by Figure 7 is that there are two independent determinants of the long-term arterial pressure level. These are:

1. The function curve relating arterial pressure and salt and water intake.
2. The function curve relating arterial pressure and salt and water output.

Two other principles of pressure control can also be derived from the infinite gain principle as follows:

A. The long-term level of arterial pressure can be changed only by altering one of the two determinants of the long-term pressure level; that is, by altering the curve relating pressure and intake or the curve relating pressure and output.
B. If a change in either one of the two function curves occurs, then the arterial pressure will automatically readjust over a period of several days to several weeks to the pressure level of the new equilibrium point.

An experimental example showing the effect on the arterial pressure caused by altering the two determinants of arterial pressure control. Figure 8 illustrates a 3-month-long record of the average changes in arterial pressure in four dogs during the following manoeuvres[23]. First, the two poles of one kidney were removed at point A, and then the second kidney was removed at point B. Following this, for a period of 2 weeks, the dogs had approximately 30% normal renal mass, but their average arterial pressure had increased only very slightly, from a normal mean value of 100 mmHg up

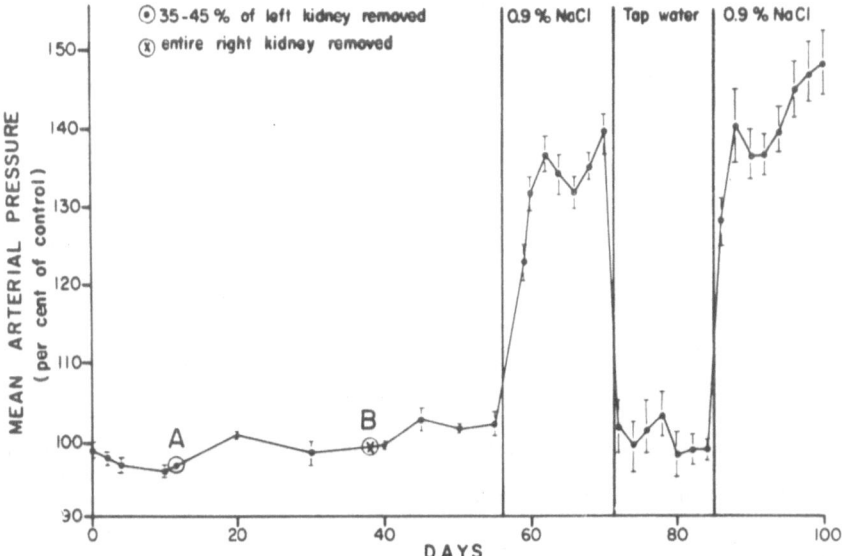

Figure 8 Effect on the mean arterial pressure in four dogs, caused by drinking 0.9% sodium chloride instead of normal drinking water, illustrating two 2-week periods of marked elevation of arterial pressure caused by drinking the saline solution. (Reprinted from Langston *et al.*[23] by permission of the American Heart Association)

to 106 mmHg. At this time the dogs were made to drink salt water instead of normal tap-water. Because the salt water made the dogs very thirsty, they drank about three and one-half times as much fluid as normally. The record shows that the average arterial pressure now rose approximately an additional 35 mmHg and remained elevated for 2 weeks while the dogs continued to drink the salt water. Then the dogs were placed on tap-water again, their intake diminished back to normal, and their pressure also fell back to the normal level. At the end of 2 weeks, a second bout of salt water drinking caused essentially the same effects as the first time.

The experiment of Figure 8 can be analysed graphically in the manner illustrated in Figure 9. Note that the two solid curves are the normal pressure-output curve and normal intake curve. These cross each other at Point A, or at a mean arterial pressure level of 100 mmHg. Reduction of the kidney mass to 30% then changed the output curve to the dashed curve. This new curve now crossed the normal intake curve at Point B, showing a pressure rise of 6 mmHg, the same rise that occurred in the experiment of Figure 8. Next, the animal's salt and water intake were increased to approximately three and one-half times normal, as illustrated by the upper high intake curve in the figure. This crosses the reduced kidney mass output curve at Point C, illustrating an increase in the arterial pressure to approximately 140 mmHg.

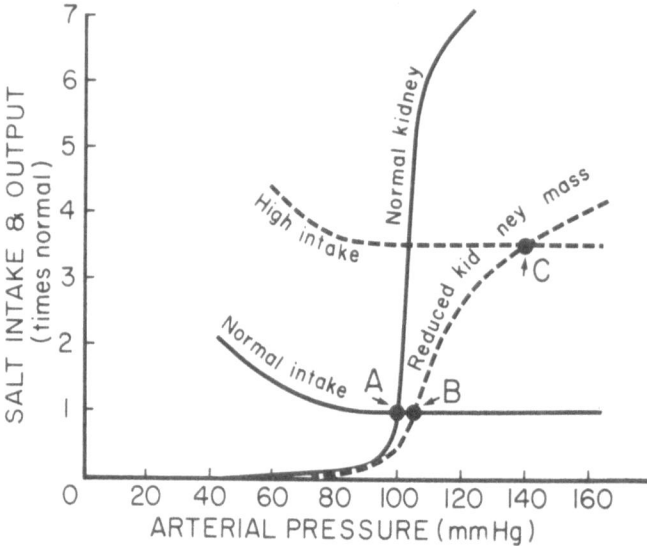

Figure 9 Analysis of the arterial pressure changes, utilizing a standard salt intake–output diagram, for the experiment illustrated in Figure 8. Note that drinking the salt solution caused the pressure to go from point B to point C as explained in the text

Roles of cardiac output and total peripheral resistance in the renal-body fluid mechanism for pressure control
From the foregoing discussions we have been able to see how alterations in body fluid volume can play a major role in pressure control. Yet, thus far,

we have not discussed the mechanisms by which fluid volume changes can cause these effects. The overall mechanism is given by the diagram in Figure 10 which shows the following sequence of events: when the arterial pressure increases, this causes increased renal output of salt and water, which leads to decreased extracellular fluid volume, decreased blood volume, decreased degree of filling of the circulation, decreased venous return, and decreased cardiac output, thus returning the arterial pressure back towards normal. Conversely, when the arterial pressure falls below normal, salt and water output falls below the intake so that the fluid volumes increase, and the venous return and cardiac output also increase until the arterial pressure once again returns to normal.

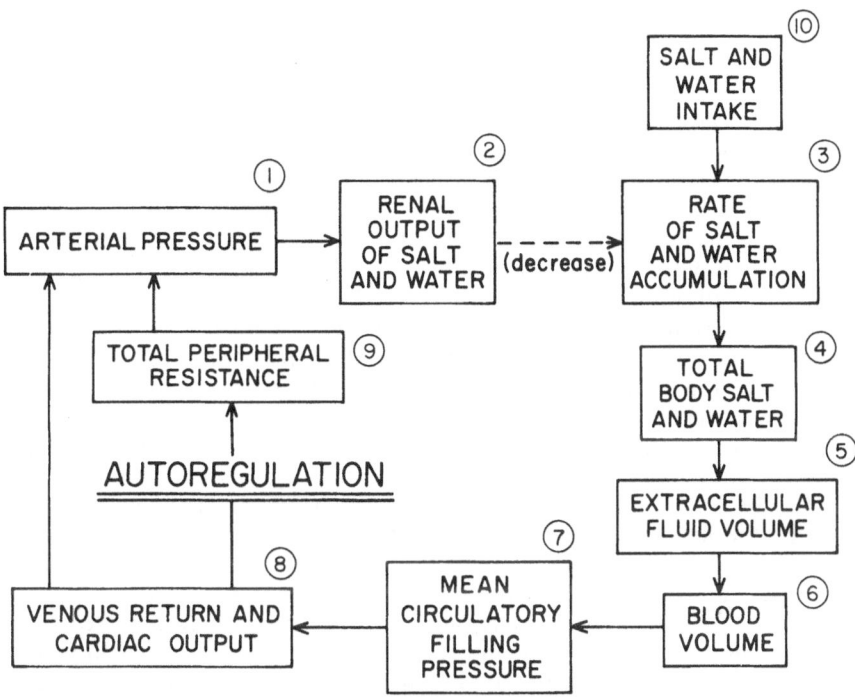

Figure 10 Diagram showing the essential steps in the renal-body fluid mechanism for arterial pressure control

However, there is still another important step in this sequence of events: this is the effect of the cardiac output on total peripheral resistance. Note in Figure 10 that an increase in cardiac output is shown to cause an increase in total peripheral resistance and, by the same token, a decrease in cardiac output to cause a decrease in total peripheral resistance. This phenomenon is known as *autoregulation* because the change in resistance automatically returns the cardiac output towards its normal level. However, this effect occurs only slowly, over a period of days or even several weeks.

Thus, when the blood volume increases and this in turn increases the cardiac output, the arterial pressure is increased in two different ways: (1) the increase in cardiac output directly increases arterial pressure; and (2) the effect of increased cardiac output to increase the total peripheral resistance indirectly increases the arterial pressure. Immediately after an acute change in blood volume, essentially all of the early increase in arterial pressure results from cardiac output. On the other hand, the available evidence indicates that over several days to several weeks the direct component of the increase in arterial pressure becomes very little, while the indirect effect acting through increased total peripheral resistance becomes by far the more important way in which the increase in cardiac output increases arterial pressure. To illustrate this point let us discuss an actual experiment in which fluid accumulated in the body of an animal and the arterial pressure increased by utilizing both the direct and the indirect methods for increasing arterial pressure.

Transient changes in cardiac output, total peripheral resistance, and other factors following an acute increase in body fluid volume. Figure 11 illustrates an experiment performed in a similar manner to that discussed for Figure 8[24]. That is, the kidney mass was decreased to 30% of normal in a group of six dogs, and the dogs were then overloaded with water and salt. However, these experiments were different from those in Figure 8 in the following way: instead of allowing the dogs simply to drink salt water, saline solution was infused intravenously at a rate of approximately 2 litres per day for the first 6 days of the experiment and then at a rate of 3 litres per day for the remaining 7 days. Figure 11 illustrates the sequential changes in right atrial pressure, stroke volume output, cardiac output, arterial pressure, heart rate, and total peripheral resistance. Note that the right atrial pressure increased 3–4 mmHg, and the stroke volume output increased an average of 70%. On the other hand, the total peripheral resistance and the heart rate actually decreased during the first few days; in subsequent experiments of this same type in which the baroreceptor nerves had been removed, neither the decrease in heart rate nor the decrease in total peripheral resistance occurred, indicating that both of these effects were attempts by the baroreceptor feedback mechanism to prevent the rise in pressure. Note also in Figure 11 that after the first few days of decreased total peripheral resistance, the total peripheral resistance then began to rise while the cardiac output returned towards normal. At the end of 2 weeks, the total peripheral resistance had risen 30%, and the cardiac output was then only 5% above normal. In other similar experiments we showed that extracellular fluid volume and blood volume increased about 30% during the first few days, but at the end of 2 weeks both of these were so near to normal that it was difficult to prove a significantly elevated extracellular fluid volume or blood volume[25,26].

Thus, in this experiment it is clear that the initial rise in arterial pressure was caused entirely by an elevated cardiac output. Then the total peripheral resistance increased while the cardiac output returned towards normal. Therefore, the increase in total peripheral resistance occurred *after* the rise in pressure and not before the rise. Or, to express this in terms of control system principles, the rise in total peripheral resistance *lagged* the rise in

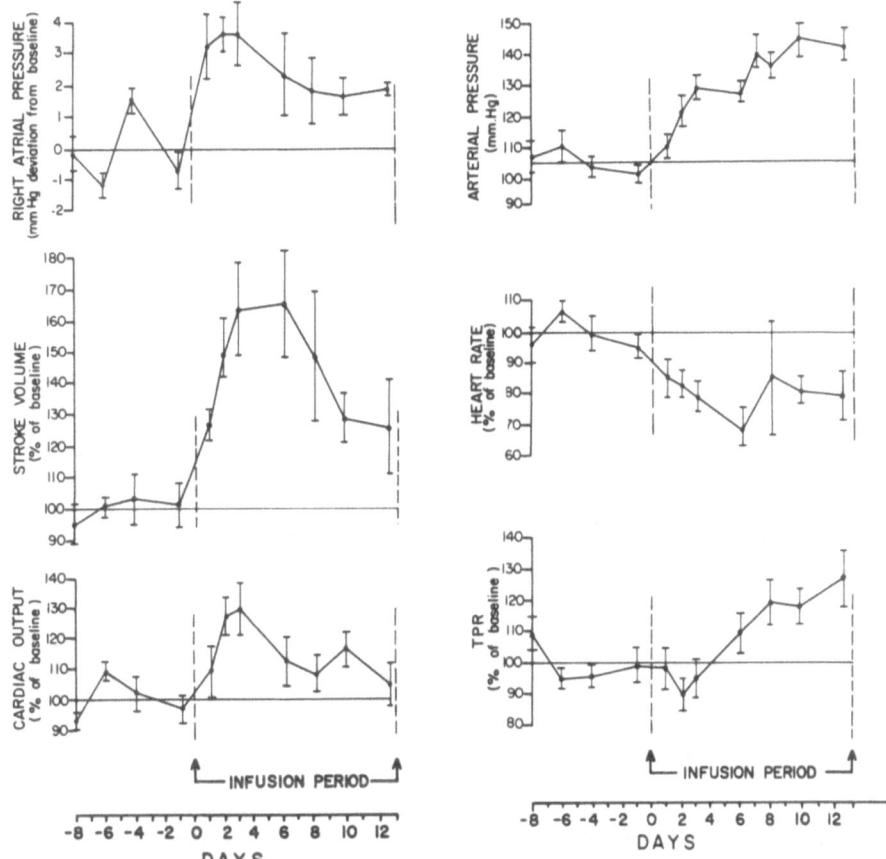

Figure 11 Changes in six circulatory variables in a series of six partially nephrectomized dogs during the course of infusion of isotonic saline solution; approximately 2 litres per day were infused for the first 6 days and then approximately 3 litres per day for the remainder of the experiment. Note the early transient rise in stroke volume output and cardiac output when the arterial pressure first rose but the late sustained rise in total peripheral resistance. (Reprinted from Coleman and Guyton[24] by permission of the American Heart Association)

arterial pressure rather than leading the arterial pressure. Therefore, the evidence from these experiments shows that the rise in total peripheral resistance was not the cause of the rise in arterial pressure. Instead, the importance of the rise in total peripheral resistance was that it caused the blood flow through the tissues to return essentially to normal after the hypertension had developed. Had it not been for this rise in total peripheral resistance, the cardiac output would have remained elevated indefinitely and the tissues would have been perfused indefinitely with more blood than they actually required for their nutritive or other needs. It is this decrease in cardiac output to the normal level which is called autoregulation.

Another feature of the autoregulation phenomenon is that, at the same time that it occurs, the extracellular fluid volume and the blood volume both decrease to a point so near to normal that the available measurement methods usually cannot show abnormal blood volume nor abnormal extracellular fluid volume by 2 weeks after the onset of volume loading hypertension.

Volume loading hypertension is a high resistance type of hypertension. One of the lessons to be learned from the above experiment is that after volume loading hypertension has become fully developed, neither the blood and extracellular volumes nor the cardiac output are elevated to abnormal levels but are distinctly within the normal ranges. On the other hand, the total peripheral resistance is greatly elevated. Thus, volume loading hypertension is a high-resistance type of hypertension. Consequently, when one studies a person who is already hypertensive when first seen and finds a high total peripheral resistance, there is no way to be sure whether this high resistance was a primary event in the development of the hypertension or a secondary effect of the hypertension and subsequent autoregulation.

The autoregulation mechanism multiplies the effect of cardiac output on arterial pressure. Let us assume that the cardiac output increases 10%. This by itself could directly increase the arterial pressure also by 10%, or from 100 mmHg up to 110 mmHg. But, now let us assume that the 10% increase in cardiac output causes a 40% increase in total peripheral resistance (which is approximately what did occur in the experiment illustrated in Figure 11). Then this would cause still another 40% increase in arterial pressure. And 40% increase times 110% gives a total increase to 154% of normal. That is, a 10% increase in cardiac output would thus result in a rise in pressure from 100 mmHg to 154 mmHg.

To what extent can the autoregulation phenomenon multiply the pressure effect of increased cardiac output? Thus far, no experiment has definitely proved how much the autoregulation mechanism can contribute to the rise in pressure when the cardiac output is increased. However, there is one very significant natural experiment in human beings that indicates that the autoregulation effect can be extremely powerful. This is the natural occurrence of coarctation of the aorta. Wakim found that the blood flow in the arms of patients with coarctation of the aorta was almost exactly identical to that in normal human beings despite the fact that the blood pressure in the upper part of the body of patients with coarctation was about 50% greater than in the normal persons[27]. He also found that the blood flows in the lower part of the body were also essentially the same as in normal persons. Thus, his results indicated that the autoregulation phenomenon is almost perfect in adjusting the blood flow to the needs of the tissues, irrespective of what happens to the arterial pressure. If this be true, then it means that the rise in cardiac output that is required to increase the arterial pressure very large amounts would be almost infinitesimal, and would certainly be unmeasurable. Thus, one can easily understand from such results as these why the renal-body fluid mechanism for blood pressure control does not normally cause, after all adjustments have been made, either a significantly elevated cardiac output nor a significantly elevated blood volume. The failure to find elevations of these two factors in many types of hypertension, therefore, seems to have been a delusory effect in leading many investigators in the hypertension field to ignore fluid volume as a powerful factor in pressure control.

Some examples of abnormal pressure control by the renal-body fluid mechanism: some mechanisms for the causation of hypertension

Let us now return to the infinite gain principle discussed earlier in this paper for the renal-body fluid mechanism of pressure regulation. This states that the arterial pressure will always adjust itself to exactly that point where the output curve crosses the intake curve, as illustrated by the intake–output diagram shown in Figure 7. Keeping this principle in mind, let us see what would happen to the arterial pressure should either the output curve or the intake curve or both become abnormal.

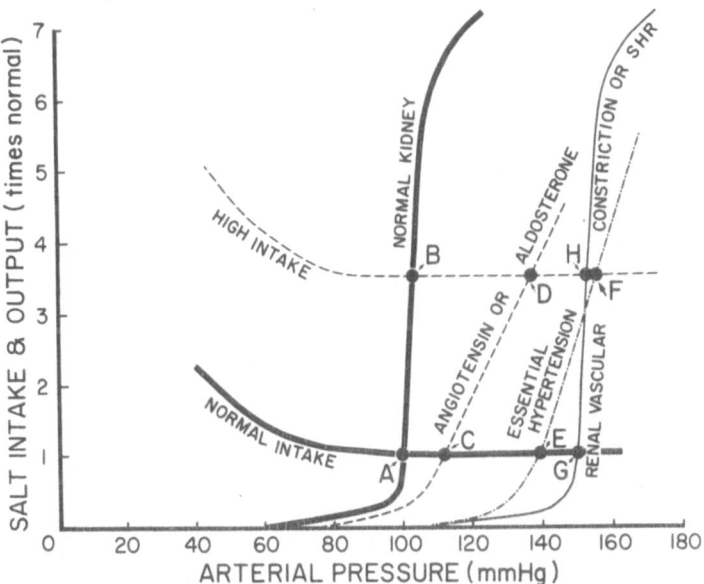

Figure 12 Analysis of several different types of hypertension using the standard salt intake–output diagram. Explained in the text

Figure 12 illustrates several different salt output curves and two different salt intake curves. Comparable curves representing water intake and output can also be drawn, and the principles are the same as for the salt curves because the water curves usually change in similar ways. The very dark curves are the normal salt output curve and the normal salt intake curve. In addition, there are three additional output curves labelled, respectively: 'renal vascular constriction or SHR'[28], 'Essential hypertension'[21], and 'angiotensin or aldosterone'[18]. These curves illustrate the manner in which each one of these conditions alters the relationship between arterial pressure and salt output. Also, the 'reduced kidney mass' curve of Figure 9 depicts the effects of loss of kidney tissue. All of these curves have been measured in the same way as that described for Figure 7 except for the curve labelled 'essential hypertension'. This curve has instead been drawn from data in the literature. Note that all of the curves are either rotated or shifted towards high-pressure levels. However, note also that one of the curves is very steep, the 'renal vascular constriction' curve, while the 'angiotensin or aldosterone' curve slopes upwards more gently. Because of the steep nature of the curve in Goldblatt animals (vascular constriction) and spontaneously hypertensive rats (SHR), the output and intake curves equilibrate with each other at hypertensive levels with both normal and high intake levels, 150 and 154 mmHg respectively (Points G and H). On the other hand, in animals receiving small amounts of angiotensin or large amounts of aldosterone the arterial pressure is normal (Point C) when the fluid and salt intake is normal but is quite hypertensive, 138 mmHg (Point D), when the salt intake increases.

Thus, one can see that if the nature of the renal function curve is known in each abnormal condition and the fluid intake level is also known, one can predict from the intake–output diagram what the eventual level of the arterial pressure will be. This diagram does not state how the pressure will get to the level at which the two curves cross, it simply states that it will get there or otherwise the animal will die. The increase in pressure might result from increased cardiac output alone. It might result from increased cardiac output followed by autoregulation that leads to increased total peripheral resistance. It might result from some hormonal change such as excess activity of the renin–angiotensin system or of the aldosterone mechanism. Or it might result from nervous stimulation of the peripheral vessels.

Failure of increased total peripheral resistance per se *to cause hypertension.* It is now clear from a considerable number of clinical conditions, as well as from experimental animal studies, that a primary increase in total peripheral resistance that does not involve changing either the intake curve or the renal function curve will not cause hypertension. For instance, opening or closing arteriovenous fistulae causes only temporary changes in arterial pressure. Thus, in a large series of human beings in which large arteriovenous fistulae were closed surgically, Warren and his colleagues were unable to find a significant change in arterial pressure[29]. Likewise, in human beings with all four limbs removed, the arterial pressure does not change even though the total peripheral resistance increases to about 160% of normal. And in several clinical conditions in which the total peripheral resistance is decreased far below normal – thyrotoxicosis, Paget's disease, pregnancy, and beriberi – the arterial pressure is not decreased below normal. Indeed, in some of these, if anything, it might be slightly increased.

On the other hand, when the kidney vessels are constricted at the same time that the peripheral resistance elsewhere increases, this often leads to an altered renal function curve and at the same time leads to persistent hypertension. As examples, infusion of either angiotensin or noradrenaline continuously over a period of many days leads to persistent hypertension. Also, it has been shown that infusion of either of these into the renal artery causes considerably more hypertension than does infusion intravenously. Therefore, once again, the principle that either the fluid intake curve or the renal function curve must be changed before hypertension can develop still holds true.

Role of the renin–angiotensin system in arterial pressure control
Thus far we have spoken hardly at all about the role of the renin–angiotensin system in arterial pressure control. However, this mechanism is well known to be exceedingly important in many instances of renal hypertension as well as perhaps in some patients with essential hypertension, particularly so-called 'high renin' hypertension.

In certain renal vascular abnormalities, in certain other types of renal lesions, in dehydration, and in salt deprivation, the kidneys secrete large amounts of renin which in turn cause the production of large amounts of angiotensin. And the angiotensin in turn has several important effects on arterial pressure.

Most investigators in the field of arterial pressure regulation have suggested that angiotensin causes hypertension as a result of its primary effect of increasing total peripheral resistance. However, we pointed out earlier that very severe changes in total peripheral resistance caused by such effects as arteriovenous fistulae, beriberi, thyrotoxicosis, Paget's disease, or removal of all four limbs of a person do not in any one of these instances alter the arterial pressure significantly. Therefore, we now know that it is naive to believe that a simple increase in total peripheral resistance alone will cause chronic hypertension. In fact, if the kidney blood vessels are not involved in the increased resistance, the long-term pressure level will not rise at all because any attempt of the pressure to rise will cause pressure diuresis and natriuresis and return of the arterial pressure to normal.

On the other hand, there is another effect of angiotensin that can explain its effect of causing long-term elevation of the arterial pressure. This is an effect of angiotensin on the kidney itself. Figure 13 illustrates experimental results which show the effect on the renal function curve caused by continuous infusion of only 5 ng/kg/min of angiotensin, an amount of angiotensin that increased the circulating angiotensin level approximately three-fold[18]. This amount is often exceeded many times over in pathological states in which the renin–angiotensin system is activated. Note the marked shift of the renal function curve to the right, which indicates that at all levels of salt intake, but especially at high levels of intake, hypertension would result.

Experiments have shown this effect of angiotensin on the kidneys to be caused about seven-eighths by a direct effect on the kidneys to decrease salt excretion and about one-eighth by the effect of angiotensin in stimulating aldosterone secretion, which then in turn also decreases sodium excretion[30,31].

Circulatory effects of arteriolar constriction when the renin–angiotensin system is activated. If the increase in peripheral vascular resistance is not a final *determinant* of the pressure level when hypertension results from activation

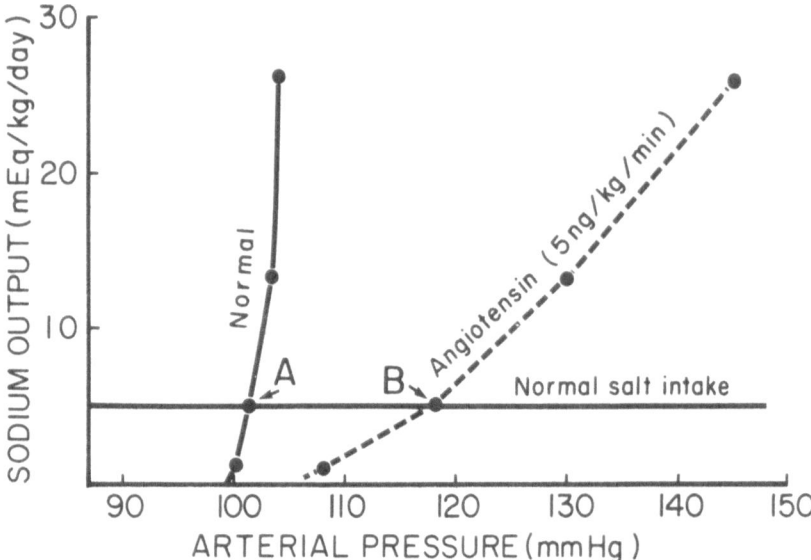

Figure 13 Effect of infusing angiotensin at a very low rate on the relationship between arterial pressure and renal sodium output. (Drawn from data in DeClue *et al.*[18])

of the renin–angiotensin system, what then is the role of the arteriolar constriction? The answer to this seems to be the following:

When angiotensin is infused for long periods of time into an animal, it causes a considerable amount of continued increase in peripheral arteriolar constriction. At first, this will increase the arterial pressure. Thus, the angiotensin-induced arteriolar constriction is a *modus operandi* for causing pressure increase. Yet, it is important to differentiate between a *modus operandi* and a *determinant* of the final level at which the pressure will stabilize. If the angiotensin should not in any way affect kidney function or salt and water intake, then the initial rise in pressure caused by arteriolar constriction would quickly cause pressure diuresis and natriuresis, which would return the arterial pressure to the normal level. However, the angiotensin also shifts the renal function curve to a higher pressure level as illustrated in Figure 13 at the same time that it constricts the peripheral arterioles, and this is the effect of the angiotensin that determines the level at which the pressure will eventually stabilize. Thus, even though the renin–angiotensin system provides the *modus operandi* for the initial rise in pressure by constricting the peripheral arterioles, it *determines* the eventual pressure level by shifting the renal function curve. If the arterial pressure rise resulting from the initial arteriolar constriction is high enough to provide balance between intake and output as required by the intake–output pressure diagram after shift of the renal function curve, then no further adjustments are required. But, if the pressure level provided by the arteriolar constriction is either too low or too high, then the volume mechanism will make whatever final adjustments are required to stabilize the pressure at the equilibrium point. Thus, the eventual blood volume may be low or high, depending on the ratio of (a) the arteriolar vasoconstriction to (b) the shift of the renal function curve[32].

An important principle is thus illustrated: the renal-body fluid mechanism for pressure control is the final arbiter of the level to which the arterial pressure will stabilize. Yet, on the other hand, this mechanism does not care how the pressure gets to the required level. It may get there by renin-angiotensin peripheral vasoconstriction or in any other way. But, if the pressure fails to get there, fluid volume will be readjusted automatically until such time that the pressure does reach that required level, or until such time that the person dies of oedema or dehydration. In other words, the renal-body fluid mechanism stands in the background awaiting the results of whatever other mechanisms might make initial adjustments in the arterial pressure. Then it provides the final adjustments that are necessary. These adjustments may be very minor if the other mechanisms have subserved the role of pressure control satisfactorily, in which case there will be essentially no changes in fluid volume, or the role of the renal-fluid volume system might be very considerable if the other controls play no role or play too much role. *Yet, still, it is the fluid intake–fluid output pressure control system that makes the final determination of the eventual stable pressure level, because of its infinite gain feature.*

Pumping capability of the heart as a limiting factor to the upper level of arterial pressure control

The reader should be already well aware that all we have said about the renal-body fluid mechanism for pressure control has presumed that the heart is capable of achieving whatever pressure level is required by the control system. Obviously, if the heart is not capable of pumping the required amounts of blood against the required pressure level, then, of course, the pressure control system will fail. But let us now stop for a moment to consider what this means: it means simply that the circulation has gone into the state of decompensated failure. That is, the pressure control system is demanding that the arterial pressure rise to a certain level before the fluid output will become equal to the fluid intake. If this pressure level cannot be reached, then the output will remain indefinitely below the intake, and fluid will accumulate progressively in the body until death occurs or until some therapeutic procedure is instituted to achieve balance. One of the best-known therapeutic procedures is administration of a diuretic. And if one will think for a moment one will realize that a diuretic shifts the renal function curve to a lower pressure level, thus allowing the circulatory system to achieve a balance between output and intake.

Capillary fluid balance as a limit to the upper level for arterial pressure control – role of the interstitium as a safety factor against excessive arterial pressures

Another factor that limits the level to which arterial pressure can rise is the limited ability of the tissue capillaries to retain fluid in the blood despite a rising arterial pressure. This is illustrated by the experiment of Figure 14 which shows the effect of massive blood transfusion into three separate

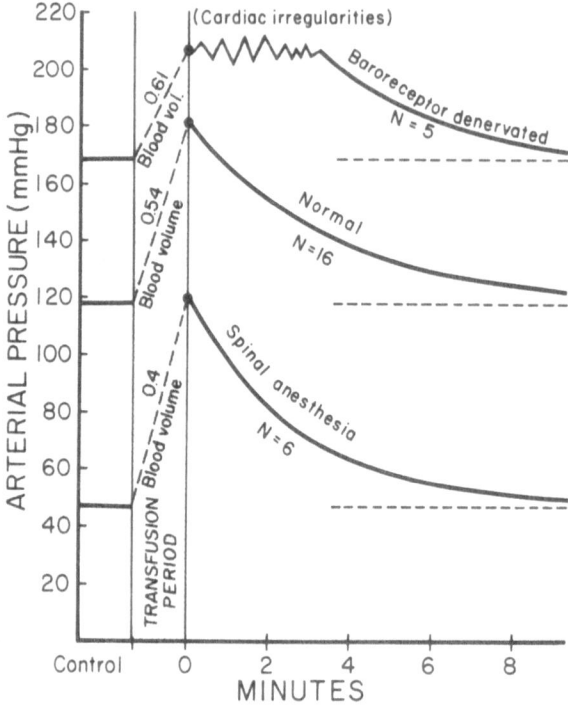

Figure 14 Effect of massive transfusion of blood into each of three different groups of dogs, each having a different level of sympathetic tone. This figure illustrates that the degree of sympathetic tone determines the maximum level at which the pressure stabilizes despite massive volume loading. (Drawn from data in Guyton *et al.*[33])

groups of dogs in three different physiological states: (1) the normal dog; (2) the dog after acute denervation of the baroreceptors so that the sympathetic nervous system was highly activated and the arteriolar tone was great; and (3) after institution of total spinal anaesthesia so that the sympathetic nervous system was totally inactivated and the arteriolar tone was greatly reduced[33]. Note that after administering the massive transfusions up to about 50% of the original blood volume the arterial pressures at first rose far above the control level in each instance. However, during the next 10 or more minutes, the arterial pressure returned essentially to the original control level. In each instance the cause of the return to the previous pressure level was rapid filtration of fluid outward through the capillary membranes and into the interstitium. Note especially that the more the capillary was protected from the arterial pressure by increasing arteriolar tone, the greater was the level at which the arterial pressure stabilized.

It is very clear from the experiment of Figure 14 that it is impossible to maintain a greatly elevated arterial pressure in the absence of a significant degree of arteriolar tone to protect the capillaries from the excess pressure. Therefore, whatever has been said about the renal-body fluid mechanism for regulating arterial pressure applies only to the long-term regulation of the arterial pressure below this limiting pressure level set by the capillary-fluid 'overflow' phenomenon.

Significance of the capillary-fluid overflow phenomenon in acute volume overload. It is well known that acute volume overload rarely causes a significant elevation of arterial pressure. What happens instead is that the arterial pressure remains elevated for only a few minutes after an instantaneous massive infusion of fluid, because most of the fluid leaves the circulation within minutes, overflowing into the interstitium while the arterial pressure returns essentially to normal[34]. Then, during the following few hours, the kidneys normally excrete this volume so that the pressure never rises more than a few mmHg. On the other hand, in animals in which the kidneys are not present to excrete this extra fluid volume, the blood pressure slowly rises during the next 24 h up to very hypertensive levels, sometimes rising as much as 40 mmHg in the 24 h period. The secondary rise in pressure is caused by several factors: first, the lymph flow from the tissues increases markedly, which subsequently transfers large quantities of protein from the interstitial spaces into the blood. The increased plasma colloid osmotic pressure provided by this extra protein now makes it possible for the circulation to retain much more fluid than previously, thus helping to promote hypertension. Second, adaptation of the baroreceptors nullifies the initial baroreflex dilatation of the arterioles that occurs when the blood volume is first increased. This allows increased arteriolar tone which therefore further protects the capillaries from the rising pressure and increases the upper limit to the arterial pressure before fluid spills into the interstitium. Third, autoregulation of local tissue blood flow with its attendant increase in arteriolar resistance also makes it possible to retain considerably larger quantities of fluid in the circulation.

In other words, the limitation on the arterial pressure level caused by the capillary fluid overflow mechanism is very important to prevent an initial rise in arterial pressure every time a person ingests large amounts of water and electrolytes. Yet, if the excess fluid volume persists for longer than a few hours, this limit itself increases for several reasons, and the arterial pressure does then rise.

SUMMARY OF ARTERIAL PRESSURE CONTROL

From the above discussions, one will see that we have emphasized very strongly the role of body fluid volumes in the long-term regulation of arterial pressure. Yet, on the other hand, we have also emphasized that acute regulation of arterial pressure during the first few minutes or even few hours of stressful states is almost entirely a nervous phenomenon. There are also special reflex mechanisms and a capillary fluid overflow mechanism to prevent acute changes in fluid volume from affecting the arterial pressure very much. For these reasons, it is only over a period of several hours to several days that fluid volume changes have very significant effects on arterial pressure. Yet, the renal-body fluid mechanism for pressure control still remains in the background as the principal long-term controller of arterial pressure because of its eventual infinite gain feature.

Control of blood flow in the local tissues: the second essential for circulatory regulation

Nearly all physiologists and clinicians are familiar with the fact that blood flow in each different tissue is controlled very precisely in accord with that tissue's physiological needs. However, certain quantitative aspects of local blood flow control are not so widely known. Therefore, let us discuss a few of these.

Basically, there are two different mechanisms for control of tissue blood flow in relation to the physiological needs of the body. One of these is extrinsic regulation of tissue blood flow by either nervous or hormonal influences. The other mechanism is intrinsic regulation of flow by the local needs of the tissues themselves – this is the phenomenon called tissue blood flow autoregulation which we have already alluded to in relation to pressure control. Let us first discuss this autoregulation mechanism of the tissues themselves to control their own blood flows.

TISSUE BLOOD FLOW AUTOREGULATION

In numerous studies of tissue blood flow it has been shown repeatedly that the blood flow in each tissue almost invariably is barely that amount which will perform the necessary physiological role of the flow – almost never excess flow and almost never a deficit of flow in relation to the tissue needs[35]. Obviously, a deficit could lead to serious disruption of tissue function. On the other hand, an excess of tissue flow would lead to excess return of blood to the heart, excess cardiac output, and excess workload on the heart. Thus, it seems to be an essential principle of cardiovascular regulation that the tissues protect themselves against deficit of blood flow but at the same time protect the heart against unnecessary excess blood flow.

Metabolic control of local blood flow – metabolic autoregulation. In most tissues the physiological need for blood flow is mainly to supply nutrients to the tissues and also to remove excreta. Therefore, it is very significant that experiments have shown these metabolic needs of the tissues to be among the most important of all controllers of local tissue blood flow. In most tissues, the need for oxygen is the most potent of the control effects[36,37]. Whenever there is a deficiency of oxygen, the blood vessels automatically dilate within a few seconds and therefore allow greatly increased blood flow to the tissues with consequent delivery of increased quantities of oxygen.

However, oxygen deficiency is not the only nutritional deficiency that can lead to increased blood flow. Experiments have even shown that decreased glucose in a perfusion medium of an isolated perfused tissue will lead over a period of 5–15 min to vascular dilatation and consequent increased blood flow, presumably for the purpose of delivering increased glucose or other metabolic substrates to the tissues[38]. It is also very significant that tissues deprived of vitamin B, as occurs in the disease beriberi, develop extreme vasodilatation, presumably also for the purpose of relieving the deficiency state[39]. Also, administration of cyanide to an animal will cause marked peripheral vasodilatation[40].

The mechanism of the increased blood flow in nutritionally deficient tissues is still questionable. Some investigators believe that the deficiency state itself simply allows relaxation of the arterioles because of insufficient nutrients to maintain contraction[36]. Other investigators believe that deficiency leads to generation of vasodilator substances in these tissues (such as release of adenosine in oxygen deficient tissues) which in turn causes active vasodilatation[37]. In either event, the result is the same: the deficiency sets into play a typical negative feedback control system to try to relieve the deficiency.

Another aspect of metabolic autoregulation is the ability of various cellular excreta to cause vasodilatation. For instance, excess carbon dioxide or hydrogen ions in the tissues will lead to vascular dilatation; and perhaps other substances will as well, such as urea, uric acid, and so forth. As an example, carbon dioxide excess is the major metabolic controller of blood flow in the brain[41], even though oxygen deficiency is the more important excitant for blood flow control in most other tissues.

The special autoregulatory mechanism of the kidneys. Under normal resting conditions, approximately one-fifth of the cardiac output flows through the kidneys. Also, it is significant that the autoregulatory mechanism of the kidneys is considerably different from that elsewhere in the body. In general, this mechanism hardly responds to local metabolic changes in the kidneys. Instead, it responds primarily to the need of the kidneys to excrete certain substances. For instance, prolonged elevation of urea, amino acids, and other nitrogenous products will lead to progressive increase in renal blood flow. An increase in sodium intake will do the same, and certain hormones, such as aldosterone, will alter the long-term level of renal blood flow. In each instance, this seems to be related to the rate at which the renal tubules can process the electrolytes and waste products while forming urine. When the glomerular filtration rate is too little or too great, the concentrations of these substances at the macula densa in the initial portion of the distal tubule change, and feedback responses to the afferent and efferent arterioles automatically control both renal blood flow and glomerular filtration rate. Recent studies indicate that there are at least two separate feedbacks, one of which controls the afferent arterioles and the other the efferent arterioles[42,43]. Without at this time going into the nature of these feedback controls, one can readily see that, once again, the control of blood flow is primarily in response to the local physiological needs of this tissue to perform its homeostatic functions for the body.

Autoregulation of blood flow during increased tissue activity. One of the important features of local tissue blood flow autoregulation is that this mechanism provides for automatic increase in blood flow whenever local tissue activity increases. Thus, even increased brain activity can increase brain blood flow as much as 50%; most significant of all, increases in muscle activity can often increase blood flow in local muscle areas as much as 10–20-fold.

Presumably the mechanisms that adjust blood flows when the arterial pressure changes, are the same mechanisms that make the blood flow adjustments during increased tissue activity. For instance, when the tissue activity increases, the metabolic needs of the tissues increase so that a relative deficiency of oxygen develops immediately. This could easily be the initiating stimulus for the increase in blood flow. Yet the detailed mechanisms, in general, are still a matter of dispute.

Feedback gains of the autoregulatory control mechanisms
The potency of the local blood flow control mechanisms to maintain the tissue blood flows at the levels required for proper tissue function can be expressed in terms of feedback gains. If the blood flow is maintained precisely at the level required despite extraneous factors tending to change the flow, such as a change in arterial pressure, then the feedback gain of the system is said to be infinity. If the control system is capable of decreasing the flow variation in response to a change in pressure to one-half the uncontrolled variation, then the feedback gain is 1·0. If it can decrease the variation to one-third of the uncontrolled variation, then the feedback gain is 2·0, and so forth in accordance with the equation that was presented earlier in this paper.

Many studies of the autoregulatory feedback gain of renal blood flow have shown that this gain approaches infinity when the arterial pressure is altered within the normal operating range[15-17,42,43]. That is, the changes in arterial pressure have almost no measurable effect on renal blood flow. On the other hand, in most tissues of the body, an acute change in arterial pressure will cause an acute change in blood flow almost proportional to the change in pressure. Yet, over a period of many minutes[44], and especially over a period of many days, the long-term autoregulatory mechanisms will eventually adjust the blood flow almost completely to its original control level despite the pressure change. For instance, Folkow and his co-workers have shown that constriction of the femoral artery in a rat leads, over a period of several weeks, to marked peripheral vasodilatation, thus returning the blood flow in the limb towards normal[45]. And the studies quoted earlier in this paper regarding coarctation of the aorta[27] have shown that the blood flow in the high pressure area of patients with coarctation of the aorta is almost exactly normal, as is also true of the flow in the low-pressure area. Thus, the data that are available at present suggest that local blood flow control by the mechanism of autoregulation operates in almost all instances at very high feedback gains.

EXTRINSIC CONTROL OF TISSUE BLOOD FLOW
We are all so familiar with the extrinsic controls of tissue blood flow mediated through nervous and hormonal systems that we need to say very little about these. But again, some aspects of their quantitative importance need to be emphasized.

Nervous controls
The nervous controls of local blood flow generally subserve some function that is especially important to the entire body rather than to the local tissues. Among these functions are the following:

1. Control of body temperature mediated by signals from the hypothalamic area of the brain to the skin blood vessels.
2. Acute control of arterial pressure initiated by the baroreceptors or other nervous receptors that elicit sympathetic reflexes.
3. Sympathetic vasoconstriction throughout the body in response to such effects as exercise, rage, excitement, anxiety, haemorrhage, and so forth.
4. Strong vagal stimuli to the heart in certain types of fainting.

The nervous signals to the peripheral circulation can be very powerful for many hours at a time. However, in most tissues the local autoregulatory mechanisms can eventually override or at least partly override the nervous signals, particularly when the nervous signals cause serious local dysfunction. For instance, strong sympathetic stimulation of the intestine leads immediately to almost total cessation of blood flow. But, within a matter of minutes, the blood flow returns essentially to normal, despite continued sympathetic stimulation[46]. Likewise, strong sympathetic stimulation to the kidneys can decrease renal output to as little as 10% of normal activity, but over a period of half an hour or more, the renal blood flow returns almost to normal despite continued sympathetic stimulation[47]. Also, the local autoregulatory vasodilator response that occurs in muscles when they are activated during exercise can entirely or almost entirely override the sympathetic vasoconstrictor effect.

Yet, despite the ability of local autoregulatory mechanisms to override the vasoconstrictor signals, the fact that these signals can constrict some blood vessels, such as the skin blood vessels and some of the splanchnic vessels for many minutes, or perhaps even hours, at a time allows temporary diversion of blood flow from these areas to areas that have more immediate need. For instance, during exercise, blood flow is diverted into the muscles; and during circulatory shock, a major share of the blood flow is diverted to the heart and brain.

Hormonal Controls
Among the more important hormonal controllers of the circulation are the catecholamines and angiotensin. In general, the catecholamines play almost the same role as the sympathetic nervous system in circulatory control. In experiments in our laboratory we have found that circulating noradrenaline under some conditions will increase the cardiac output, but at other times will have little effect or will even decrease the cardiac output. The reason for these differences seems to be that noradrenaline has two effects on tissue blood flow each opposing the other. That is, a direct effect on the blood vessels tends to constrict the vessels, but noradrenaline also increases local tissue metabolism which induces a secondary vasodilatation. These often balance each other, or at other times one of them prevails.

In the case of angiotensin, Young and his associates have demonstrated that prolonged infusion of angiotensin over a period of a week will decrease cardiac output by as much as 30%[32]. Thus, the vasoconstrictor effect of angiotensin seems to be a potent one that can lead to long-term depression of local blood flow despite the undoubted attempts of the local autoregulatory mechanisms to overcome the vasoconstrictor effect of angiotensin. Therefore, in the case of angiotensin, and perhaps also in the case of other vasoconstrictor substances, the long-term level of local blood flow can be decreased below the normal control level. This does not mean that the autoregulatory mechanisms are not still functional. Without these mechanisms, one would reasonably expect that the vasoconstrictor effects might decrease blood flow much more. For instance, acute infusion of noradrenaline or angiotensin into an isolated tissue can sometimes decrease blood flow to as little as a few per cent of normal. Yet, even massive infusion of either of these two hormones intravenously over a period of days to weeks will rarely decrease the total body flow – the cardiac output – more than 30%. Consequently, one can be quite certain that the local tissue autoregulatory mechanisms are still functioning. However, what has happened is that the continual vasoconstrictor effect of the hormone has *biased* the control blood flow to a lower than normal control level. When this occurs, increased activity of the tissues will increase the blood flow to a level above this new control value, but when the tissue activity returns to normal the autoregulatory mechanism will bring the flow back to this depressed control level. Conversely, a decrease in blood flow below the depressed control level will elicit autoregulatory feedback to bring the flow up to the depressed control level but not up to the normal level.

To state this principle still another way, hormones can change the control level to which the autoregulatory mechanism adjusts the local blood flow, sometimes in a downward direction and sometimes in an upward direction, depending on the nature of the hormone.

CONTROL OF CARDIAC OUTPUT

At the beginning of this chapter, it was pointed out that the two essentials of cardiovascular control are: (1) control of arterial pressure; and (2) control of local tissue blood flow. But nothing was said about control of cardiac output. Fortunately, if both of the two essentials are met, then cardiac output will automatically be controlled. Let us examine this more fully:

Cardiac output as a sum of the local tissue blood flows. It is a simple mathematical axiom that cardiac output is equal to the sum of the blood flows in all the local tissues. Therefore, one can also state that cardiac output control is equal to the sum of all the controls of all of the blood flows in all the local tissues. And this control results from, first, maintenance of an adequate arterial pressure by the arterial pressure control mechanisms and, second, intrinsic and extrinsic control of the blood flows in the respective tissues. When the local tissues demand excessive amounts of flow, the overall cardiac output must change accordingly. This is achieved mainly by vasodilatation in the active tissues. Yet, it is absolutely essential that the arterial pressure control mechanisms play their role as well, to maintain or sometimes even to elevate the arterial pressure if the cardiac output is able to rise high enough to supply the demands of the tissues. Therefore, let us examine the role of arterial pressure control as a permissive factor in cardiac output control.

Importance of arterial pressure control when excesses of cardiac output are required

When large proportions of the body tissues vasodilate simultaneously, the total peripheral resistance becomes greatly decreased. Consequently, under these conditions it is absolutely impossible for the arterial pressure to be maintained at a high level by increasing the total peripheral resistance. Consequently, the pressure to be maintained at a high level by increasing the total peripheral resistance. Consequently, the pressure must be maintained in another way. The mechanism by which this is achieved is two-fold. First, sympathetic nerve signals constrict the capacitance vessels of the body, especially the vessels of the so-called blood reservoirs – the spleen, the venous plexus of the skin, and the splanchnic vessels. This causes marked transfer of blood from these peripheral vessels to the heart, tending to increase the input pressure to the heart, which thereby enhances cardiac output in accord with the Frank-Starling law of the heart. Second, nerve stimuli to the heart itself increase its effectiveness as a pump at the same time.

The importance of arterial pressure control when excess cardiac output is demanded by the tissues was beautifully demonstrated in experiments by Asker and Hamilton in which they showed that dogs could increase their cardiac outputs only a fraction as much during treadmill exercise when their sympathetic nervous system was removed than had been the case before[48]. A study in our laboratory, illustrated in Figure 15, also demonstrated the same principle when the cardiac output was increased by the metabolic

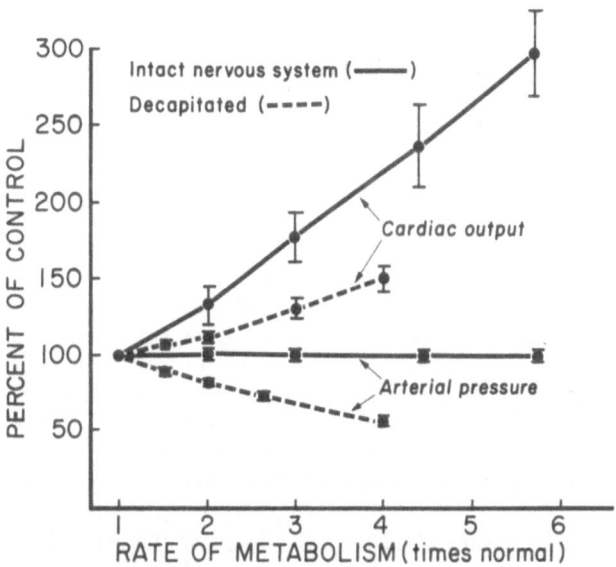

Figure 15 Effect of increased rate of metabolism on cardiac output and arterial pressure in normal dogs and decapitated dogs. This illustrates that when the arterial pressure falls, as it does when reflex control of pressure is blocked, the cardiac output cannot increase as much as it normally does. (Drawn from data in Banet and Guyton[49])

stimulant dinitrophenol[49]. Maximal stimulation by this compound in the normal dogs, as illustrated in the figure, increased the cardiac output up to 300% of the normal level before the circulatory system failed and caused death of the animal. On the other hand, in animals that had received total spinal anaesthesia to block the sympathetic nervous system, the arterial pressure fell markedly, as illustrated in the figure, and the cardiac output increased only to 150% of normal, at which time the circulatory system failed and the animals failed to survive.

Thus, both the experiments of Asker and Hamilton and the one from our laboratory have demonstrated the extreme importance of the arterial pressure control mechanisms as a necessary adjunct to increasing the cardiac output in response to tissue need.

Lack of 'feedback' control of cardiac output per se
It is very significant that there is no sensor in the body that can detect the cardiac output itself. Therefore, in the absence of an appropriate sensor, there also is no built-in mechanism for feedback control of cardiac output. This is quite different from the arterial pressure controls, where there are several separate sensors, all of which play important roles in maintaining the arterial pressure. This difference between the feedback control of arterial pressure and cardiac output is demonstrated in Figure 16, which shows the effect of transfusing two separate series of dogs with 400 ml of blood in a period of 5 min. The dogs in one of these groups (16A) were normal while the other dogs had had their heads removed (16B), thereby removing all of their circulatory reflexes. In both instances, the cardiac output increased approximately 2-fold, illustrating that the presence or absence of nervous controls had little effect in providing feedback control of the cardiac output. On the other hand, note that the arterial pressure rose only an insignificant amount in the animals with intact nervous systems in comparison with a tremendous increase in the dogs without nervous systems.

'Feed-forward' control of cardiac output
Though there is no known mechanism for feedback control of cardiac output, in a sense there is at least one mechanism for 'feed-forward' control that occurs at the onset of exercise in the following way:

When an animal or a human being anticipates exercise, the sympathetic nervous system usually becomes activated even before the exercise begins, and this leads to increased constriction of the capacitance vessels of the body, increased heart rate, and perhaps even stimulation of vasodilator nerve fibres in the muscles (though this is questionable). All of these effects together can increase the cardiac output at least to a slight to moderate amount even prior to the exercise[50]. Thus, these extrinsic signals provide an increase in cardiac output in anticipation of the need for increased blood flow through the tissues. And they also increase the arterial pressure at the same time. Thus, this mechanism is actually a feed-forward mechanism for increasing both arterial pressure and cardiac output. Presumably it is an intrinsic function of the nervous system itself that is built in from birth. However, it is also very possible that at least part of this mechanism can be

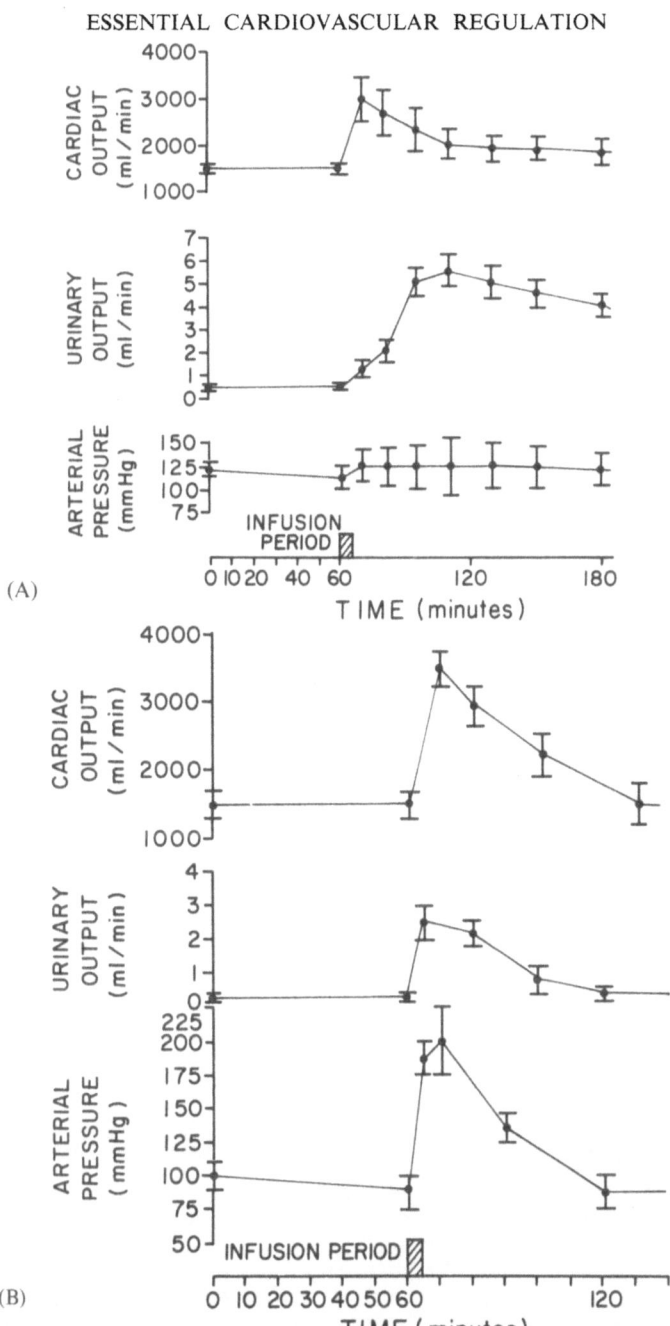

Figure 16 Effect of infusion of 400 ml of blood on arterial pressure, urinary output, and cardiac output in two separate groups of dogs: (A) normal dogs and (B) headless dogs without pressure-regulating reflexes, showing almost the same response of the cardiac output but markedly different responses of the arterial pressure. (Modified from Dobbs, W. A., Ph.D. thesis, University of Mississippi School of Medicine, 1970)

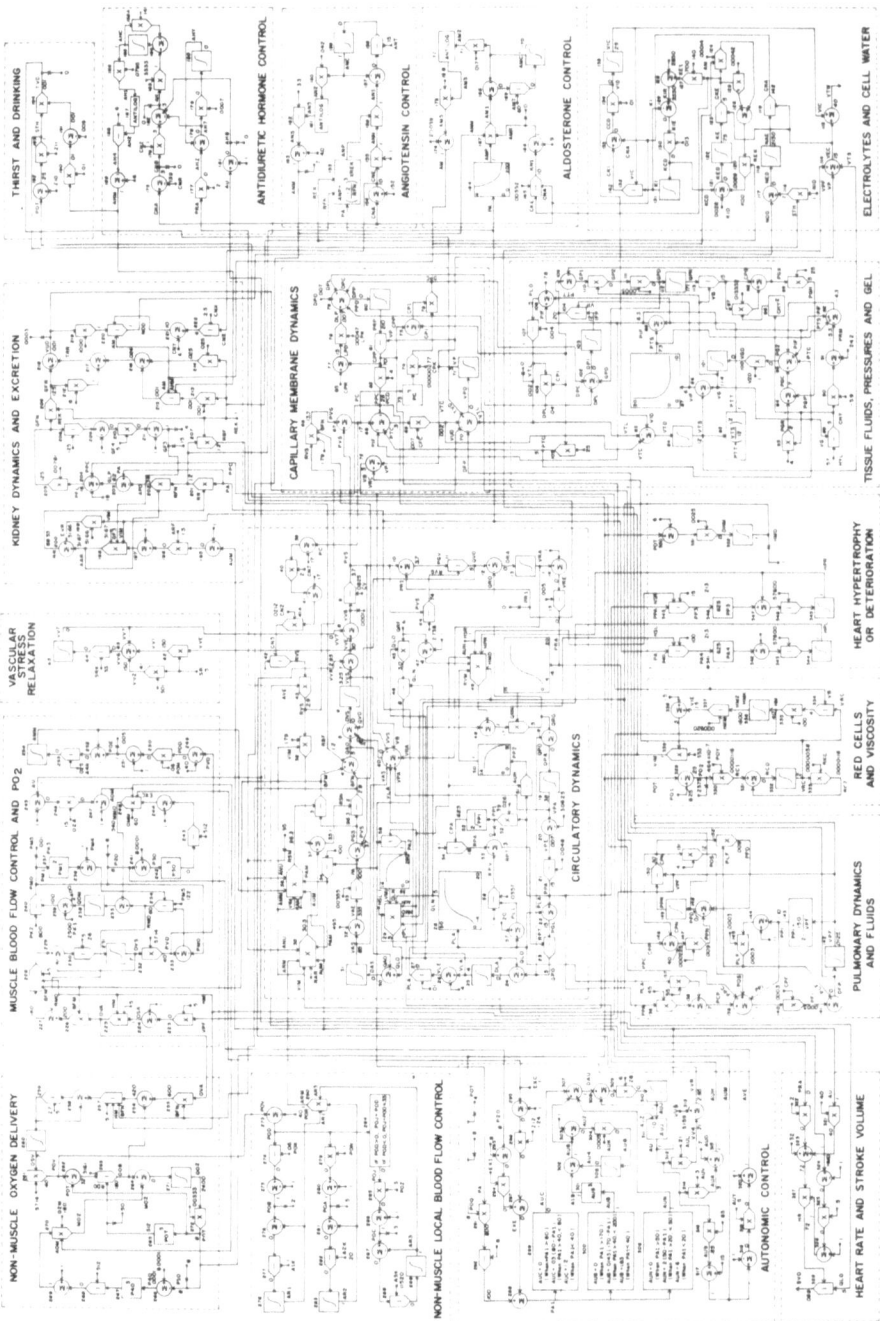

Figure 17 Analogue diagram of a computer model of the circulation that can be used to show the interdigitating functions of the different portions of the circulatory system. (Reprinted from Guyton et al.[52] by permission of *Annual Review of Physiology*, vol. 34; © 1972 by Annual Reviews Inc.)

298

learned, because the process of anticipation is a learned behavioural manifestation. This would fit well with the data from both temperature regulation and respiration regulation studies showing that animals and human beings can indeed establish learned mechanisms of vegetative control.

A complex analysis of circulatory control

In recent years it has been possible to build mathematical models of the circulation that embody all the principles of circulatory control that have been discussed in the present paper[19,20,51,52]. Figure 17 illustrates the analogue circuit diagram of such a model. Each of the blocks in this diagram represents a mathematical equation. This diagram embodies 352 equations, while others that have been developed have embodied as many as 600 equations. Models such as these can be programmed on a computer to determine the effect on the circulation of changing any single parameter of circulatory function. For instance, what is the effect of acute cardiac failure on circulatory control? The computer gives the answer that circulatory readjustments begin immediately and the usual complex of reactions occur: fluid retention, angiotensin secretion, aldosterone secretion, rise in right atrial pressure, and other effects until either the fluid output rises up to equal fluid input or until the body becomes so overfilled with fluid that death ensues.

Likewise, the model can be used to study abnormalities of blood pressure control. Thus, any factor that alters the renal function curve, as expressed in the equations of the kidney portion of the model, will lead to a necessary change in the level of arterial pressure.

Clearly, even within the complexity of a model such as that illustrated in Figure 17, the two basic essentials of overall circulatory regulation are still very apparent: first, the system maintains an adequate arterial pressure in the face of almost any normal circulatory stress; and, second, blood flow in each individual tissue is controlled in accord with physiological needs. As these two essentials are met, the cardiac output also is automatically regulated, for the cardiac output is simply the sum of the regulated blood flows through the individual tissues.

References

1. Guyton, A. C., Cowley, A. W., Jr. and Coleman, T. G. (1972). Interaction between the separate control systems in normal arterial pressure regulation in hypertension. In J. Genest and E. Kiow (eds.), *Hypertension '72*, pp. 384–398. (New York: Springer-Verlag)
2. Cowley, A. W., Jr., Liard, J. F. and Guyton, A. C. (1973). Role of the baroreceptor reflex in daily control of arterial blood pressure and other variables in dogs. *Circ. Res.*, **32**, 564
3. Liard, J. F., Cowley, A. W., Jr., McCaa, R. E., McCaa, C. S. and Guyton, A. C. (1974). Renin–aldosterone, body fluid volumes and baroreceptor reflex in the development and reversal of Goldblatt hypertension in conscious dogs. *Circ. Res.*, **34**, 549
4. McCubbin, J. M., Green, J. H. and Page, I. H. (1956). Baroreceptor function in chronic renal hypertension. *Circ. Res.*, **4**, 205

5. Kezdi, P. and Spickler, W. (1967). Baroreceptor and sympathetic activity in experimental renal hypertension. *Circulation*, **17**, 785

6. Kreiger, E. M. (1970). Time course of baroreceptor resetting in acute hypertension. *Am. J. Physiol.*, **218**, 584

7. Sagawa, K. and Watanabe, K. (1965). Summation of bilateral carotid sinus signals in the barostatic reflex. *Am. J. Physiol.*, **209**, 1278

8. Scher, A. M. and Young, A. C. (1963). Servoanalysis of carotid sinus reflex effects on peripheral resistance. *Circ. Res.*, **12**, 152

9. Heymans, C. and Neil, E. (1958). *Reflexogenic Areas of the Cardiovascular System*. (London: J. and A. Churchill, Ltd)

10. Sagawa, K., Ross, J. M. and Guyton, A. C. (1961). Quantitation of cerebral ischemic pressor response in dogs. *Am. J. Physiol.*, **200**, 1164

11. Gauer, O. H., Henry, J. P. and Behn, C. (1970). The regulation of extracellular fluid volume. *Ann. Rev. Physiol.*, **32**, 547

12. Linden, R. J. (1973). Function of cardiac receptors. *Circulation*, **48**, 463

13. Mancia, G., Lorenz, R. R. and Shepherd, J. T. (1976). Reflex control of circulation by heart and lungs. *Internat. Rev. Physiol.*, **9**, 111

14. Granger, H. J. and Guyton, A. C. (1969). Autoregulation of the total systemic circulation following destruction of the central nervous system in the dog. *Circ. Res.*, **25**, 379

15. Selkurt, E. E., Hall, P. W. and Spencer, M. P. (1949). Influence of graded arterial pressure decrement on renal clearance on creatinine, p-amino hippurate and sodium. *Am. J. Physiol.*, **159**, 369

16. Thompson, D. D. and Pitts, R. F. (1952). Effects of alterations of renal arterial pressure on sodium and water excretion. *Am. J. Physiol.*, **168**, 490

17. Thurau, K. and Deetzen, P. (1962). Diuresis in arterial pressure increases. *Pflugers Arch.*, **294**, 567

18. DeClue, J. W., Guyton, A. C., Cowley, A. W., Jr., Coleman, T. G., Norman, R. A., Jr. and McCaa, R. E. Subpressor angiotensin infusion, renal sodium handling, and salt induced hypertension in the dog. *Circ. Res.* (In press)

19. Guyton, A. C. and Coleman, T. G. (1967). Long-term regulation of the circulation: Interrelationships with body fluid volumes. In E. B. Reeve and A. C. Guyton (eds.). *Physical Bases of Circulatory Transport: Regulation and Exchange*, pp. 179–201. (Philadelphia: W. B. Saunders Co.)

20. Guyton, A. C. and Coleman, T. G. (1969). A quantitative analysis of the pathophysiology of hypertension. *Circ. Res.*, **24**, 1

21. Guyton, A. C., Coleman, T. G., Cowley, A. W., Jr., Scheel, K. W., Manning, R. D., Jr. and Norman, R. A., Jr. (1972). Arterial pressure regulation: overriding dominance of the kidneys in long-term regulation and in hypertension. *Am. J. Med.*, **52**, 584

22. Guyton, A. C., Coleman, T. G., Cowley, A. W., Jr., Manning, R. D., Jr., Norman, R. A., Jr. and Ferguson, J. D. (1974). A systems analysis approach to understanding long-range arterial blood pressure control and hypertension. *Circ. Res.*, **35**, 159

23. Langston, J. B., Guyton, A. C., Douglas, B. H. and Dorsett, P. E. (1963). Effect of changes in salt intake on arterial pressure and renal function in nephrectomized dogs. *Circ. Res.*, **12**, 508

24. Coleman, T. G. and Guyton, A. C. (1969). Hypertension caused by salt loading in the dog. III. Onset transients of cardiac output and other circulatory variables. *Circ. Res.*, **25**, 152

25. Douglas, B. H., Guyton, A. C., Langston, J. B. and Bishop, V. S. (1964). Hypertension caused by salt loading. II: Fluid volume and tissue pressure changes. *Am. J. Physiol.*, **207**, 669

26. Manning, R. D., Jr. (1973). Hemodynamic and humoral changes during the initial phase of salt-induced, renoprival hypertension. Ph.D. thesis, University of Mississippi

27. Wakim, K. G., Slaughter, O. and Clagett, O. T. (1948). Studies on the blood flow in the extremities in case of coarctation of the aorta: determination before and after excision of the coarctate region. *Proc. Mayo Clin.*, **23**, 347

28. Norman, R. A., Jr., Enobakhare, J., DeClue, J. W., Douglas, B. H. and Guyton, A. C. (1978). Arterial pressure-urinary output relationship in hypertensive rats. *Am. J. Physiol.*, **234**, R98

29. Warren, J. V., Nickerson, J. L. and Elkin, D. C. (1951). The cardiac output in patients with arteriovenous fistulas. *J. Clin. Invest.*, **20**, 210

30. Waugh, W. H. (1972). Angiotensin. II: Local renal effects of physiological increments in concentration. *Can. J. Physiol. Pharmacol.*, **50**, 711

31. Lohmeier, T. E., Cowley, A. W., Jr., DeClue, J. W. and Guyton, A. C. Failure of chronic aldosterone infusion to increase arterial pressure in dogs with angiotensin-induced hypertension. (Submitted for publication)

32. Young, D. V., Murray, R. H. and Bengis, R. G. Experimental angiotensin II hypertension. (In preparation)

33. Guyton, A. C., Batson, H. M., Jr. and Smith, C. M., Jr. (1951). Adjustments of the circulatory system following very rapid transfusion or haemorrhage. *Am. J. Physiol.*, **164**, 351

34. Manning, R. D. and Guyton, A. C. (1978). Fluid volume, plasma protein and hemodynamic changes during experimental hypertension in conscious, anephric dogs. *Fed. Proc.*, **37**, 294

35. Johnson, P. C. (1964). Review of previous studies and current theories of autoregulation. *Circ. Res.*, **14** and **15** (Suppl. 1): I—2

36. Guyton, A. C., Ross, J. M., Carrier, O., Jr. and Walker, J. R. (1964). Evidence for tissue oxygen demand as the major factor causing autoregulation. *Circ. Res.*, **14**, 60

37. Berne, R. M. (1964). Regulation of coronary blood flow. *Physiol. Rev.*, **44**, 1

38. Haddy, F. J. Personal communication

39. Burwell, C. S. and Dexter, L. (1947). Beri-beri heart disease. *Trans. Assoc. Amer. Physicians*, **60**, 59

40. Guyton, A. C., Jones, C. E. and Coleman, T. G. (eds.) (1973). *Circulatory Physiology: Cardiac Output and Its Regulation*, 2nd ed. (Philadelphia: W. B. Saunders Co.)

41. Rapela, C. E. and Green, H. D. (1964). Autoregulation of canine cerebral blood flow. *Circ. Res.*, **25**: I–205.

42. Hall, J. E., Guyton, A. C. and Cowley, A. W., Jr. (1977). Dissociation of renal blood flow and filtration rate autoregulation by renin depletion. *Am. J. Physiol.*, **232**, F215

43. Hall, J. E., Guyton, A. C., Jackson, T. E., Coleman, T. G., Lohmeier, T. E. and Trippodo, N. C. (1977). Control of glomerular filtration rate by renin-angiotensin system. *Am. J. Physiol.*, **233**, F366

44. Granger, H. J. and Guyton, A. C. (1969). Autoregulation of the total systemic circulation following destruction of the central nervous system in the dog. *Circ. Res.*, **25**, 379

45. Folkow, B., Gurevich, M., Hallback, M., Lundgren, Y. and Weiss, L. (1971). The hemodynamic consequences of regional hypotension in spontaneously hypertensive and normotensive rats. *Acta Physiol. Scand.*, **83**, 532

46. Folkow, B., Lewis, D. H., Lundgen, O., Mellander, S. and Wallentin, I. (1964). The effect of graded vasoconstrictor fibre stimulation on the intestinal resistance and capacitance vessels. *Acta Physiol. Scand.*, **61**, 445

47. Norman, R. A., Jr. Personal communication
48. Asker, E. and Hamilton, W. F. (1963). Cardiovascular response to graded exercise on the sympathectomized-vagotomized dog. *Am. J. Physiol.*, **204**, 291
49. Banet, M. and Guyton, A. C. (1971). Effect of body metabolism on cardiac output: role of the central nervous system. *Am. J. Physiol.*, **220**, 662
50. Guyton, A. C., Douglas, B. H., Langston, J. B. and Richardson, T. Q. (1962). Instantaneous increase in mean circulatory pressure and cardiac output at onset of muscular activity. *Circ. Res.*, **11**, 431
51. Dickinson, C. J., Sackett, D. L. and Goldsmith, C. H. (1973). MacMan: A digital computer model for teaching some basic principles of haemodynamics. *J. Clin. Computing*, **2**, 42
52. Guyton, A. C., Coleman, T. G. and Granger, H. J. (1972). Circulation: Overall regulation. *Ann. Rev. Physiol.*, **34**, 13

Part VII
History

19
Medicine in the court of Charles I

H. TREVOR-ROPER

William Harvey, whose birth we celebrate this year, is the greatest physician in our history. He was also physician-in-ordinary to Charles I, who was, to say the least, one of the more interesting of our kings. He was closely associated with the person of the king, both in prosperity and in adversity. In the years of peace, he accompanied the king personally on his journeys, travelling three times into Scotland: for his coronation in 1633; on the military expedition of 1639; and in the summer of 1641 when the king sought to raise a royalist party in Scotland to resist the Parliament of England. He was also present at the first battle of the Civil War, the battle of Edgehill on 23 October 1642. He did not of course take part in the battle—he was then 64 years old—but spent the time reading a book behind a hedge while the bullets whizzed past his ear. For the next 4 years he was at the court at Oxford, experimenting in the hatching of eggs in Trinity College, and in 1646, when the king had fled from that falling capital to the protection, as he supposed, of the Scots at Newcastle, Harvey joined him there. It was only when he was transferred from Scottish to English custody that the king was parted from his chosen doctors, as from his chosen chaplains. Meanwhile, in all his works, Harvey showed devotion to the king. In 1628, as royal physician extraordinary, he dedicated to him his greatest work, on the movement of the heart; in 1642 as a committed royalist, he suffered the sack of his official lodgings at Whitehall and thereby lost all his papers—the most crucifying grief of his life, he afterwards said; and it was to raise his spirits in the total collapse of the royal cause in 1648 that he was persuaded to publish his last work, on the generation of animals.

This being so, the subject 'medicine at the court of Charles I' seems natural enough for the opening lecture at a Harveian conference, and at first I thought that I knew well enough how to handle the topic. However, on closer consideration, I am not so sure. For what in fact is the distinctive character of Charles I's medical patronage? Who, apart from Harvey, were his court doctors, those physicians whom he drew together round his person and his family? Once we ask this question we encounter difficulty. The court of Charles I was certainly distinctive. It was an elaborate, correct, aesthetically oriented society, very different from that of James I or Elizabeth. But his physicians—or at least the most distinguished of them—were not discovered by him. They were all inherited from his father. In fact, we find that it was James I, not Charles I, who was the great innovator. Harvey himself came to court under James I, and it was in that reign that the foundations of his great work were all laid.

This being so, I think it is best to speak of medicine and the court in the time not of Charles I but of Harvey. In this way we can see how James I, by his personal patronage, temporarily altered the pattern of English medicine, giving a new impulse to heretical ideas, and passing those ideas on to the next generation. We can then see how, beneath an apparent continuity, Charles I, by the subtle shift of his patronage, quietly put the clock back; and we can see where, in this process, Harvey fits in.

Of course the court did not operate in a vacuum. There were other, less personal, more continuous, and therefore in the long run stronger institutions beside which the patronage of the court had an accidental, almost whimsical character. In particular there was the Royal College of Physicians, founded by Henry VIII in 1518 and now well established; well organized; sure of itself. The college set out to maintain the standards of medicine, and protect the public, by licensing those physicians whom it approved, banning those whom it did not approve, and keeping the subordinate technicians of the profession —apothecaries and surgeons—in their subordinate place. Its discipline may not have been very effective. Unlicensed practitioners throve in London, protected by powerful patrons, and the apothecaries remained the physicians of the poor. However, by 1600 the college had established itself as the central organ and the club of the profession, the arbiter of medical standards and medical fashion. Its Fellows knew each other, had similar ideas, and a common base of proper academic training.

Theoretically, all Fellows had to have degrees from English universities; however, in fact many of them had studied abroad. The English universities did not have organized medical schools, and although Henry VIII had founded regius chairs of medicine, and Dr Caius, in the mid-sixteenth century had introduced the study of anatomy at Cambridge, the best training was still to be found in Continental universities; after which English degrees could always be obtained by incorporation. The most admired foreign university at the time was the university of Padua, with its famous anatomy theatre. Thomas Linacre and John Chambre, the founders of the Royal College in London, were both doctors of Padua, so was its reformer, John Caius. Padua was also the model for the new university of Leiden, founded in 1575 during the Dutch revolt against Spain. Padua and Leiden were the centres of experimental anatomy within a conservative, Aristotelean tradition. There were also other traditions, as we shall see.

Compared with the dignified Fellows of the Royal College of Physicians, the English court physicians of the sixteenth century, it must be admitted, were a miscellaneous lot, picked out by personal accident or personal whim. Some of them were reputable enough, but some would never have qualified for membership of the college. Some were foreigners. Henry VIII had had two Italian doctors—a Genoese, Giovanni Battista Boerio, whom he had inherited from Henry VII and who would employ Erasmus as travelling tutor to accompany his sons to Rome, and a Venetian, Agostino de Angustinis, whom he took over from Cardinal Wolsey. Queen Elizabeth had at least two foreign doctors. The first was an Italian, Cesare Adelmare from Treviso, a doctor of Padua, whom she inherited from her sister Mary. He prospered in England, and his son Giulio Cesare Adelmare would make a great career in the law, ending as Sir Julius Caesar, Master of the Rolls. The second was a Portuguese Jew, Rodrigo Lopez, who had worked for ten years at St Bartholomew's Hospital, the training-ground of so many doctors, including Harvey. Dr Lopez too made his mark, in a way: in 1594 he was hanged on a charge of seeking to poison the Queen in the interest of the king of Spain. Such conspiracies were a constant source of worry in Renaissance courts, and court doctors were expected to keep up to date, especially in the subject of poisons and their antidotes.

Other court doctors were eccentric in other ways. Some of them were regarded by respectable physicians as quacks. Certainly some of them were medical heretics. In the sixteenth century there was one great medical heresy, and the history of medicine, at that time, is largely conditioned by its impact. That heresy was Paracelsianism, alchemical medicine, 'introchemistry'.

The new chemical medicine was in some ways a direct protest against, and challenge to, the Galenic orthodoxy of the established physicians. As such it was popular among their rivals, the depressed classes of the medical profession, the surgeons and apothecaries; but it was condemned by almost all the institutes of higher learning. However, by the end of the century certain universities—Basel, Montpellier, Nantes—had begun to make tentative compromises with it. At the same time certain princely courts began—not always for disinterested scientific reasons—to welcome chemical doctors. The English court, under Elizabeth, remained conservative, but several European rulers—the Emperor Rudolf II, the King of Denmark, the Landgrave of Hesse and other German princes—patronized the new medicine and founded laboratories and academies to promote it. This royal patronage sometimes placed the court doctors in frontal opposition to the established medical corporations.

The most spectacular of such confrontations occurred in 1603, the year of the accession of James I. It occurred in Paris and I shall return to it shortly, for it had a direct influence on the medical history of the English court. Meanwhile I shall prepare my ground by stating that at that time there were two main lines of progress in experimental medicine. On the one hand there was the anatomical school of Padua and Leiden, conservative, Aristotelean, Galenist. On the other hand there was the chemical school of Paracelsus which had been made reputable by Peter Severinus in Denmark and had penetrated the universities of Basel, Montpellier and Nantes. Both movements had their extremists. In Paris, where passions had been sharpened by ideological civil war, the Medical Faculty was as extreme in its Galenism as the Theological Faculty, the Sorbonne, in its Catholicism. In Germany the Paracelsians ran riot in alchemical fantasies. But we are in England, and in

Elizabethan England, in medicine as in religion, there was compromise. The doctors from Padua and Leiden, and the new medical reformers from Basel and Nantes, met amicably in the College of Physicians, and the royal doctors, a race apart, did not influence either medical science or, except in the *cause célèbre* of Dr Lopez, public events.

On one occasion indeed, it seemed that the Royal College itself might quietly yield to the chemical reformers. In the 1580s a committee of the Royal College was set up to plan an official English pharmacopoeia. At the same time a Physic Garden was established under the direction of the famous herbalist John Gerard, much to the alarm of the Apothecaries, who were hampered by the incorporation in one body with the Grocers, and who protested in vain against this encroachment on their preserves. It looked as if the Royal College was about to extend its activities, liberalize its philosophy, and admit chemical remedies. This movement coincided with the admission into the College of an active Paracelsian reformer, who enjoyed aristocratic patronage, Thomas Muffet. Muffet was a doctor of Basel, who had been to Denmark and had known the scientific innovators patronized by the Danish court: the astronomer Tycho Brahé and the reformer of Paracelsian medicine Peter Severinus. He was himself an experimental doctor who had made a special study of insects. He also wrote a didactic poem on silkworms and enjoys perpetual fame because of his little daughter's encounter with a spider.

However, this first reforming period, in the end, came to nothing. After 1594 the project of a pharmacopoeia ran out of steam. The old queen, conservative in everything, gave no encouragement, and when she died in 1603, nothing had been done. Her court physicians followed her quickly to the grave: Dr Gilbert, the great philosopher of magnetism, in 1603; Dr Lancelot Browne, her first physician and the father-in-law of Harvey, in 1605. The way was now open for the new king to exercise his patronage, if he wished, in a new way.

King James had already given some hint of his ideas. As king of Scotland he had chosen, as his court doctor, one John Craig, whom he had picked up in Denmark when he went there, in 1589, to collect his wife. Craig was an interesting man. Like Muffet, he had taken his doctorate at Basel, and again like Muffet, he had become friendly with the Danish scientists, Peter Severinus and Tycho Brahé. When King James moved to London, he brought Craig with him and kept him as his first court doctor there. It can be seen as a sign that Muffet's enterprise was to be resumed. Next year, another sign pointed in the same direction. The king sent a personal doctor to Scotland to attend to his second son, Prince Charles, now 4 years old and ill in Dunfermline, and to bring him to London. The doctor he chose was Henry Atkins. Atkins was a doctor of Nantes, another 'Paracelsian' university. In the 1580s he had been on the committee of the Royal College to devise a new pharmacopoeia. In 1593 he had volunteered to sail as a ship's doctor on the Earl of Essex's expedition to Cadiz. This too showed an interest in practical experiment. Most of the Paracelsian doctors, like Paracelsus himself, had sought experience as army doctors, and Muffet himself had accompanied Essex's earlier expedition to France in 1591. When Atkins returned from Scotland with the Prince, King James made him his first English physician in ordinary.

Later, another doctor of Basel, Matthew Lister, who had succeeded Muffet as physician and agent of Mary Countess of Pembroke at Wilton, was appointed court doctor to the new queen. Thus the new reign was signalized, in medicine and at court, by something of a Paracelsian invasion. James I, it is well known, was an extravagant king. The court, its cost, offices, honours—all were inflated in his reign. So were the court doctors. At the end of the reign, a cry was raised against them. Queen Elizabeth, it was observed, had been content with three physicians, one surgeon and one apothecary, at a total cost of £416 per annum, while King James, at his death, was retaining seven physicians, six or seven surgeons, and two or three apothecaries[1]. One of King James's physicians alone cost more than the whole Elizabethan establishment. Most of these doctors are mere names to us, but those whose personality and tastes can be discovered have something in common. Like Craig and Atkins they are unorthodox, experimental, chemical doctors. Sometimes their unorthodoxy seems to verge on charlatanism. But that was in keeping with the character of the court.

For the court of James I was very different from that of Elizabeth. From the beginning, conventional observers were shocked by its undignified, even disorderly character, so different from the hieratic regularity of the old queen's court. But this unconventionality had another side to it too. Intellectually the new court was remarkably open to new ideas. It became the resort, and the refuge, of adventurers, fortune-seekers, charlatans, but also of philosophers, scholars, scientists of unorthodox genius. In the world of medicine it welcomed both types. James I positively disliked respectable physicians. He liked eccentrics.

For instance, there was Leonard Poe. The Royal College knew Dr Poe only too well. It condemned him, again and again, as an ignorant charlatan. But he was protected by noble patrons, supported by Privy Councillors, consulted as a scientist by Francis Bacon, who also disliked the established physicians and believed in open-ended experiment. In 1609 James I appointed Poe to be physician in ordinary to the royal household, and the Fellows of the Royal College found themselves obliged to admit him as a colleague. They did so with reluctance, and changed their rules in order to be able to resist next time[2]. And then there was a strange Scotsman who wrote his name, in Latin, as Macollo. I suspect it was really McCulloch. He had taken a degree at the new university of Franeker in Holland and had been chief physician to the Grand Duke of Tuscany. Afterwards he was also described as 'physician in ordinary' to the Emperor Rudolph II*. He was a baroque character and wrote books of Paracelsian chemical medicine in a flamboyant Latin style.†
James I made him his physician in ordinary in 1620, together with another

* The claim is made by the editor of Macollo's posthumously published *XCIX Canons or Rules . . . for Practitioners in Physick* (1659). It is not mentioned in Macollo's funeral inscription in St Margaret's, Westminster, quoted by Munk, which describes him as 'Magni Hetruriae ducis Archiater quondam'. But he may have treated the Emperor, who was the Grand Duke's brother-in-law. In Arthur Johnston's *De litiae Poetarun Scotorum* (1637) there are some Latin poems by Macollo (then called James Macallo), addressed to various members of the Medici family.

† He published two books on the chemical treatment of *Lues Venerea, Theoria Chymica* (Florence 1616) and *Iatria Chymica* (London 1622).

Scotsman, Dr Chambers, who was denizened for the purpose and succeeded Dr Craig, who had just died. We know little about Dr Chambers, except that he was once so enraged by anti-Scottish remarks in a pub in Kenilworth that he pulled down the pub-sign and threatened to burn it[3]. The English physicians evidently thought little of him. He was not made a member of the College.

Those were the less distinguished of King James's physicians-in-ordinary. Better known was another foreigner who arrived in 1611 from the still smouldering medical battlefields of Paris. This was Theodore Turquet, who preferred to be known as Theodore de Mayerne.

Mayerne was the youngest of a triumvirate of chemical doctors, all Huguenots from Geneva, who held court appointments under Henri IV of France, and had aroused the furious opposition of the orthodox Galenist Faculty of Medicine, dominated by two powerful figures, both called Jean Riolan, father and son. The son would afterwards draw attention to himself again by attacking Harvey's theory of the circulation of the blood. Indeed, he was the only critic whom Harvey would deign to answer. For 5 years, from 1603 to 1608, the Paris Faculty, led by the Riolans, had attacked the heretical court doctors, anathematizing them as ignorant charlatans, forbidding them to practise, patients to resort to them, or apothecaries to make up their medicines. But the battle did not damage them in the least. The heretical doctors continued to practise without fear, and Mayerne, who in 1609 was the sole survivor of the trio, enjoyed a splendid practice in Paris. All the *beau monde* went to him, Protestant and Catholic alike: the king's mistress, the Comtesse de Moret; his financier Sébastien Zamet; the old *mignons* of Henri III; the young Bishop of Luçon, afterwards Cardinal Richelieu, whom he cured of *lues venerea*; the dukes of Bouillon and Rohan, rival leaders of Huguenot revolt; the entire *haute société protestante*. He cured them by Paracelsian, alchemical methods, by patient observation, by strange hermetic formulae, and by an irresistible bedside manner; and in his spare time he was diligent in his chemical laboratory, distilling essences, making projections, seeking to transmute metals, to discover the philosopher's stone.

However, although he was not afraid of Riolan and the Paris faculty, Mayerne was frightened of one thing: the loss of royal protection. In 1606, at the height of the Paris battle, he had reinsured himself by visiting England and had scored a great success at the court of James I. He had also taken the precaution of being incorporated as a doctor of Oxford University. Two years later, Henri IV had offered him the highest medical post at his court— but on condition that he became a Catholic; for by now the Catholic reaction was in full swing. After some agony, Mayerne refused the terms. Two years later, Henri IV was assassinated, and Mayerne decided to act. Through the English ambassador in Paris, he made excellent terms for himself. He was to be first physician to the king of Great Britain with a salary of £600 a year, board and lodgings at court, allowances for apothecaries and servants, and exemption from all taxes. At the same time, he was allowed to keep his titular position at the French court, and a retaining fee: the French ministers, on their side, were ready to pay this price. In the heart of a rival court, Mayerne, they thought might be useful, as their spy.

So began the phenomenal career of Mayerne in England. His coming was well timed. James I was naturally well disposed; so was his most intellectual minister, Francis Bacon. To Bacon the old Galenic physicians, with their traditional, academic theories were as distasteful as the Schoolmen in philosophy, and he called for a revival of 'the ancient and serious diligence of Hippocrates'—that is, observation and therapy[4]. He was also interested in chemistry and therefore, as he would write, 'partial to policaries'[5]. To both king and minister Mayerne was thus a welcome visitor. Moreover, in the Royal College of Physicians, the ground had been prepared for him by the influence of men like Muffet and Atkins. In 1616, as royal physician, he was admitted as Fellow of the Royal College. His reception there astonished him. The grandees of the college accepted him not, as he had expected—for it was, after all, the equivalent of the Paris Faculty—'with hostile faces and oblique glances'—but with open, welcoming arms. He was particularly delighted by the friendship of Sir William Paddy, a cultivated high anglican, who had been one of the projectors of the English pharmacopoeia under Queen Elizabeth and was now one of the royal doctors. He also learned all about Muffet and his work. Afterwards, from Muffet's apothecary, Mayerne obtained Muffet's manuscripts and published Muffet's beautifully illustrated work on insects, with a dedication to Paddy. Thus, thanks to Mayerne, Muffet was more fortunate than Harvey, whose work on insects would perish in the sack of his lodgings in 1642.

One of the public effects of this new Jacobean spirit, and of the rise to prominence of a new group of royal doctors, was the success of the apothecaries in emancipating themselves from the control of the grocers, and the resumption, and realization, of the Elizabethan project of a British Pharmacopoeia. Both these results were achieved in 1618, and the moving spirits in the Royal College were the royal physicians, particularly Atkins, Mayerne, Craig and Paddy. The physicians did not, of course, intend to set the apothecaries free—only to free them from the hampering control of the grocers, in order that they might be more closely linked with, and subordinate to, themselves. But it was a welcome change nevertheless, and as the new pharmacopoeia included a whole section on chemical medicine, the victory for the experimental doctors was obvious. That victory was largely due, as the King himself stated, to the initiative of 'our well beloved physicians Theodore de Mayerne and Henry Atkins'.

Once established in the court of James I Mayerne soon built up a huge practice in England. He also retained his foreign patients. With his courtly manners he was acceptable everywhere and James I used him as an agent in numerous delicate affairs, literary and diplomatic as well as medical. Mayerne thoroughly enjoyed dabbling in international politics. From his position in the English court, he planted a sister in the court of James's daughter the Electress Palatine, Queen of Bohemia; his first wife was the sister of the Dutch ambassador in Paris, his second the daughter of the Dutch ambassador in London. Nearly all English ambassadors abroad, and nearly all foreign ambassadors in England, even including the Spaniard Gondomar, were his patients; and he was adept in combining medicine with politics. He was the unofficial emissary of French Huguenot grandees and of the city of Geneva. In 1620 he bought a feudal castle in Switzerland, and set up as Baron d'Aubonne in the Pays de Vaud; as such he became the trusted agent of the canton of Berne, leader of the Swiss Confederation. He had princely patients in Germany. He made regular visits to the Continent to see his patients, and took with him secret instructions. On one occasion he was arrested in Paris and ordered out of the country. That caused a great rumpus, but no explanation was ever offered. There can be no doubt that he was regarded as a Huguenot spy. When the Thirty Years War broke out, he was at the centre of the international Protestant alliance. He advised on treaties, received ambassadors, recommended generals, handled secret intelligence and instructions. His castle of Aubonne was well placed as a listening post and his friend, the old Huguenot hero Agrippa d'Aubigné, now exiled at Geneva, invented a special 'telephone' for long-distance secret communication with him.

In the autumn of 1624 Mayerne set out to revisit his chateau of Aubonne. Before leaving London he wrote out, for the other royal doctors, a full psychosomatic case-history of the king: to us an invaluable document. Unfortunately the king became gravely ill during his absence, and the royal deathbed was attended, in his absence, by the physicians in ordinary and by some other doctors, including William Harvey, who was now physician extraordinary. All that Mayerne could do was to convey the congratulations of the city of Geneva to Charles I on his accession. By his absence he had missed an unedifying episode which perhaps he could have prevented; for the amateur and infelicitous medication of the Duchess of Buckingham led one of the subordinate royal doctors—a Scotsman called George Eglishem—to declare that the Duke of Buckingham had poisoned the king. This charge would afterwards prove very useful. Extended to embrace Charles I, it would be solemnly repeated in the Grand Remonstrance of 1641 which precipitated the Civil War and in the Remonstrance of the Army of 1648 which precipitated the king's execution; and it would be faithfully publicized by the revolutionary hack-writer, John Milton.

I have described the court of James I as open to ideas, tolerant of heresy, encouraging experiment. Behind its apparent disorder and occasional absurdity, it was a Baconian court. In medical matters, the reign was unique in its opposition to the monopoly, the privileges, and therefore the dogmatism of the established physicians. Of course, the established physicians themselves were not caste-bound, as in Paris. It is noteworthy that not one of them had studied in Paris, although the medical faculty there was renowned for anatomy and Mayerne himself would send his son to study there. But royal patronage undoubtedly encouraged the success of the more liberal, experimental physicians within the college. The liberal atmosphere and the medical achievements of the reign—the incorporation of the Apothecaries and the publication of the London pharmacopoeia—were undoubtedly facilitated by the character and patronage of the court.

What then of the new reign? Outwardly on the accession of Charles I, there was a great difference. As Lucy Hutchinson, the widow of the regicide Colonel Hutchinson—no friendly critic—would put it, 'the face of the court was changed' and 'the bawds and catamites' of the previous reign disappeared, or at least practised their vices in corners, out of royal sight. The court of

Charles I was chaste, correct, orderly, hierarchical. It was also much more conservative. It was conservative in politics. It was conservative in medical affairs too. It saw the reinforcement of the power of the physicians over the apothecaries and the surgeons, the eclipse of chemical innovations, the return to orthodoxy: fortunately, in the person of Harvey, to the orthodoxy not of Paris but of Padua.

Outwardly, indeed, there was apparent continuity. The medical establishment at court remained intact: most positions, after all, had been granted for life. But gradually the inflated court of James I was reduced by death or retirement and new doctors appeared. The first of them was a Scotsman, David Bethune, doctor of Padua, who became the king's physician in ordinary. He was joined by Matthew Lister, who had been physician to the late Queen Anne. The new queen, Henrietta Maria, acquired a new physician, the Roman Catholic Thomas Cadyman. He too was a doctor of Padua, though not a very good one: he was evidently more concerned to exhibit his stylish horsemanship than to advance his science. We have a fine account of him, with whip and groom, putting his horse through its paces*. As for Mayerne, his exceptional position as medical supremo was explicitly confirmed, but he soon became aware of a gentle wind of change.

The first blow was the Duke of Buckingham's war with France on behalf of the French Huguenots. This naturally embarrassed Mayerne, who was officially retained by both crowns and had important contacts on both sides. He was now suspect on both sides. In England some saw him, most unjustly, as another Dr Lopez. In France, he suffered an even greater blow. The French government took advantage of the war to cancel his office and retaining fee. Long and loud Mayerne protested. He wrote to Richelieu, he mobilized royalty, ambassadors, apothecaries, but it was no good. From now on, he was physician to the English court only.

Nor was that all. Charles I took the opportunity to forbid him ever to leave England again. Mayerne was very mortified. He was a cosmopolitan. He loved to dabble in international affairs. He had invested in a castle in Switzerland. But Charles I was firm. Mayerne's medical services, he said, were indispensable to him: he did not wish to be stranded without them, like the dying James I. It is probable that this was not the king's real, or at least his only, reason. After all, he would allow Harvey to go on a long journey to Vienna and Italy in 1636. But Mayerne had too many political interests, and his politics were not those of the new court. After 1628 Charles I had had enough of the Protestant International, and he was determined to keep this incorrigible busybody under control. To compensate him for the blow, he promised Mayerne anything that he might ask. A few years later, Mayerne cashed this blank cheque. He requested and obtained, with his colleague the equestrian Dr Cadyman and a courtier, Sir William Brouncker, a monopoly of distilling. We may thus honour him as a founder of the Distillers' Company. But he never saw Aubonne again.

Instead, he concentrated on his experiments: medical experiments, chemical experiments, botanical experiments. Around him, in London as in

* See the account in Munk, from Baldwin Hamey's MS, 'Bustorum Aliquot Reliquiae'. in the Royal College of Physicians.

Paris, buzzed a swarm of empirics, apothecaries, technicians, many of them *émigrés* like himself. He devised new instruments for the distillation of essences and elixirs, extracted and mixed opiates and unguents, experimented with plants, exchanging rare seeds with foreign enthusiasts, produced cosmetics and perfumes for royal and noble ladies and fumigations for costly funerals. He extended his patronage to immigrant goldsmiths and native gardeners: it was on his recommendation that John Parkinson, the famous herbalist, was made botanist royal to Charles I. He also studied the technology of art, patronizing enamellists from Geneva, discovering new colours, inventing new inks for miniaturists, rescuing Protestant goldsmiths from the Inquisition in Milan, questioning great artists—Rubens, who painted his portrait, Van Dyck, Mytens, van Somer—on the secrets of their technique. He wrote, but never published, or even finished, treatises on all branches of medicine. He enjoyed food and wine: he was, it was remarked, 'of somewhat more than liberal diet'. He is even credited with a cookery book: one of the many desperate attempts by foreigners to improve our English cuisine; and at one time he tried, unsuccessfully, to corner the English oyster beds. But this may have been out of chemical rather than gastronomic interests, as he was interested in the manufacture of pearls.

At one time—in 1638, when he was 65 years old—the court of France tried to lure Mayerne back to Paris. He expressed great appreciation of this gesture, but declined to come. He hoped one day to revisit France, 'my dear country', he replied; but he was now too old to transplant, and 'all my designs and hopes, in this winter of my age, are confined within the bounds of this most happy island', an oasis of peace in warring Europe, where the king and queen were so kind to him and insisted on his presence. No doubt they were, and did. Nevertheless, in a sense, this very Jacobean figure was always an outsider in the court of Charles I. He remained always a Huguenot, always a cosmopolitan, always interested in that 'Rosicrucian enlightenment', as it has been called, which was the intellectual world of the Protestant International. He had no sympathy with the policies of Charles I, which cut England off from Europe, or with the style of the court, and although he conformed with the Church of England, he positively disliked the clericalism of Archbishop Laud, which severed that Church from the Protestant cause in Europe*.

So, when the great crisis came in 1642, and the court left London, Mayerne did not follow it. Physical immobility, professional convenience, love of metropolitan life conspired to keep him in the capital. It is difficult to imagine him, like Harvey, continuing his experiments in the ultra-royalist atmosphere of embattled Oxford, or as the head of an Oxford college. So he stayed in his handsome house in Chelsea, which had formerly belonged to Sir Thomas More. His chief concern, in those years, was to preserve his income. At one time, the Parliament stopped his royal salary. At another it threatened him with war-taxation. On each occasion Mayerne reacted forcefully. He rehearsed the terms of his contract with James I. He threatened to emigrate. He

---

* Neither Strafford nor Laud used Mayerne as his physician, although Strafford's doctor, Sir Maurice Williams, took professional advice from Mayerne when Strafford was ill at York in September 1640. Laud's physician was Sir Simon Baskerville.

ostentatiously packed his bags and made preparations to leave for Holland. He forced full-scale debates in both Houses of Parliament. His patients in the Lords and Commons extolled his services to the country, lamented the possible drainage of such a brain, and hinted that he might prove politically useful, since he had influence in the canton of Berne. In the end, he stayed in London, exempt from all taxes, appointed by Parliament to care for the health of the royal children. On one famous occasion he was obliged to displace himself. Queen Henrietta Maria was ill in childbirth at Exeter, and a desperate message was sent from the king in Oxford through the diplomatic bag of Mayerne's father-in-law the Dutch ambassador: 'Mayerne, pour l'amour de moy, allé trouver ma femme'. The Parliament gave the necessary leave, and the 71-year-old Mayerne, for all his corpulence, and his 80-year-old colleague Dr Lister, set out, by coach, with a parliamentary safe conduct, to ease the birth of Princess Henrietta, 'la belle Stuart', afterwards Duchess of Orléans.

Mayerne never saw the king or queen during the civil wars and revolution. At court, he was replaced by his colleague William Harvey, who in the 1630s had gradually acquired the personal favour of the king and in 1639 had succeeded Bethune as physician-in-ordinary. For in manner at least, Harvey was much more in tune than Mayerne with the chastened character of the Caroline court. It was not that Harvey himself subscribed to the aggressive new royalism or its neo-stoic philosophy. Certainly he was conservative in his personal habits. He would ride out to see his patients with brocaded foot-cloths on his horse—a 'very decent' fashion, as Aubrey admitted, but 'now quite discontinued'. But intellectually, in many ways, he was a 'libertine', a sceptic. His closest friends, in the intellectual world, were the sceptical lawyer John Selden and the materialist philosopher Thomas Hobbes. Neither of these could be described as traditional royalists: one was a parliamentarian, the other a radical, outside all parties. Harvey's mind was open to all ideas, but he was careful in those that he expressed. His own religious views, and his greatest work was, as he realized, implicitly heretical. However, anatomy, unlike Paracelsian chemistry, was a conservative discipline; Aristoteleanism covered a multitude of sins; and Harvey's staid manner, his refusal to involve himself in politics, and his quiet devotion to research made him more attractive personally to Charles I than the flamboyant medical heretic and political *intrigant* Mayerne.

So, in the 1630s, we seem to witness the growing personal ascendancy of Harvey at the king's court, while Mayerne, increasingly, is concerned with the French queen and the royal children. It was not a change of personnel, but a shift within personnel, since Jacobean times. In 1617 it was Mayerne who had accompanied James I to Edinburgh, and had received, together with many others, the freedom of that then lavish city. In 1633, it was Bethune and Harvey who took that journey and shared that honour. In the same happy decade, while Mayerne was conducting his chemical experiments in his private laboratory in London, Harvey was regularly dissecting the red and fallow deer which the king had hunted and illustrating their anatomy and generation to 'my royal master, whose physician I was and who was himself much delighted in this kind of curiosity, being many times pleased to be an eye-witness and to assert my new inventions'. It is less easy to envisage Charles I attending the arcane, alchemical conjurings of Mayerne.

Indeed, there is a sharp distinction between Harvey and Mayerne: a distinction that was emphasized by their physical appearance. Harvey was small and quick—'that little perpetual movement called Dr Harvey' as the Earl of Arundel described him. Mayerne—see Rubens' portrait of him—was immobilized by corpulency. In medicine Mayerne's great strength was in chemistry and therapy. He was essentially a Baconian, distrustful of orthodoxy. Harvey was Baconian in his respect for experiment, but in every other way he differed from his colleague. 'All his profession', says Aubrey, who was his patient, 'would allow him to be an excellent anatomist, but I never heard of any that admired his therapeutique way. . . . He did not care for Chymistry and was wont to speak against them with an undervalue'. As for Bacon, who was also one of his patients, Harvey does not seem to have admired him. His remarks on him are disparaging. He esteemed him much, says Aubrey, for his wit and style, but would not allow him to be a great philosopher. 'He writes philosophy like a Lord Chancellor', said he to me, speaking in derision'; and Bacons' 'lively hazel eye' he described, unflatteringly, as 'like the eye of a viper'.

Being so different, how did Mayerne and Harvey agree together at court? It seems that they agreed to differ, and since both were men of great tact they differed amicably enough. We know only one communication between them: a letter from Mayerne in London to Harvey, who was attending the court at Newmarket, on the health of the king's nephew, the Elector Palatine. It is an urbane but somewhat magisterial *consilium*. In a private note, Mayerne observed of one of his patients that he had been 'guasté par D. Harvey'[6]. Of Harvey's views on Mayerne, apart from his general 'undervalue' of chemistry, we know nothing. Here too, as in everything, he was discreet.

Harvey was a man of genius and it is impossible to generalize from him. He does not fit into the pattern of the court, either of James I or of Charles I. The other physicians whom he joined at the court of King James were often interesting men, with advanced ideas, but except for Mayerne they were not profound researchers and some of them were pure adventurers. All of them were on the make. We find them perpetually begging and scrounging for lands and leases, patents and perquisites, confiscations, wardships, fines. They speculated in forfeitures, cornered coal, garbled tobacco. When Charles I succeeded the throne, the character of the court physicians changed. The new arrivals are perhaps more respectable than their predecessors but they are less interesting and they made no contribution to science at all. Their learning was conservative, decorative and thin. Arthur Johnston, the Scot who succeeded Harvey as physician extraordinary, was a connoisseur and editor of Latin poetry. John Wedderburn, another Scot, began as professor of philosophy at St. Andrews. Walter Charleton was a light-weight reactionary littérateur. Appropriately, it was in the Bodleian Library, not the new Jacobean Physic Garden or Anatomy School, that the king chose to knight Simon Baskerville. Harvey is quite different, from these as from those. His speculations were purely intellectual. He was a researcher, content with his lot. He was never knighted. He did not need such 'wooden legs'. Perhaps his conservatism made him more at home in the chaste, correct, archaizing court of Charles I than in the swinging court of James I; but it was conservatism with a difference: superficial conservatism only, the conservatism once recommended by one of the greatest teachers at his own university, the university of Padua, *extra ut moris est, intus ut libet*: outward conformity, inner freedom*.

References

1. Hist. MSS Comm. Cowper MSS II 291–5
2. See Sir George Clark, *The Royal Society of Physicians in London*, I, 196
3. *Cal. S. P. Dom. 1623–5*, pp. 330, 349
4. *Advancement of Learning* (1605) pp. 38 ff
5. Spedding J. (1857). *Life and Letters of Francis Bacon*
6. BM.MS Sloane 2072 f.2 v. For other critical judgments of Harvey's therapy, see Keynes, A. *The Life of William Harvey*, 393–4. (Oxford: Clarendon Press)

* Harvey's intellectual radicalism, which contrasts with his social conservatism, is well brought out in the work of that greatest of all historians of medicine, Walter Pagel, *The Biological Ideas of William Harvey* (Basel, 1967).

20
William Harvey—the man and his work

G. WHITTERIDGE

It was around Christmas 1648 that Dr George Ent visited Harvey who was then living outside London, probably in the house of his nephew Daniel at Combe near Croydon. In the preceding January Harvey had been compelled to leave his royal master, Charles I, at Newcastle when the Parliamentary army had taken possession of the king's person. In November the decision had been reached that the king should stand his trial, a trial which began on 20 January 1649 in Westminster Hall and ended ten days later with the king's execution. Ent found Harvey deeply searching into natural things for, he said, 'if the comfort of my studies and the remembrance of many things long since fallen under my observation were not some solace to my mind, I know not what could prevail upon me to wish to survive the present time.' And so they fell to talking of Harvey's interests. 'It has always been my delight to make strict inspection into animals themselves. And I have been of the opinion that from thence we might acquire not only the knowledge of the lesser secrets of Nature but some adumbration of the great Creator himself. And although many things have been discovered by the learned men of former times, yet do I believe that far more still remains concealed in the darkness of uncharted Nature.' Harvey had then passed his seventieth birthday and his investigations of natural phenomena had been the chief interest of his whole life. This interest had undoubtedly been stimulated by Fabricius of Aquapendente under whose guidance he had learned at Padua the importance of dissection as the only method by which any true knowledge of anatomy could be acquired. At Padua dissection of the human cadaver was regularly practised in public, and private anatomies and dissections, and vivisections of animals were also frequently performed to supplement the knowledge of the human body. At Padua too Harvey learnt to love Aristotle, all of whose writings on natural philosophy were read and studied. In addition, all the medical students were trained in Aristotelean logic, and formal disputations were a necessary and integral part of the curriculum which ended in a private and a public examination at which the candidate for a doctor's degree disputed with his examiners a thesis which they had proposed. The patient investigation of biological phenomena, insatiable curiosity, an Aristotelean cast of thought and a strict regard for logical argument remained with Harvey as the chief characteristics of his works throughout his life.

When Harvey accompanied Thomas Earl of Arundel in 1636 on his Ambassadorial journey to Vienna, the artist Wenceslas Hollar, who was also with them, said of Harvey that 'he would be making of excursions into the woods, making observations of strange trees and plants, earths and so forth, and sometimes like to be lost, so that my lord Ambassador would be really angry with him, for there was not only danger of thieves, but of wild beasts.' When, in the summer of 1633 on the occasion of the king's coronation in Edinburgh, Harvey had accompanied King Charles to Scotland he took the opportunity to visit the Bass Rock, and his description of it and of its birds is one of the most celebrated digressions in his book on the generation of animals:

> The surface of this island in the months of May and June, is almost entirely covered over with nests, eggs and chicks so that for their very great numbers you can scarcely anywhere set your foot in an empty space, and such a mighty flock hovers over the island that, like thick clouds, they darken and obscure the day. And such a cry and noise they make that you can hardly hear the words of those that stand next to you. If you look down into the sea beneath, as from some high tower or steep precipice, you will see it all spread over with an infinite variety of birds, swimming to and fro in pursuit of their prey; just as some ponds in spring time are paved with frogs, and open hills and steep mountains are studded all over with countless flocks of sheep and goats. If you sail around the island and look up at the towering cliffs, you will see in each and every of their clefts and crannies innumerable colonies of birds of every kind and size, more indeed than on a clear and moonless night there are stars in the sky. And if you observe those that fly off and those that fly back, you would think them to be a vast swarm of bees.

From this book too, it is clear that Harvey was not, in the words of his friend John Aubrey, 'stiff, starcht, and retired, as other formall Doctors are', but would talk to all and sundry, knowing that something could be learned from every one, from the wise man and from the fool. Like Chaucer's Clerk of Oxenford, 'gladly wolde he lerne, and gladly teche'. And so he tells of the huntsmen whom he knew who could distinguish by the sound of its voice what any particular hound in the whole pack was doing at any moment in the chase, and who could recognize any individual stag or hind in the herd by its footprints or its cast antler. With evident delight and wonder he tells the story of the shepherd who took one lamb out of forty penned together and carried it to its mother as she was grazing with the whole flock on the hillside.

Of all Harvey's writings, the one which best reveals the wide scope of his interests is the first, his Lectures on the whole of Anatomy, *Prelectiones anatomiae universalis*. In 1607, he had been admitted as a Fellow of the College of Physicians, and in 1615 he was appointed as its Lumleian Lecturer with the obligation of delivering lectures on anatomy, lectures which took the form of a commentary on the dissection of a human cadaver. These lectures Harvey delivered for the first time on 16, 17 and 18 April 1616 on the bodies of two men who had been hanged for theft at the end of the preceding week. These lectures were not published during his lifetime and they remain as they were written in note form, but as the subject of them was the anatomy of the whole male human body they provided Harvey with the opportunity to range widely over a great diversity of problems, to quote his own observations or to mention case histories in confirmation or refutation of disputed opinions, with the result that from them we can have a clear picture of his manner of work, of the extent of his reading and of his knowledge, of the quality of his observations and of his judgements.

When Harvey gave these Lectures for the first time, he was already 38 years old, physician to King James I and to members of the Court, physician to St Bartholomew's Hospital, and a man of maturity and experience. The knowledge which he had acquired of the animal kingdom was vast. In these Lectures there are references to more than one hundred different kinds of birds, beasts, fish and insects. Only a few of these, such as the elephant, the whale and the walrus, he had not himself dissected, but for the rest his remarks concerning them are based on his own observations and his own dissections. Some of the rarities had come from the king's collection, such as the ostriches which he mentions several times. (It was from this source that he obtained the cassowary which he describes in his *De generatione animalium* and which had been sent from the East Indies to Holland and given to James I as a present by Prince Maurice of the Netherlands.) He seems to have been one of the first anatomists to work on the guinea pig and on the seal, for his remarks on the anatomy of the seal predate the first known description of it published by Marcaurelio Severino in 1655. He worked on dogs and rats, but only twice in the Lectures refers to the cat. He was interested in the optic nerves of the mole and in the respiration of the otter. He was interested in birds of very many different kinds, their song, their brain and their viscera. He discovered their air-sacs and thought he was the first to do so. Though he does not refer to their behaviour in the Lectures it is clear from *De generatione animalium* that he had spent much time in watching them. In the Lectures he says of some men that they waddle like a puffin and he remarks that the flesh of cormorants is not delicate to eat; doubtless he had tried. He refers to a parrot that could grasp things with its toes, presumably the celebrated parrot owned by his wife which he describes at length in *De generatione*, and he reveals the fact that he once owned a pet monkey which unfortunately died of tuberculosis.

However entertaining these Lectures may be for the wide diversity of scraps of information they contain, their chief importance lies in the fact that they reveal the state of Harvey's ideas at that date in the areas of his future work, the movement of the heart and blood, and the generation of animals, and in addition the numerous other topics and problems which engaged his attention. Scattered through his published works there are a number of references to other writings which he one day intended to publish, notably a treatise on respiration and on the physiology of the lungs, a collection of medical observations and perhaps an account of his pathological findings and a treatise on the spleen. Not even the notes for any of these are now known to exist. As Harvey himself explained, many of his papers including all his work on insects were stolen from his lodgings in Whitehall by the Parliamentary soldiery during the Civil War, he being absent in attendance on the king. Those that remained, he bequeathed at his death to the library of the College of Physicians along with his books, his rare collections, his best Persian carpet and other household stuff. But the College was burnt in the Great Fire of London in 1666 and only a small proportion of the books in the library was rescued.

In the Anatomical Lectures we can find something of Harvey's views on respiration in 1616. Without the knowledge of the existence of oxygen and without the facilities for microscopical examination, it is obvious that he was unlikely to have made any lasting contribution to the subject, had he written the book which he intended. Nevertheless, it is also clear that he knew as much about respiration as any of his contemporaries, if not more. With regard to its mechanical aspects, he knew of the various kinds which are to be met with in man and he had some idea of the muscles involved and of the parts played by each. He knew that there were two kinds of respiration, in the first of which the belly was expanded in inspiration and contracted in expiration and in the second the belly was contracted in inspiration, the thorax lifted up and the shoulders raised, and he said that this kind of respiration occurred when the first was impeded. He thought that the action of the diaphragm in respiration was that of a secondary agent, seeing that it was not to be found in birds which nevertheless 'sing and modulate their voice'. With regard to the intercostals he was, not surprisingly, in error for their true action has only been discovered within the last half-century. He knew that they had some part to play but decided that the external and internal intercostals acted in tonic motion and both contracted and relaxed simultaneously to move the ribs upwards and downwards. Although later in his Letters to Riolan he was concerned to demonstrate that it was the same blood which circulated from the arteries into the veins and so let it appear as though he did not know of the distinction between venous and arterial blood, and although in *De motu cordis* he does not mention the subject, a note in the Lectures proves that he was well aware of the distinction between them:

> through the lungs passes incessantly all the nutriment of the body and the whole mass of the blood; which explains why arterial blood is redder.

The knowledge that air was somehow necessary for respiration and respiration for life was a commonplace notion from remote antiquity, but one remark of Harvey's on this subject is of interest:

> Why and how air is requisite for all animals that breathe, as how also air is necessary for a candle and for fire, I have seen.

That unsuitable air killed by suffocation had been known from Galen's time. That fire died from too much air or too little was also known and written about, but it is tempting to think from his remark 'I have seen' that Harvey knew a little more on this subject. By 1660 Boyle had proof of this necessity by his experiments with his suction pump. Did Harvey see the experiments performed by Robert Fludd in 1617 when he enclosed a flame in an inverted glass vessel over water? did he see the flame go out? and did they substitute a bird for the flame? There is unfortunately no possible answer. The only other indication that Harvey thought the air to contain something necessary for life comes from the conversation with him reported by John Greaves at the end of his treatise on the Pyramids.

> That I and my company should have continued so many hours in the pyramid and live . . . was much wondered at by Dr Harvey, his Majesty's learned physician. For, said he, seeing we never breathe the same air twice, but still new air is required to a new respiration (the *succus alibilis* of it being spent in every expiration) it could not be, but by long breathing we should have spent the aliment of that small stock of air within and have been stifled; unless there were some secret tunnels conveying it to the top of the pyramid whereby it might pass out, and make way for fresh air to come in at the entrance below.

To the question of the respiration of insects Harvey contributed one observation. He had seen a wasp suffocated in oil and deduced that flies breathe through their tails. With regard to plants he asked, but did not answer, the question 'Do they need air?' a question which was answered by Stephen Hales.

Harvey's knowledge of surgery and pathology was considerable, but it was not that of a practising surgeon. He was well-informed on the subject of dropsy, describes its effect on a number of the parts of the body and the post-mortem appearance of a number of organs of those who had died of it. He says that he had cured it by lenitive drugs and he knew of the dangers of paracentesis. With regard to trepanning, he warns the surgeon to exercise care because of the varying thickness of the diploë. He knows of the different kinds of hernias and of their surgical treatments. He had witnessed many post-mortem examinations in the hospitals in Italy, when he was a student, and in London at St Bartholomew's Hospital, and he had attended autopsies carried out for him on a number of his own patients. There is nothing in the Lectures concerning his obstetrical and gynaecological practice for the anatomy of the uterus and of the foetus was not discussed in them. For our information on this we have to rely on what he says in the chapter on Parturition in his *De generatione animalium* and from this it appears that he was wise and experienced, believing in the minimum of interference in most cases of childbirth.

Perhaps because of the prevalence of malaria in the region around Venice and Padua, Harvey seems to have been particularly interested in morbid conditions of the spleen, and he discusses at length the relationship between the liver and the spleen; but he comes merely to the general conclusion that the different noxious conditions which he has observed 'are the consequences of diseases and the cause of death' and that:

in the beginning it is from errors of diet and natural weakness that bad concoction follows, and from bad concoction comes bad condition and from this some kind of corruption of the viscera and thence death when the viscera are totally consumed. For it is indeed a marvel how long it is possible to live with how small a part or none remaining, like the man who lived for months after the whole of his liver was corrupted.

If we turn to the areas of Harvey's future work, it is possible to know precisely from these Lectures how far he had gone in 1616 in his investigation of the movement of the heart and blood. From the outset he had clearly been impressed by the observation published in 1559 by Realdus Columbus on the systole and diastole of the heart and arteries. At that time it was generally believed, as would indeed seem probable, that the apex beat of the heart occurred in its diastole which was thought to be an active movement by which the heart sucked blood from the vena cava into the right ventricle. Columbus had decided that this opinion was the reverse of the truth, that contraction was the active movement of the heart, that the apex beat occurred as the heart contracted to expel the blood, and that the systole of the heart therefore corresponded with the diastole of the arteries. This truth Harvey had not learnt in Padua, for Fabricius, like the majority of his contemporaries, still believed in the ancient and erroneous notion. So it would seem that Harvey began by re-investigating the movement of the heart, observing its action as it slowed down towards death in vivisected dogs and in cold-blooded creatures like snakes and fish, and he confirmed the opinion which Columbus had reached. From this Harvey probably went on to examine Columbus's further hypothesis concerning the pulmonary transit of the blood. Columbus had examined the action of the valves of the heart and had concluded that they were competent. From this it followed that blood from the right ventricle had to pass through the lungs to reach the left ventricle, and this he proved by the simple experiment of cutting the pulmonary vein to demonstrate that it contained blood and not air. By 1616, this hypothesis had won no general acceptance. In the Lectures Harvey merely accepts the validity of Columbus's findings and does not pursue the problem any further. Being convinced of the truth of the hypothesis by his own knowledge of the action of the valves of the heart, he merely concludes: 'that the action of the heart in so far as it is an instrument of movement is to send the blood from the vena cava into the lungs through the pulmonary artery and from the lungs through the pulmonary vein into the aorta'. All this work forms the basis of the first seven chapters of *De motu cordis*, that is up to the chapter in which Harvey announces his hypothesis concerning the circulation of the blood throughout the whole body. It is true that in 1628 he added more observations and gave further experimental proof of each stage of the argument, but the fundamental part of this work had been done by 1616 although the conclusion to which he would eventually come had not then been foreseen by Harvey, for the simple reason that he had not then realized the importance of the action of the valves of the veins. Fabricius claimed to have discovered these valves in 1574 and from then on he had been in the habit of demonstrating them to his students, and Harvey certainly saw this demonstration and heard Fabricius's explanation when he was in Padua. But Fabricius had no idea of their real use and thought that they were designed merely to slow the impetus of the blood as it left the heart. In the Lectures there is no discussion of these venous valves and of them Harvey merely says that their use is to break off the pulse in the veins, clearly showing that he was then unaware of the direction of the flow of venous blood. According to Robert Boyle, it was when he first realized the competence of the valves of the veins, and consequently their significance, that Harvey began to think whether the blood did not in fact move as it were in a circle throughout the body, and to this realization he may have come some time between 1619 and 1625.

With regard to the subject of animal generation, the Lectures contain many references to observations already made by Harvey on the genitalia of many different kinds of animals, on foetuses and on the growth of the chick in the egg. He knew that in the first fashioning of the foetus the lungs are 'white as snow' and that they change colour at birth. He knew the structure of the ductus arteriosus and of the foramen ovale and he says that the ventricles of the foetus are like 'twin kernels' and that the heart appears to have a double apex. All these observations are repeated in *De motu cordis*. What is more, his observations on the developing embryo had already led him to the conclusion that it grows by epigenesis and that the blood is in being before either the heart or the liver:

> nor is the heart the chief part by virtue of its origin, for I think that the ventricles ... are made from the drop of blood which is found in the egg and the heart is fashioned along with the remaining parts as sprouts come forth from an ear of corn, all together from something which is too small to be seen.

Though epigenesis is now a commonplace notion, it was far from being so in Harvey's time. Aristotle had deduced it from his observations of the developing chick in the egg, but from Aristotle's time until 1564 no one had thought of setting a clutch of eggs under a broody hen and opening one each day from the beginning of incubation till the day of hatching, and no one apparently had repeated the experiment until Harvey did so. The anatomists had concentrated their attention on the problem of mammalian reproduction. But the difficulty of obtaining sufficient material for any sequence of observations was enormous, and this problem was only solved for Harvey by the generosity of King Charles who put at his disposal the royal herds of red and fallow deer. The earlier anatomists had relied largely on human material with all its disadvantages, for they had to depend on the opportunities as they arose of dissecting abortions and still-births and all these foetuses were too old to show anything of the early stages of development. Consequently there was a wide diversity of opinion, the most important being a preformationist idea to the effect that all the parts were already present in the embryo from the beginning and merely grew in size. Harvey's achievement in observing the epigenetic development of the chick by 1616 was remarkable.

The Anatomical Lectures then are clearly of great importance in any study of Harvey's work as a whole, but before turning to his three published books we must consider also his unpublished treatise on the movement of animals, *De motu locali animalium*, written in 1627. Although it is unfinished and still little known, it is far from negligible, for it shows that Harvey knew more about the structure and action of muscle than his contemporaries. He was certain that contraction was the chief action of muscle, that contraction is most powerful in the belly of the muscle and that the essential contractile element in muscle is fleshy fibre and neither ligament, sinew nor tendon, for there are muscles in which there is not one tiny fibre of sinewy material, for example the muscles of the eyes, and yet they contract. Tendons, which were then generally believed to be the contractile element of muscle, Harvey regarded as a non-essential component only present when extra strength was required. Though he was certain that nerves do not exert any pulling force on muscles, 'they are not like reins to guide trace-horses', he was uncertain as to the part they actually played. Did they communicate sensation to the brain and did the brain then make a judgement and, as it were, order a movement? And did the same nerve convey sensation and movement? and if so were they conveyed simultaneously or alternately? And so he asks himself a series of questions which he cannot answer. The initiation of contraction he attributes to 'motive spirit', but what he really understands by 'motive spirit' is far from clear.

There is no doubt that this work on the action of muscle enabled him in 1628 to produce the correct description of the contraction of the heart. In 1616, though he knew of its muscular nature, he was still thinking of its action in terms of the alternating contraction and relaxation of its longitudinal and transverse fibres. Another point of considerable importance is that this work shows Harvey in possession of a technique by which he could perform all the animal experiments necessary to prove the hypothesis of the circulation. 'A cock's head off, the arteries being tied and artificial ventilation given, movements are seen to persist . . .'. The technique of artificial ventilation was demonstrated to the Fellows of the Royal Society by Robert Hooke in 1667 and at that time it seems to have been considered a novelty.

On the nature of muscular contraction, Harvey was, of course, at sea, for he was working without even a light microscope on a problem which no-one could solve until after the advent of the electron microscope. He did, however, take the problem of the movement of muscle to a stage beyond which no further advance was then possible. In this work, as in all his writings, it is the quality of the questions which Harvey asks of the material in front of him that is remarkable, and he touches on problems that only future generations could solve. So here he asks 'What kind of movement is involved in scratching?' and he makes the intriguing remark: 'leap out of the stern of a boat', nothing more, and one is left to wonder whether he was interested in the reaction of the boat long before Newton had asked the same question.

So much has been written and said about *De motu cordis* that there is little need to discuss it further. It is certainly the most rigidly formal and polished of all Harvey's writings. It is also in many ways the most impersonal. The form of the academic disputation which constitutes its structure imposes both the formality and the impersonality. It is as if Harvey had written the work with a tight rein on his imagination, omitting everything that did not strictly bear on the problem in hand. There is no room in it for speculation or for the digressions into other topics which engage his attention, both of which abound in *De generatione* and make it so attractive in spite of long passages of tedious and repetitive anatomical description. Yet *De motu cordis* contains some of Harvey's most brilliantly descriptive pieces of writing, equal to anything in *De generatione animalium*. For example, his description of the dying heart:

> When all things are already in a languishing condition, the heart dying away, there intercedes between these two motions a short time of stillness, and the ventricle being as it were awakened seems to answer to the motion sometimes swifter, sometimes slower, and at last, drawing towards death, it ceases to answer by its motion and only by gently nodding its head seems as it were to give consent, and moving scarce perceptibly, seems only to give a sign of motion to the beating auricle . . . And whilst by little and little the heart is dying, you may see after two or three beatings of the auricles, the heart will, being as it were roused, answer, and very slowly and with difficulty bestir itself and beat once.

Harvey's images are always vivid. He likens the heart's action to that of swallowing and conjures up the vision of a horse drinking:

> just as we may see when a horse drinks and swallows water, at every gulp the water is supped down into the belly and this movement makes a noise and yields a pulse to those who listen and touch him.

Or again to the firing of a shot from a heavy flint-lock pistol:

> where by compressing the trigger, the flint falls, strikes forcibly upon the steel and brings forth a spark which falls onto the powder which is ignited, enters the touch-hole and explodes, and the bullet flies out and pierces the mark, and all these movements by reason of their swiftness appear to happen simultaneously as in the twinkling of an eye.

Harvey's most celebrated comparison of the action of the heart with that of a pump does not occur in *De motu cordis* but in the Second Letter to Riolan. We have good reason to believe that in 1637 Harvey saw a new type of fire-engine in use at a fire near the house of his friend the Earl of Arundel, and it was the manner of action of its piston-pump that caught his attention and led him to describe the spurting of blood from a cut artery at every contraction of the heart by saying:

> Just as water, by the force and impulsion of a fire-pump is driven aloft through pipes of lead, we may observe and distinguish all the forcings of the engine, even though it be a good way off, in the flux of the water when it passes out, the order, beginning, increase, end and vehemency of every stroke.

For twenty years after the publication of *De motu cordis* controversy raged around Harvey's discovery and during this time Harvey held his peace and made no public answer to any of his critics. That he had a very real dislike of controversy is clear from a number of remarks scattered through his writings. He never indulged in the scurrilous invective or personal abuse which not infrequently found its way into the arguments of his contemporaries touching anatomical problems.

I think it a thing unworthy of a Philosopher and a searcher of the truth, to return bad words for bad words; and I think I shall do better and more advised, if with the light of true and evident observation I shall wipe away those symptomes of incivility.

He believed that truth could never lack a patron and that it was a clear sign that the cause was of no good for which its author had to contend with 'brawling and ferocity'. But there is no doubt that the attacks hurt.

Better it is at times to endeavour to grow wise at home in private, than by the hasty divulgation of such things to the knowledge whereof you have attained with vast labour, to stir up tempests that may deprive you of your leisure and quietness for the future.

I do not think that in Harvey's case this deliberate withdrawal sprang from arrogance. He does not boast of his own achievements, and except for the discovery of the circulation hardly ever claims any originality:

Know that I treat but the steps of other men who have lighted me the way.... But in chief of all the Ancients, I follow Aristotle; and of the later writers Hieronymus Fabricius of Aquapendente ....

In the margin of his own copy of Galen he remarked that the chief errors which a man can make spring from credulity and arrogant temerity, and he glossed Galen's boast that he could point the way to truth with the one word 'Arrogant'. His attitude to his predecessors and contemporaries is summed up in *De motu cordis*:

I do not endeavour nor think it fit to defraud any of the Ancients of the honour that is due to him, nor to provoke any of the moderns, nor do I think it seemly to contend and strive with those who have been excellent in anatomy and were my teachers. Moreover, I would not willingly lay an aspersion of falsehood upon anyone that is zealous for the truth, nor disgrace him with the stain of error.

This attitude was far removed from that of a man like Vesalius who lambasted Columbus's friend and colleague, the Spaniard Juan Hamusco da Valverda, because he had dared to publish in Spanish a textbook of anatomy which Vesalius chose to consider a straight plagiarism of his own writings. He describes Valverda as:

one who never put his hand to a dissection, who is totally ignorant of medicine and of the primary disciplines, and who has constituted himself the interpreter into Spanish of this our art for the sake of base gain.

That this was pure libel is clear from the fact that for many years Valverda held the appointment of master of the hospital of Santo Spirito in Rome where all the medical students of the papal university, the Sapienza, did their clinical studies. But in this kind of abuse, Vesalius was not unique.

Harvey's reply to Riolan, his *Exercitationes duae anatomicae de circulatione sanguinis*, was published simultaneously in Cambridge and Rotterdam in 1649. It was provoked by the receipt of Riolan's latest work, his *Encheiridium anatomicum et pathologicum*, published in 1648 and sent to him by the author. Riolan had returned to Paris in 1642, a sick and embittered man, thinking that he had never received the credit that was his due, and resuming his duties in the Faculté de Médecine in Paris, he immediately began publicly to criticize Harvey's discovery. But his criticisms were more emotional than rational and based on theory rather than observation. During the years that Riolan was in England in attendance as her physician on Marie de Médicis, widow of Henri IV and Charles I's exceedingly tiresome and difficult mother-in-law, Harvey and Riolan certainly met; and Harvey knew Riolan in those days for the brilliant anatomist and walking encyclopaedia of medical knowledge that he had been in his youth, and Harvey saw the change that had taken place in him. In the first of the two Letters, Harvey refutes Riolan gently but firmly on every point, and at the same time he explains why Riolan had got into such a tangle, partly admitting and partly denying the circulation, and why he was endeavouring 'to build a reeling and tottering opinion of the circulation, lest, forsooth, he should destroy the antient rules of Physic'. And so the second purpose of this Letter is to show that Harvey's doctrine of the circulation does not destroy this ancient physic, but furthers it.

The Second Letter is totally different in character from the First. Though it is addressed to Riolan in the first sentence, there is no further mention of him till the final paragraph when Harvey turns to two specific points in Riolan's criticism, his denial that blood circulated through the portal vein and his belief in arteriovenous anastomoses, and refutes both by experimental evidence. The greater part of the Letter is a restatement of his hypothesis concerning the circulation of the blood supported by further experimental evidence. In contrast to the first Letter which is as random as Riolan's book, it proceeds in an orderly and well-organized form and the points which it discusses are chosen deliberately to answer specific criticisms or to refute alternative notions. In so far as it is a reply to the criticism of any one man, it is an answer to Descartes who, although he supported Harvey's hypothesis concerning the circulation, could never agree with him on the manner of the filling of the heart and of the heart's action. Descartes did not in fact understand the muscular nature of the heart. In all probability this Second Letter was written around 1640, in any case considerably before the First Letter, which must have been written 1648/9.

Harvey's last published work, his *De generatione animalium*, which appeared in 1651 when he was 73, is certainly not the last to have been written. We know that in 1638 Sir Thomas Browne saw a draft of the book or at least some part of the manuscript. As I have already said, we know that by 1616 Harvey had already reached a conclusion concerning the epigenetic development of the chick embryo. The few dateable events mentioned in the book all occurred between 1633 and 1642, and we also know that after the outbreak of the Civil War and during the time that he was with the court in Oxford Harvey was still investigating eggs between the years 1642 and 1644. From this we may, I think, assume that immediately after the publication of *De motu cordis*, Harvey turned all his attention to this problem of the reproduction of animals. The long series of years during which he observed the process of generation in the hind and doe were somewhere between 1630 and the outbreak of the Civil War. After 1642 the king was not at Hampton Court nor did he have leisure to interest himself in Harvey's work, as he had done in the past, for Harvey says Charles 'much delighted in this kind of curiosity being many times pleased to be an eye-witness to my new discoveries'. It was this interest which without doubt constituted a bond between the two men. Harvey seems to have taken little interest in politics and his loyalty to the king sprang from personal affection.

The extent and scope of the problem which Harvey set himself to solve in *De generatione animalium* was this: how conception is effected, what is the part of the male and what of the female, how heredity is to be explained, how life is transmitted and what this living thing is, in what order the parts appear in the embryo and in the foetus and how they are nourished. Like the problem of muscular contraction, these were questions which Harvey could not answer, not from any flaw in the method which he used but because the necessary technological aids had not been invented and the necessary ancillary sciences had not been developed. All Harvey could do was faithfully to record what he could see with the naked eye or only a single lens, and the quality and accuracy of these observations is remarkable.

By his daily inspections of chick embryos and his monthly investigations of the growing foetuses of the hind and doe, Harvey demonstrated the truth of his hypothesis that both develop alike by epigenesis and in no other way.

> From our account it is plainly to be understood that the generation of the chick is accomplished by epigenesis rather than by metamorphosis; that its parts are not fashioned all together at the same time but emerge successively and in due order; that while the chick is increasing, at the same time it is being formed, and while it is being formed it is increasing; that some parts grow out from others that existed previously and are divided from them and that the beginning, increase and perfection of the chick proceeds by way of growth till finally the foetus appears . . . .

Unlike the theory of the circulation of the blood which was accepted in his lifetime, this theory of epigenesis won no general acceptance for generations to come, and after Leuwenhoek had reported in 1677 that he had seen the male spermatozoa, 'like river eels' with long tails that 'wriggled much', the eye of faith saw in many a spermatozoon, an animalcule or an homunculus, complete in all its parts. It was only the microscopical observation of the development of organs by differentiation of the cells formed by divisions of the fertilized ovum that pre-formationist views were finally made untenable.

For all its great length, *De generatione animalium* is an unfinished book. It is unfinished not simply because it is incomplete in lacking any account of the generation of insects for which all Harvey's notes had been stolen, but because Harvey never finished writing it, nor put it into its final form. The book comes to an abrupt stop at the end of Chapter 72 and there is no summing up and no final conclusion. There follow what appear to be three disconnected treatises. But on looking at them more closely, it becomes plain that these treatises were designed to fit into the latter end of the book which was never written. The last of them, 'On Conception', serves as a kind of temporary conclusion. In this Harvey sets out and supports by elaborate syllogistic argument his thesis that conception is effected by contagion after the same manner in which contagious diseases reap a carnage of mortal men; that conceptions of the womb are akin to conceptions of the brain. And yet at the same time he cannot really believe that his theory is true.

> I have invented this fable because I see that nothing more remains in the uterus after coitus to which I might ascribe the reception of the principle of generation than in the brain after sensation and experience which constitute the principle of art. . . .
> If what I have called by the common name contagion, as being derived from the spermatic contact in coitus and remaining behind in the female when the spermatic fluid itself is no longer present, is the efficient cause and artificer of the future procreation, if I repeat, this contagion, be it atoms or odour, or any other thing, be unrelated to the nature of a body, then it needs must be a thing incorporeal. And if, moreover, upon enquiry it appears to be neither a spirit nor a demon, neither the soul nor any part of the soul, nor anything having a soul, . . . what then remains, since I can imagine no other thing and no other man so far has thought of anything even in a dream, but to confess openly that I am at a stand-still.

And so he puts forward his theory only as a temporary solution.

> I only ask as my just deserts to put forward as true those things which in this whole dark business seem probable until such time only as their falsity may be proved openly before all men.

In the Introduction to *De generatione animalium*, Harvey set down the method which he had used throughout his life in investigating the various phenomena which had interested him. It contained no novelty. It was the method used by Aristotle, the method of slow and careful investigation repeated many times. It was a method which had been practised by the anatomists of Padua from at least the time of Vesalius. By precept and example they had shown that observation was the only possible method by which anatomy could be learned and that it was the only weapon with which to combat the false opinions of authority. So although Harvey takes Aristotle and Fabricius as his guides, he accepts their opinions only when his own observations show them to be true. It is only from the careful consideration of the phenomena observed, the weighing and assessing of their meaning, that correct judgements can be formed.

> Wherefore it is that our judgement errs about phantasms and appearances comprised in our minds, unless sense give a right verdict, established upon frequent observations and unerring experience.

Nor are his own writings to be taken on trust:

> Give me leave to whisper in your ear, gentle Reader, that you be sure to weigh all that I have said . . . in the steady scale of experience, and give no further credit to it than you perceive it to be securely bottomed by the faithful testimony of your own eyes.

In all his writings Harvey insists many times over that the only way to achieve any knowledge of biological phenomena is to interrogate Nature herself,

> for there is nothing mor ancient than Nature nor of greater authority . . . I do not profess to learn or to teach anatomy from books or from the maxims of philosophers but from dissections and from the fabric of Nature.

In chapter 16 of *De motu cordis* Harvey said that it was his wish that above all else his hypothesis of the circulation should be founded upon arguments based on anatomy. In his Letters to Riolan he insisted that he had endeavoured to show the truth of the circulation,

> by my observations and experiments, and not to demonstrate it by causes and probable principles, but to confirm it by sense and experience, as by a powerful authority, according to the rule of the anatomists.

Harvey's mind was entirely directed to the contemplation of the intractable problems of living biological material, and so he writes in *De generatione animalium,*

> although it be a new and difficult way to find out the nature of things by the things themselves, rather than by the reading of books to take our knowledge from the opinions of Philosophers, yet must it needs be confessed that the former is a much more open way to the hidden secrets of natural philosophy and one which leads less into error.

These were lessons which it took biologists well over a hundred years to learn and to apply. But simply because Harvey used the method of discovery which succeeding generations have recognized as being the only one that is valid, we must not forget that the content of his thought was not that of any modern scientist. For him blood was the vehicle of the soul (that is of the tripartite soul of Greek philosophy). The obscure palpitation which he discerned in the blood indicated its lifegiving faculty and accounted for the initiation of the heart-beat. The circulating blood was fraught with 'spirits' which could not be separated from it, and its innate heat ensured the functioning of all the organs of the body and the continuance of life in every part. Muscles moved at the command of the motive spirit, and the conceptions of the womb could be thought of as analogous with the conceptions of the mind. When he sounds at his most modern, these ideas are still present in his thought, and we can only arrive at the full understanding of *De motu cordis* if we have regard to all these ideas which are present in his other writings.

And so the further lesson which he has to teach is that of careful reading of any man's works, lest we impute to the author ideas and opinions that he could not and did not have.

> For whosoever they be that read the words of authors and do not by the aid of their own senses abstract therefrom true representations of the things themselves as they are described in the author's words, they do not conceive in their own minds aught but deceitful eidola and vain fancies and never true ideas. And so they frame for themselves certain shadows and chimaeras, and all their theory and contemplation, which none the less they count knowledge, represents nothing but waking men's dreams and sick men's fantasies.

21
The history of venous valves

J. B. de C. M. SAUNDERS

In the entire literature of medicine there is scarcely a more contentious or
tangled subject than the history of the discovery of the venous valves. Yet
it is a subject of great interest and importance for a deeper and fuller understanding of the reception and controversies which surrounded William
Harvey's epochal contribution to medicine. Indeed, William Harvey, in the
only conversation he had with his equally distinguished contemporary, the
chemist Robert Boyle (1627–1691), stated without equivocation that it was
consideration of the function of the valves in the veins which gave him the
clue and established the starting point from which his discovery arose[1].
Another contemporary, Hermann Conring (1606–1681), initially an opponent,
became a supporter of the new theory and was among the first to realize that
the function of the venous valves in preventing the reflux of blood was
crucial in the evolution of Harvey's thought[2]. As Gweneth Whitteridge in
her outstanding study on William Harvey has succinctly put it: 'On these
two questions, the action of the valves of the veins and the quantity of blood
in the body, rests the whole hypothesis of the circulation[3].'

The discovery of the venous valves relates not only to William Harvey's
discovery of the circulation but to the understanding and appreciation of the
great intellectual enterprise which extended over two centuries, largely from
Padua, to formulate the new scientific methodology which established the
essential beginnings of modern medicine and led to the slow initiation of a
new clinical approach to the problems of medicine. It was a simple but
subtle methodology, continuing to the present, of which William Harvey was
the conscious exemplar as expressed in the typical seventeenth-century con-
ceit. In the dedication of the *De motu cordis* Charles I is called upon to
'contemplate the Principle of Man's body, and the Image of your Kingly
power'.

Although Caspar Bauhin (1560–1624), the botanist–anatomist of Basle,
claims without citation both in a gloss and in the text of his two anatomical
works[4], that Avicenna (980–1037) had described in his great '*Canon*' the
presence of valves in the veins under the term '*cellulae*', a search through the

principal Latin editions[5] of that great work and its huge commentaries fails to reveal any mention of structures which could be so interpreted. This is not surprising, since it is doubtful that Avicenna under Mohammedan prohibitions ever carried out any first-hand anatomical investigations and, indeed, subscribed to the doctrine that the surgical art was an inferior craft.

The first unequivocal mention of the presence of venous valves is to be found in the work, *De dissectione partium corporis humani* (Paris, 1545) of Charles Estienne (Stephanus) (e. 1503–1564), a distinguished member of the great family of scholar-printers. His text was almost complete and the greater part in print by 1539 when, owing to a dispute and subsequent litigation, publication was delayed until 1545. According to the preface, the section dealing with the venous valves was completed before the work was enjoined by law. Hence, we may assume that his discovery occurred prior to 1539[6].

Estienne designated the structures which he had discovered in the hepatic veins (not the portal veins as incorrectly stated by Edward Streeter[7]) as membranes, epiphyses, apophyses and compares them to the 'valves' found in the heart[8]. He believes that their purpose is to slow down the blood in its ebb and flow, preventing engorgement of the liver and permitting the arrest and retention of the blood which, in the Galenical theory[9], is said to be manufactured in the liver for its more perfect elaboration, since blood, like new wine, needs maturing, say contemporaries[10].

Estienne's observations were of little significance, for he had reference to the relatively insignificant ostial valves seen both externally, near or at the entrance of the hepatic veins into the vena cava, and internally, at the mouths of tributary vessels, and not the more typical parietal valves. Nevertheless, we find his opinions recurring in the subsequent literature, with and without reference to the source.

The possible existence of venous valves either in the hepatic system or elsewhere had generally little meaning to the fifteenth- or sixteenth-century physician, if he knew of their presence. The focus of attention was primarily on the arrangement and distribution of the veins in connection with rationale of venesection, under the searching re-examination of its therapeutic application following the introduction of the purified classics of Greek medicine by humanist–scholars. Venesection, although the sheet-anchor of therapy especially in febrile and infectious diseases, had waxed and waned in its use since the days of Hippocrates (460–370 BC). In general, it was used both as a prophylactic and therapeutic measure. The indications for its use were elaborate, depending upon the seasons, the day of the year, astrological conditions, the patient's horoscope and maturity, the nature of the disease and many other geographical and individual differences. For our purposes it is important to recognize that in acute diseases, venesection was enjoined for the most part when the site of the disease was below the diaphragm, when the administration of a purgative was regarded as the equivalent of blood-letting[11]. Curiously, Hippocrates says little on the technique, although he warns us against the use of scarification and informs us how to take care of the wound with a dressing of wine, oil and wool. The older school at Cnidos did not accept the views of the Hippocratic school at neighbouring Cos on blood-letting. Indeed, Chrysippos the Cnidian (fl. 340 BC) totally rejected phlebotomy and, according to Galen, stated that 'it should be removed altogether from our means of cure'[12]. His pupil Erasistratos (310–250 BC) carried Cnidian opinion to the school at Alexandria where it was in conflict with that of his older contemporary, Herophilos (335–280 BC), a product of Cos and a great admirer of Hippocrates. Although Erasistratos, so Caelius Aurelianus (fl. 400) informs us[13], modified his views and practised venesection to a limited extent, his own disciples completely discarded the procedure, which may be related to Erasistratos' discovery of the venous valves as claimed by Garrison[14]. Thus arose the long and acrimonius controversies on blood-letting which were to extend through succeeding centuries long after Harvey's death. To most physicians Galen provided the indications for phlebotomy and Antyllos (fl. 140) the operative procedures.

The literary renaissance given such great impetus by Poggio Bracciolini (1380–1459) and Lorenzo Valla (1406–1459) had been in full flood for nearly a century before it had a major impact on medicine. Medical humanistic endeavour in the recovery and publication of purified Hippocratic and Galenical texts had to await the early years of the sixteenth century to have much influence on practice. Hitherto standard practice in phlebotomy, following Arabian methods, was to let blood from a part of the body as remote as possible from the seat of the affection. It was often deemed sufficient to evacuate a drop or two of blood from a finger or toe to obtain therapeutic results. Physicians trained in the newly available classical tradition found it difficult to cast aside the old mediaeval medicine. Thus we find Symphorien Champier (1472–1539), teacher of Michael Servetus (1511–1553) the martyr physician, although a pioneer in comparing Greek and Arab medicine, failing to note any discrepancy in the teachings on venesection.

When William Harvey undertook his work on the circulation the principle and rationale underlying venesection were of supreme importance. The indications in the classical Hippocratic–Galenical view for venesection was the diathesis known as a plethora ($\pi\lambda\eta\theta\acute{\omega}\rho\alpha$) or plenitude ($\pi\lambda\tilde{\eta}\theta\sigma\varsigma$), almost synonymous terms, supposedly due to a quantitative increase in the body of the four humours in their usual or normal proportions. It was regarded as being of two types[15]: the first type, sometimes known as a 'plenitude', is generalized super-abundance which overwhelms the body causing a 'weakness of strength' and is recognized by the feeling of heaviness and difficulty in movement; the second type is confined to an increase of humours in the content of the vessels which, by causing their distension, gives rise to a sense of tension, soreness, and pain. As both types may exist in health and disease and may be either local or general, venesection may be employed either prophylactically or therapeutically[16]. Finally, there is also a third type in which one or other of the humours is superabundant and this type 'is not called a plethora but a cacochymia' (a bad humour)[17].

Without going into the complicated details and differences in performing a phlebotomy in the sixteenth and seventeenth centuries, it is necessary to provide in brief a few of the general principles for an understanding of the significance of the venous valves in the thinking of Harvey's immediate predecessors and contemporaries. Hippocrates is said by Galen[18] to have invented the two techniques used for the evacuation of the redundant humours, although they are referred to very obscurely in the Hippocratic corpus. Indeed, the precise meaning of the terms employed led during the Renaissance to a controversial literature of massive proportions. The first method was called 'revulsion' (*revulsio*), by which was meant that the site for bleeding was chosen as remote as possible from the suspected seat of the affection. 'Revulsion' was chosen in the early stages of the disease or as prophylaxis. The idea of revulsion, as Leonard Fuchs (1501–1566) put it, is to draw back the blood about to press upon and slip into some part of the body 'and which therefore should be used to guard against future disease'[19]. In revulsive bleeding a vein in the foot was often selected as being remote, with the concurrent idea that the pathological and toxic humours would be carried away from the more 'noble' or vital organs such as the heart. However, bleeding must be made *e directo* (or in Hippocratic terms κατ'ἴξιν)[20], 'in a straight line'; that is, the line of the natural direction of the veins upon which the direction of the current of blood depends in its ebb and flow. Under the latter proviso, since the right and left sides of the body possess distinct vessels, 'revulsion' must be performed on the same side as that of the presumed affection. Apparently, this idea arose from the Hippocratic observation that if a patient with an enlarged spleen bleeds from the nostril of the opposite side, the omen portends death[21].

The second method is to bleed by 'derivation' (*derivatio*). This meant that once the humours had settled in a specific part, organ, or tissue of the body, causing corruption with the formation of pus or fluid, then one bled from the nearest vessel to the lesion. Again, there had to be some direct anatomical relationship[22].

The re-introduction into actual practice of the principles and procedures of Hippocrates and Galen on an extensive scale occurred in 1514 during an epidemic of 'pleurisy'. A scholarly physician, Pierre Brissot (1478–1522), professor of medicine at Paris, condemned Arab practice as absurd and pointed to the brilliant results which could be obtained by returning to the views of Hippocrates. He was promptly banished for his audacity by the Paris Faculty and retreated to Portugal where, in 1518, he was again presented with the opportunity of applying the recently rediscovered principles. He was again attacked under the leadership of Denis, the Royal physician, but proceeded to protect himself by writing a book on his experiences[23]. This book went through several editions and served primarily to widen the controversy which waged back and forth for many years among sixteenth-century authors.

In 1538 Andreas Vesalius (1514–1564) tentatively entered the dispute by adding to an illustration of the vena azygos distributed to his students at Padua the observation that, owing to the origin and arrangement of this vein, the basilic vein of the right side should be opened when pleural pain spreads downwards from the third or fourth rib on either side[24]. Vesalius' mentor, Nicolaus Florenas (fl. 1540), Archiater to the Emperor Charles V, wrote requesting Vesalius to develop his thought more extensively. This resulted a year later in the publication of Vesalius' *Bloodletting Letter* of 1539[25]. In this epistle Vesalius introduced an entirely new dimension to the venesection controversy. He saw clearly that to carry out the reclaimed Hippocratic–Galenical principles required an accurate and detailed knowledge of the venous system and, in cases of pleurisy or pleuro-pneumonia, information on the precise drainage of the walls of the thorax by way of the azygos system. Since this system drains into the superior vena cava on the right side, obviously phlebotomy in 'revulsive' and in 'derivative' bleeding in diseases of the chest should be carried out through the right basilic vein at the elbow to fulfil the maxims laid down by the fathers of medicine. Vesalius was fully aware of the strength of his position for he could only be challenged by those who were willing to use, not polemical abuse, but the dissecting knife. Furthermore, he forced a detailed inspection of the vessels to determine structurally the arrangement of the finer fibres supposed to form their walls. By analogy with the muscle fibres of the walls of the stomach, oesophagus, and other organs the venous fibres were presumed to exist in three layers: longitudinal, oblique and transverse, and were responsible for the so-called 'natural action and motion' of the body humours, to attract, retain, and expel the excess[26]. It was these fibres which were responsible for the flux of blood to the exterior or the interior, producing the normal and abnormal physiological responses of health and disease. The outward movement of one or more of the humours would give rise to the flushing of the face, increase of surface temperature, sweating etc. as in exercise, emotion, fever, and other outward signs or symptoms of disease. Inward movement of the humours, directed by these fibres and retained, led to the local accumulation of fluids, anasarca, cardiac irregularities, local inflammation, and abscession.

The concept of fibres gave rise to such terms as textures or tissues which might be closely or openly interwoven to harbour a greater or lesser quantity of one or other of the humours. The idea that the fibre constituted the fundamental structural unit survived for a very long time, until displaced by the cell theory of Schleiden and Schwann and the introduction of the achromatic microscope in the nineteenth century. As Rudolf Virchow (1821–1902) put it: 'the fibre is to the physiologist what the line is to the geometrician'[27]. Following the criticism of Gabriel Falloppius (1523–1562), Vesalius later recanted, denying the existence of the three layers of fibres in the veins with the statement 'that the fibres had come rather from the imagination of authors than that they existed in the nature of things'[28].

The challenge to Vesalius' ideas on blood-letting were not long in coming; and on his own terms. In June or July 1546, Vesalius, now attached to the Court of the Emperor Charles V, arrived at Ratisbon having been detained at Nimwegen over the illness of the Venetian ambassador. He was now called in consultation over the illness of Francisco d'Este (1516–1578), Marquis of Massa-Lombara, who was being attended by the famous anatomist Giambattista Canano (1515–1579), professor at the medical school of Ferrara and principal physician to the d'Este family. At the bedside of the patient, Canano informed Vesalius that he and his colleague, Amatus Lusitanus (Juan Roderigo) (1511–1568), had observed valves similar to those found at the origins of the pulmonary artery and the aorta in the azygos and other veins of the body and that those valves would prevent the reflux of the blood, thus vitiating the Vesalian thesis on blood-letting in diseases of the chest[29]. This conversation, reported by Vesalius himself, was followed the very next year by Amatus Lusitanus' published report in which Vesalius' argument is described as being 'utterly erroneous'. Amatus states that in 1547 'dissections of twelve human cadavers and of animals, and in the presence of a large assembly of learned men', the parietal venous valves were demonstrated, and that when air was forced upward in the azygos vein, as was also observed by Canano, it was 'unable to escape on account of the aforementioned ostiola or opercula which it possesses at its junction with the vena cava. Hence, it is certain that if air cannot be derivated from the vena azygos to the cava, *a fortiori*, neither can there be a reflux of the blood which is thicker than air'[30]. There can be no doubt that Amatus saw the venous valves, although his technique of inflating air misled him as to their functional direction.

Vesalius was compelled to respond to Amatus Lusitanus' published attack. He did so in the more sumptuous second edition of his monumental work *De humani corporis fabrica* of 1555. Here, seemingly as an after-thought, he appended inappropriately a passage to a very short chapter in the first edition dealing primarily with the vessels related to the pancreas and mesentery to suit more the convenience of the publisher rather than the arrangement of the text. Characteristically, no names are mentioned; but the passage is clearly directed at Canano and Amatus, to whom he refers as 'certain individuals of faulty judgement who shamefully declare that not even air can pass from the azygos vein into the stem of the cava'. Curiously, almost every writer has declared that Vesalius failed to find the venous valves and even denied their existence. Nevertheless, both in the text and in the marginalia of the elaborate cross-reference system with the illustrations he compares the structures found in the lumina of veins (which he variously calls *protuberans, substantia eminens* or *extuberationes* rather than by the common contemporary term *ostiola*) to the leaflets of the pulmonary and aortic valves. 'In fact', he says, 'when the veins are emptied of blood and divided lengthwise while flacid, this thicker substance is seen hanging down within the vessel and thus closes the lumen'[31]. Obviously, Vesalius observed the collapsed valves adhering to the venous walls. His serious error lay in his assumption that these structures served to strengthen the walls of the veins and, dominated as he was by the Galenical physiology, they could play no dynamic part in the ebb and flow of the blood.

Jacobus Sylvius (1478–1555), at one time teacher of Vesalius at Paris and whom he later attempted to destroy with a frenzied publication in which his pupil is referred to as *Vaesanus* (madman)[32], immediately saw in the criticism of Amatus a further opportunity to attack his enemy. In his last work, *The Isagoge*, published in the year of Sylvius' death, he wrote: 'membranous epiphyses (valves) are also to be found in the mouth of the vena azygos and frequently in other large veins, such as the jugular, the brachial, the crural, and the trunk of the cava [*sic*] as it emerges from the liver'[33]. Clearly the observations are taken from Amatus published a few years earlier and the error a misreading of cava for hepatic vein, which can easily have been made by one who did little or no dissection, from the involved passage in Estienne's work. E. T. Withington would have liked more credit to be given to Sylvius but examination of other contemporary sources would negate his opinion.

Realdus Columbus (c. 1516–1559), successor to Vesalius in the chair of anatomy at Padua in 1544, an anatomist of great competence, whose discoveries on the pulmonary transit were so important for William Harvey, made further contributions to knowledge of the venous valves. Columbus was a meticulous dissector and well-read. Internal evidence reveals that he was entirely familiar with the new revised edition of Vesalius' *Fabrica*. He had read, or knew by hearsay, the opinions of Canano and Amatus and was fully familiar with the observations of Estienne on the valves in the hepatic vein. Their findings apparently inspired him to search for venous valves in the portal system to determine the mechanism controlling intestinal absorption. As is well known, valves are not found in the trunk of the portal or splenic vein; however, they are present in the smaller radicles. Anatomists have been very careless, says Columbus, 'because they have neglected to follow these veins [mesenteric] to their end where they might easily have observed the great industry of nature, that is to say, with what great art she contrived matters so that these veins could easily receive the chyle, but so that these little membranes [valves] would prevent its escape'[34]. Columbus' eye and hand must have been exceedingly steady to reveal and observe these fine mesenteric valves. In view of Columbus' clear statement that these small valves had been overlooked and can only be found by pursuing the mesenteric radicles to their termination, it is odd that an anatomist such as Edward Streeter[35] should dismiss Columbus' findings as an 'error of observation', and K. J. Franklin in his history of the venous valves should say that we cannot be certain of Columbus' findings of valves in the portal system[36]. Doubtless the latter was thinking of the intrahepatic radicals of the portal system instead of its origin in the mesenteric and splenic veins. However, Juan Valverde (fl. 1550), a pupil of Columbus and the first to publish his teacher's discovery of the pulmonary transit, also comments on Vesalius' theory of phlebotomy[37].

The successor to Realdus Columbus at Padua was Gabriel Falloppius (c. 1523–1562) who together with Franciscus Valesius (ob. 1592) and Bartolomaeus Eustachius (1520–1574), anatomists all, denied the existence of venous valves in the vena azygos. All seem to have had little regard for Amatus, possibly because he was a *marrano* who had been forced to accept Christian baptism (which he later rejected) under the persecution of the Spanish Inquisition. One suspects that they confined themselves to inspection of the entry of the azygos vein into the superior vena cava where valves are often imperfect or absent. Falloppius had difficulty in believing that Amatus had correctly reported Canano whose 'irreproachable character and flawless teaching' he so greatly admired[38]. He states in an aside that perhaps Canano was joking when he discussed the subject with Vesalius; an aside with which Vesalius was unable to agree when he replied to Falloppius in the *Examen*. Indeed, Archangelo Piccolomini (1521–1605) who succeeded his teacher Canano at Ferrara where Falloppius started his academic career, was also fully aware of the venesection dispute and of the venous valves, and provided in 1586 a full account of the matter[39].

341

From the time of Charles Estienne, the existence of venous valves was well known by almost every major anatomist teaching at Padua, Ferrara, Rome[40], and elsewhere. The dispute was primarily not as to their existence in the hepatic, azygos, mesenteric, brachial and crural veins but whether they would obstruct the Galenical ebb and flow of blood, especially those in the azygos system, or whether they constituted, as Vesalius said, simply reinforcements to the venous walls especially in regions where smaller radicles debouched upon larger vessels. The essential clinical problem affected the rationale and technique of phlebotomy, especially in pleurisy or pleuro-pneumonia which had become epidemic throughout Europe since the beginning of the sixteenth century and possibly related to outbreaks of influenza. The latter was often called the English sweating sickness, as described on his fifth visit to England by John Caius (1510–1573) in 1552[41] and a subject of grave import to the members of the Royal College of Physicians, but the disease was given at least a dozen other names according to Crookshank[42].

Following the death of Falloppius in 1562 no permanent appointment was made to the chair of anatomy and surgery at Padua for over two years. Lectures and demonstrations were given by temporary appointees, Franciscus Lendinara, Prosper Borgarucius and others[43], which proved to be a most unsatisfactory arrangement. On April 10, 1565, the Venetian Senate formally appointed Hieronymus Fabricius of Aquapendente (c. 1533–1619) to the vacant chair[44]. Although Fabricius' academic career was a brilliant one, his courses in anatomy over the years were not altogether satisfactory. There were numerous interruptions and difficulties. Not all were of his own making but were due to lack of bodies, student unrest, plague, inclement weather and his own frequent illnesses, which were noticeable from 1573/4 onwards. Nevertheless, he frequently delayed the opening of his course out of pique, evaded his teaching duties, and in a number of years failed to teach at all. These difficulties led to student petitions and decrees from the *Riformatori* forcing him to teach, which he did *non adeo exactam* (not very thoroughly). In the academic year 1606/7 no anatomy was taught because, so it is said, his course on surgery was so profitable that students urged him to continue at the expense of anatomy[45], but hardly a responsible action for a surgeon. Professor Howard Adelmann in his study of Fabricius[46] points out that he gave repeated emphasis on certain topics which reflected his research interests and on almost all of which he prepared manuscripts for publication.

One of Fabricius' research publications was the small tractate, *De venarum ostiolis* of 1603, which was to become famous as a primary source from which William Harvey drew in developing his *De motu cordis*. According to the preface, the pamphlet was intended to be part of a series, which together would constitute a major anatomical contribution[47]. He wrote that such intermittent, uniform publications would not only serve the convenience of students, and their pocketbooks, but would ensure greater accuracy, since more time could be given to the revision of individual tractates. Admirable though the intention was, the project was abandoned leaving future bibliographers with the problem of trying to determine which of his many pamphlets belonged together.

For the number and excellence of its illustrations on the venous valves and their approximate position, and for the brevity and clarity of its text, the *De venarum ostiolis* leaves little to be desired. Nonetheless, it presents many puzzling features. First of all, Fabricius claims that the function of the venous valves is to prevent venous distension in the extremities, especially the lower, which they do by 'slowing' venous flow; yet he implies that they must be incompetent since at the same time he accepts the Galenical ebb and flow theory. Then, he covertly espouses Vesalius' notion that they strengthen the walls of the vein. Finally, he believes that the slowing of venous flow assists nutrition by allowing time for tissue exchange. This last idea he takes from Charles Estienne whom he contradicts, again covertly, by denying 'the statements handed down by one who wrote before me'. Yet Fabricius illustrates the very ostial valves[48] described by Estienne as lying in the hepatic veins, but which Fabricius mistakenly thought Estienne, 'one who wrote before me'[49], had placed in the portal system.

Even more difficult to understand is Fabricius' unequivocal statement that none of 'the more recent anatomists' had mentioned the venous valves and that he was the first to see them 'in 1574 when, to my great delight, I observed them during dissection'[50]. Nevertheless, Fabricius in the Dedication to his *De venarum ostiolis* commends the professor of anatomy at Wittenberg, Salomon Alberti (1540–1600), 'who had written most learnedly on the valves of the veins'. Alberti's essay on the venous valves appeared in his *Tres Orationes*, published at Nuremberg in 1585[51], and contains the first specific illustrations of the venous valves derived from a dissection of the brachial and crural veins and demonstrated before his students in the year 1579. In acknowledging his debt to Fabricius, Alberti states that he 'acquired knowledge of the valves partly by hearsay [*auditione*], and partly from a letter [*schaeda*] containing the observations of Fabricius which, the Honourable Senator of the Republic and illustrious physician, George Palm, my very dear friend, sent to me at Nuremberg'. He states, further, that his own demonstration was carried out a little later than that of Fabricius in the same year[52]. Furthermore, Alberti's essay is prefaced by an extensive discussion of the venesection controversy in relationship to the venous valves, mentioning by name all the major participants and their opinions, Vesalius, Cananus, Amatus, Falloppius, and Eustachius. If Fabricius' *De venarum ostiolis* is read in the context of those who preceded him in the blood-letting controversy, it is obvious from his statements that he was entirely familiar, not only with Alberti's work, but with prior theories on the function of the venous valves. Indeed, Fabricius' treatise is a fundamental contribution to the dispute which occupied the minds of all physicians and surgeons (such as himself) for nearly a century, producing so vast a literature that one can do no more than touch upon it. Although K. J. Franklin finds it surprising that Fabricius 'regarded himself as the first discoverer of these structures', he excuses Fabricius on the grounds of a faulty memory and ill-health; nevertheless, in view of his reference to Alberti's work in the dedication of the *De venarum ostiolis* and oblique reference to Estienne, 'it was open to him [Fabricius] to give more credit to earlier workers'[53]. In an age dominated by the appeal to authorities, it is strange, although excusable on the grounds that Fabricius' pamphlet was no more than a chapter in what was to be a larger work. On the other hand, there may have been other reasons; certainly Fabricius' own statements are unreliable.

A further complication must be introduced in the history of the venous valves. Throughout contemporary literature there are frequent statements that the discoveries described by Fabricius on this subject were in reality made by his friend and intimate the Servite friar, Fra Paolo Sarpi (1552–1628) of Venice. Sarpi was one of the most remarkable figures in Europe at the end of the sixteenth and beginning of the seventeenth century. Theologian, statesman, philosopher and scientist, who has been called 'The Greatest of the Venetians', Sarpi is well known to historians of the Reformation for his History of the *Council of Trent*, but is seldom mentioned in histories of science and medicine. Yet Galileo Galilei (1564–1642) described him as 'my father and my master' and wrote of him 'No man in Europe surpasses Master Paolo Sarpi in his knowledge of the science of mathematics'. He carried on an extensive correspondence with the 'father of modern algebra' and famous cryptographer, Francois Vieta (1540–1603), and the Scottish mathematician, Alexander Anderson (*c.* 1582–1620) and was called upon to revise their works[54]. He communicated with William Gilbert (1544–1603) on the magnet, advised and assisted Santorio Santorio (1561–1636) in his work on the measurement of metabolism[55]. Sir Henry Wotten (1568–1639), the British Ambassador to Venice who knew Sarpi well, commented not only on his mathematical ability, but added that he was 'so expert in the history of plants, as if he had never perused any book but nature'[56]; and Robert Sanderson (1587–1663), Bishop of Lincoln, lamented to Isaak Walton his regret at not accompanying Sir Henry as chaplain for he lost the opportunity of meeting 'one of the late miracles of general learning, prudence and modesty . . .'[57].

In 1570, aged 18, the youthful Fra Paolo Sarpi was called to Mantua by its Duke, Guglielimo Gonzago (fl. 1570) who became his patron. Here, apart from literary, theological, linguistic and mathematical studies, he pursued with great passion anatomical and physiological investigations in which he continued for most of his life. Next to mathematics, anatomy had the greatest fascination for him. This common interest brought him on his return to Venice in 1574 in close relationship with Fabricius of Aquapendente and Santorio Santorio and they became intimate friends. This is the very year in which Fabricius claims to have first seen the venous valves. Following an attempted assassination in 1607 at the instance of Pope Paul V, these physicians were called to attend him. The Doge and the Venetian Senate rewarded the attending physicians with valuable gifts, and Fabricius was ennobled for his surgical services[58].

Although there is an extensive literature on Fra Paolo Sarpi, it deals primarily with his life[59], his service as Chief Councillor to the State, his influence on foreign affairs, and his historical contributions[60,61]. He published very little on science but was more than generous in communicating the results of his work and experiments freely to leading scientists throughout Europe. Unfortunately many of his manuscripts, especially those dealing with scientific subjects, were destroyed in a fire at the Servite monastery in

1769. Fortunately many of these manuscripts were excerpted in 1740, before the fire, for Marco Foscarini, Doge in 1762–1763, and occupy some twenty-nine folio volumes in the state archives.*

The relationship between Fabricius and Paolo Sarpi in matters scientific was very close, as acknowledged by Fabricius himself. In his monograph *De visione* (Padua, 1600), Fabricius draws attention to the assistance he has received from Fra Paolo of Venice, distinguished philosopher and great student of optics, and praises him as the discoverer of the important light reflex and methods of dilating the pupil to determine changes in the lens[63]. Sarpi's biographer, Fulgenzio Micanzio, goes on to say that Fabricius was niggardly of praise and acknowledgment in that work which contains much more derived from Paolo Sarpi 'of which I am a witness, and others ought at least to have attributed praise to whom it is due, so also in respect to the blood'. Micanzio then announces that Paolo Sarpi discovered the venous valves. Thus, says Micanzio, 'There are many eminent and learned physicians still living, and of these Santorio Santorio and Pietro Asselineo, who knew that it was neither the speculation nor invention of Aquapendente but of the Padre, who on considering the gravity of the blood came to the following conclusion: 'it could not remain stationary in the veins without there being some barrier which would retain it, and by opening and closing should afford that current which is necessary to life'. Therefore, for this reason, he dissected with still more care, and found the valves. He gave an account of them to his medical friends, especially to Aquapendente, who acknowledged it in his public lectures, and it was afterwards acknowledged in the writing of many illustrious authors'[64]. There is much evidence that Sarpi, while in Mantua prior to 1574, had engaged in dissection and had worked on the specific gravity of fluids.

Further, there is an undated letter preserved among Sarpi's notes (*Schaedae Sarpianae*) in which Fra Paolo expresses regrets at having to give up animal experimentation. 'I must tell you that I am no longer in a position to be able, as before, to relieve my hours of silence by making anatomical observations on lambs, kids, calves, or other animals. If I were, I should now be more than ever desirous of repeating some of them, on account of the noble present you have made me of the great and useful work of the illustrious Vesalius. There is a very close similarity between the things I have already noted and written down on the motion of the blood in the animal body and the structure and use of the valves. It is with pleasure I observe that my findings are indicated in book VII, Chap. xix, but with less clarity'[65]. Evidently Sarpi had been reading the final chapter of Vesalius' *De humani corporis fabrica* on experimental physiology. He concludes the letter with some interesting observations on the restoration of respiration and expresses the opinion that the air we breathe contains some principles or agent capable of vivifying the blood and re-establishing its motion. Sarpi's letter substantially supports the statements made by Fra Fulgenzio Micanzio, but it is also responsible

* Of great importance is the biography written by his secretary, friend and successor, Fra Fulgenzio Micanzio. This was published anonymously soon after Sarpi's death and suspected as a plagiarism. However, the original autograph, but with many important differences, was discovered in 1849 in the Venetian Archives.

for the spurious claims made by some[66] that Sarpi had anticipated Harvey in the discovery of the circulation, and that he had attempted to keep his findings secret (*secretum nulli relevandun*). This error seems to have arisen through translators in post-Harveyan times rendering 'movement of the blood' (*sanguinis motus sive motio*) as 'the circulation of the blood'.

The French 'amateur' Claude Peiresc (1580–1637) (who was the first to observe the lacteals in humans while dissecting the body of a man executed soon after a heavy meal), resided at Venice or Padua from 1599 to 1602; that is while Fabricius' *De venarum ostiolis* was in process of publication. He was a close friend of Fabricius, attended his lectures and demonstrations, and often dissected with him. Pierre Gassendi (1592–1655) in his *Life of Peireskius* tells us that when they discussed the newly published 'and brilliant book of William Harvey on the passage of the blood ... and that, among other pieces of evidence, he had corroborated it by means of the venous valves', Peiresc replied 'he heard [*inaudierat*] something about the venous valves from Aquapendente who mentioned [*meminerat*] that the Servite, Sarpi, was their first discoverer'[67].

Then we have the letter of Thomas Bartholin (1616–1680) written from Padua on October 30, 1642 and addressed to Jan de Wale (*Walaeus*) (1604–1649) at Leiden in which he reports an important conversation with Johann Vesling (1598–1649), who was a student at Padua since 1628, and who in 1632 became Professor of Anatomy, Surgery and Botany. The conversation is as follows: 'On the Harveyan circulation Vesling disclosed to me a secret revealed to none: namely, that the discoverer was Fra Paolo of Venice (from whom Aquapendente received knowledge of the venous valves) as he saw from Sarpi's original writing that Fra Fulgentius, Sarpi's disciple and successor, had preserved in Venice'[68]. Thomas Bartholin seems to have been sure of his ground on the question of the venous valves since he reverts to the matter twice in his later publication[69], but more importantly he recognizes that there is a distinction between Sarpi's presumption, though based on observation, and Harvey's hypothesis (*promulgatio*) and proof (*probatio*) 'by various arguments and experiments', and thereby tempers his original speculative statement. Jan de Wale, one who following experimentation vigorously defended Harvey's views, supports Bartholin. In his *Epistolae duae*, said to have been written almost simultaneously around 1641/2, de Wale says: 'At that time Paul of Venice, the Servite, a man beyond compare, observed the structure [*fabrica*] of the valves in the veins more accurately than the great anatomist Fabricius of Aquapendente later published, and deduced from the construction of the valves and other experiments the motion [*motum*] of the blood is claimed in an extraordinary manuscript that I understand is still preserved in Venice'[70].

Despite the contemporary evidence to the contrary on Sarpi's influence on Fabricius, Giovanni Battista Morgagni (1682–1771), himself writing more than a century later[71], aware of most of the existing literature, and in opposition to his own contemporaries, such as Haller and Eloy, asserts that no one during Fabricius of Aquapendente's life attributed the discovery of the venous valves to Sarpi. Morgagni's opinion was picked up by the early medical historian, Kurt Sprengel[72] (1792–1803), from whom it passed to others.

The history of the venous valves to the time of William Harvey presents itself in a series of steps extending over a century, and knowledge of their presence was virtually a Paduan tradition involving every major figure concerned with the teaching of anatomy and surgery at that school during the sixteenth century. The controversy which surrounded the subject primarily related to the effect of the presence of valves in the veins in the pursuit of Hippocratic principles in the use of phlebotomy as a major therapeutic procedure. Almost every suggestion, save one, as to their function was made to harmonize their presence with the Galenical theory of the ebb and flow of the blood. One could deny their presence, regard them as a sort of stiffening for the walls of the veins, look upon them as agents to retard blood flow allowing a degree of stagnation to facilitate metabolism. Unquestionably the stagnation theory literally held the field as the term *ostiolae* (little doors), the contemporary word used in language of agricultural irrigation was the most popular; to conceive of them as competent valves would destroy not only Galenical theory but the very rationale of venesection. As the Letters to John Riolan and his son testify, William Harvey became fully conscious of how destructive his theory would be to the whole intellectual basis and context of contemporary practice. He saw his contribution clearly in relationship to venesection[73], and soon became aware of the depths of the controversy he would stir up. 'But since the birthday of the Circulation of the Blood, almost no day has past, nor the least space of time, in which I have not heard both good and evill [*sic*] of the Circulation of the Blood which I found out'[74]. Once Harvey's hypothesis had been established when, as he told Robert Boyle, the valves in the veins gave him the first clue, then it was inevitable that a long period of delay would ensue as he sought by experiment the final proof. It would take more than the advice of Horace to withhold publication until the ninth year[75], to account for Harvey's delay. The only figure who was not entirely held in bondage by orthodox Galenical teaching seems to have been Sarpi who, from what little we know about his contribution, carried over his interest in the specific gravity of fluids, which he communicated to Galileo[76], to advance a new inductive conception as to the necessity of venous valves to support the weight of the blood; nothing was made of it save the series of distortions promulgated by Fabricius.

There are many who, when they view William Harvey's *De motu cordis* as expressing the clear beginning and having achieved the acme of the modern scientific method in biology, are struck with amazement when on reading Harvey's *De generatione* that he was and remained fundamentally an Aristotelian, although he would differ with their tenets on occasion. However, as Dr Gweneth Whitteridge points out, it could hardly have been otherwise since, as a product of Padua, 'it was there that he found a philosophical approach to learning which fitted his own personality, the rational, unemotional attitude of the Aristotelian'[77]. Beginning with Pietro d'Abano (1250–1315), the Great Lombard, and the publication of his *Conciliator differentiarum philosophorum et praecique medicorum*, written in 1310 (printed in Venice 1471), Padua was provided with a brand of medical Aristotelianism which was to receive progressive refinements. These refinements continued without break to the time of Giacomo Zabarella (ob. 1589), Cesare Cremonini (ob. 1631), to Galileo and seventeenth-century science. Harvey, as a graduate in philosophy and medicine, could not escape the echoes of the great debate of the 1580s and Zabarella's brilliant exposition on scientific method. The debate was carried forward by Cremonini, Harvey's teacher, who went still further in his appeal to experience. Professor John Randall has pointed out that 'It has become a recent fashion to view the whole "Renaissance" and indeed the very "birth" of modern science itself, as philosophically a turning from the Aristotle of the schools to Platonism; and Italian thought of the fifteenth century has been represented as dominated by that turning. But it must not be forgotten that the vigorous life of the Italian universities remained loyal to the Aristotelian tradition'[78], and especially so in medicine.

In interpreting Aristotle, Zabarella deposes logic from a theory of science to a mere tool, 'sought not for its own sake, but for its utility in furthering science'[79]. Logic and method become interchangeable since observation alone is inadequate, and can only lead to planless collections from which principles cannot be derived. Observation from a few well chosen instances should proceed to some principle from which the observed effects can be deduced. In the technical terms of the age this is the passage from observation through the resolutive and composite methods, as used by Galileo, to scientific truth.

This is precisely what Harvey does in constructing the *De motu cordis*. The keys to the discovery of the circulation, as Harvey tells Robert Boyle, were the venous valves and the quantity of the blood. From the observations, although the valves are scarcely mentioned in the *De motu cordis*, comes the composite method (*methodus compositiva*) setting up the hypothesis to be proved by the demonstrative or regressive method (*methodus resolutiva*) of experiment (*experientia*, often but erroneously translated as 'experience') which leads to discovery. Harvey follows the Paduan tradition in its simplest form, or, if you will, is an Aristotelian empiricist to the end.

References

1. Boyle, Robert (1772). *A disquisition about the final cause of things*, in the *Works*, vol. V, p. 427. (London)
2. Conringius, Hermannus (1646). *De sanguinis generatione et motu naturali*. (Leyden and Amsterdam)
3. Whitteridge, Gweneth (1971). *William Harvey and The Circulation of the Blood*, p. 115. (London and New York)
4. Bauhin, Caspar (1592). *Institutiones anatomicae*, p. 158. (Basle)
5. Avicenna, *Liber canonis revisus . . .*, Venice, 1505 and other editions (Milan, 1473, Pauda 1476, (Giunta) Venice, 1523); also de Koning, P. (1903). *Trois traites d'anatomie arab* (Leyden)
6. Estienne, Charles (Stephanus) (1545). *De dissectione partium corporis humani*. (Paris; Prefatio; French ed. Paris, 1546)
7. Streeter, Edward (1925). in Joannes Batista Canano, *Musculorum humani picturatio dissectio*, intro. and p. 44. (Florence) (Facsimile edition ed. Harvey Cushing and Edward Streeter)
8. Estienne, Charles (1545). *De dissectione partium corporis humane*, Lib. II, cap. IX, p. 182 (French edn., p. 182)

9. Estienne, Charles: *De dissectione partium corporis humane*, Lib. III, p. 357 (French edn., p. 384)
10. Paré, Ambroise (1634). *The Works*, Lib. I, Cap. VI. (London)
11. Hippocrates. See especially *Regimen in Acute Diseases; Airs, Waters and Places; Aphorisms III*, for much on venesection
12. Galen, C., *De curandi per venae sectione*, sect. 2
13. Aurelianus, Caelius (1567). *De acutis morbus*, Lib. II, Cap. 13. (Paris)
14. Garrison, Fielding H. (1929). *An Introduction to the History of Medicine*, p. 223. (Philadelphia)
15. Galen, C., *De plenitudine*, 2
16. Galen, C., *De plenitudine, passim.*
17. Galen, C., *Methodus modendi*, XIII, 6
18. Galen, C., *Meth. Med.* V, 3; *Ad Glauconen*, II, 4
19. Fuchs, Leonhardt (1605). *Institutiones medicinae*, Lib. II, sect. 5, cap. 5. *passim.* (Basle)
20. Galen, C., *Ad Glauconen*, II, 4; *Comm. on Hum.*
21. Hippocrates, *Prorrhetics* I; Galen, C., *Comm. III in Prorrh.*
22. Galen, C., *De usu partium*, XIV, 8; *Comm. in Aphor V.*
23. Brissot, Pierre (1525). *Apologotica disceptatio, qua docetur per quae loca sanguis mitti dobeat in viserum inflammationibus, presertim in pleuritide.* (Paris)
24. Vesalius, Andreas (1538). *Tabulae Sex*, No. II, Marginalia B. (Venice)
25. Vesalius, Andreas (1539). *Epistola, docens venam axillarem dextri cubiti in dolove secandam*, Basle, (English tr. Saunders, J. B. de C. M. and O'Malley, C. D. *The Bloodletting letter of 1539*. New York, 1940)
26. Vesalius, Andreas (1539). *Epistola docens* etc., p. 19 ff. (Basle)
27. Virchow, R. (1860). *The Cellular Pathology*, p. 25. (New York)
28. Vesalius, Andreas (1564). *Anatomicarum Gabrielis Falloppii observationum examen*, p. 81. (Venice)
29. Vesalius, Andreas (1564). *Examen*, p. 82 ff. (Venice)
30. Amatus Lusitanus (Rodriguez, Juan) (1620). *Curationum medicinalium centuriae*, VII, Centuria I, p. 81 ff. (Burdigalae) (1st edn., 1547)
31. Vesalius, Andreas (1555). *De humani corporis fabrica* (2nd edn.), Lib. III, cap. IV, pp. 442–443. (Basle)
32. Sylvius, Jacobus (1551). *Vaesani cuiusdam calcumniarum in Hippocratis Galonique rem anatomicam depulsio.* (Paris)
33. Sylvius, Jacobus (1555). In *Hippocratis et Galeni physiologiae partem anatomicam isagoge*, cap. V. (Paris)
34. Columbus, Realdus (1559). *De re anatomica*, Lib. IV, p. 165. (Venice)
35. Streeter, Edward (1925) in Joannes Batista Canano, *Musculorum humani picturatio dissectio*, intro. and p. 44. (Florence) (Facsimile edition ed. Harvey Cushing and Edward Streeter)
36. Franklin, K. J. (1927–8). *Proc. Royal Soc. Med.*, **21**(1), 12
37. Valverde, Juan (1556). *De la composition del cuerpo humano*, Lib. VI, cap. 7, f. 122a. (Rome)
38. Falloppius, Gabriel (1561). *Observationes Anatomicae*, f. 118a, b, 119a. (Venice)
39. Piccolomini, Archangelo (1586). *Anatomicae praelectiones explicantes mirificam corporis humani fabricam.* (Rome)
40. Eustachius, Bartholomaeus (1564). *Oposcula anatomica* . . ., cap. V., *Tractatus de Vena, passim.* (Venice)
41. Caius, John (1552). *Boke on Counseill against The Disease Called The Sweate* (London)
42. Crookshank, F. G. (1922). *Influenza*, pp. 36, 72. (London)

43. Tosoni, P. (1844). *Della anatomia degliantichi e della scuola anatomica padovana*, p. 95 ff. (Padua)

44. Favaro, G. (1909). *Memorie e Documenti por la Storia della Universita di Padova*, vol. 1, p. 301 ff.

45. Favaro, G. (1911/12). *Atti della nazione gemanica artista nello Studio di Padova*, vol. 2, p. 262. (Venice)

46. Adelmann, H. B. (1942). *The Embryological Treatises of Hieronymus Fabricius of Aquapendente*, p. 25. (New York)

47. Fabricius, Hieronymus (1603). *De venarum ostiolis, dedicatio.* (Padua) (K. J. Franklin, tr. Springfield, Ill., 1933, p. 45 ff.)

48. Fabricius, Hieronymus (1603). *De venarum ostiolis*, Tabula tertia at R.S.

49. Fabricius, Hieronymus (1603). *De venarum ostiolis*, Tabula secunda, fig. V, *explanatio*.

50. Fabricius, Hieronymus (1603). *De venarum ostiolis*, f. A. recto, p. 1.

51. Albertus, Salamon (Christianus) (1585). *De valvulis membraneis quorundam vasorum*, etc. In his *Tres Orationes*, etc. f. L 7 verso ff. (Nuremberg)

52. Albertus, Salamon (1585). *De valvulis membraneis quorundam vasorum*, etc. In his *Tres orationes*, etc., f. Ma, recto. (Nuremberg)

53. Franklin, K. J. (1933). In his translation of the *De venarum ostiolis* of Fabricius, p. 22. (Springfield, Ill.)

54. Vieta, Francois (1646). *Opera mathematica, passim.* (Leyden)

55. Santorio, Santorio (1614). *Ars de Statica medicina.* (Leyden)

56. Wotton, Sir Henry (1903). *Reliquiae Wottonianae*, Letter to Dr. Collins, Provost and Regius Cambridge, in Izaak Walton's' *Lives*', (Ed. G. Sampson) (London)

57. Walton, Izaak (1678). *The Life of Dr. Sanderson, Late Bishop of Lincoln*, 2 vols. (London)

58. Campbell, Arabella G. (1869). *The Life of Fra Paolo Sarpi*, p. 171. (London)

59. Bianchi-Giovini (1826). *Biografia di Fra Paolo Sarpi*, 2 vols. for extensive bibliography. (Zurich)

60. Mazzini, P. (1838). *Westminster Review*, pp. 146–193

61. Sarpi, Paolo (1789–90). *Opera*, (Ed. Giovanni Seliaggi). (Naples)

62. Campbell, Arabella G. (1869). *The Life of Fra Paolo Sarpi*, Intro. p. v. (London)

63. Fabricius, H. of Aquapendente (1600). *De visione, voce, aditu*, p. 93, M. 73 recto. (Venice)

64. Micanzio, F. (n.d.) *Vita di Fra Paolo Sarpi*, Venice, MS.

65. Sarpi, P. (n.d.) *Schedae Sarpianae*, MS., n.d., quoted by Bianchi-Giovini, q.v. (Venice)

66. Haller, A. van (1774–7). *Bibliotheca anatomica*, vol. 1, p. 308. (Tiguri)

67. Gassendi, P. (1657). *The Mirror of True Nobility and Gentility*, Book IV, pp. 28, 29. (London)

68. Bartholin, Thomas (1740). *Epistolarum medicinalium a doctis vel ad doctos scriptarum, Centuria I.*, Epist. XXVI, pp. 113–115. (Hague)

69. Bartholin, Thomas (1641). *Anathomia reformata*, etc. (Leyden)

70. Wale, (Walaeus), J. de (1669). *Epistolae duae de motu chyli et sanguinis* appended to Bartholin, T. *Anatomia* (Amsterdam).

71. Morgagni, Giovanni Batista (1740). *Espistolae anatomicae*, vol. 2, Epist. XV, Sect. 68–69, pp. 155 ff. (Venice)

72. Sprengel, Kurt (1803). *History of Medicine*, vol. IV, p. 32. (Halle)

73. Harvey, William (1928). *The Anatomical Exercises of Dr. William Harvey, excitatio prima*, p. 137 ff. (London)

74. Harvey, William (1928). *The Anatomical Exercises of Dr. William Harvey*, p. 145. (London)

75. Horatius Flaccus, quintus: *Ars poetica*, 1. 386 ff.
76. Grisellini, F. (1758). Memoire aneddote . . . . (1759), *passim*, appended to Holmstadt, *Del genio di Fra Paolo* . . . , Venice, 1785, vol. 2.
77. Whitteridge, Gweneth (1971) *William Harvey and the Circulation of the Blood*, p. 3. (London and New York)
78. Randall, John H. (1940). *Journal of the History of Ideas*, vol. 1, p. 182.
79. Randall, John H. (1962). *The Career of Philosophy*, vol. 1, p. 292. (New York and London)

22
Harvey's conception: 'De generatione animalium', 1651

R. V. SHORT

Unlike the fame of *De motu cordis*[1], Harvey's *De generatione animalium*[2], published in Latin towards the end of his life in 1651, and translated into English two years later[3], had little impact on the development of our ideas about reproduction. In contrast to his clear, logical and methodical approach to an understanding of the circulation of the blood, his attempts to unravel the complexities of avian and mammalian reproduction by a similar process of observation and experiment left him with an insoluble riddle:

> And for my owne particular, since I plainly see that nothing at all doth remaine in the uterus after coition, whereunto I might ascribe the principle of generation; no more then remaines in the braine after sensation, and experience, whereunto the principle of Art may be reduced; but finding the constitution to be alike in both, I have invented this Fable. Let the learned and ingenious flock of men consider of it; let the supercilious reject it: and for the scoffing ticklish generation, let them laugh their swinge. Because, I say, there is no sensible thing to be found in the uterus, after coition; and yet there is a necessity, that something should be there, which may render the female fruitful. (Ref 3, pp. 546–547)

Harvey's conclusions were soon made to seem foolish, and were forgotten in the light of subsequent discoveries[4]. In contrast to the Aristotelean view that the 'female testicles' of mammals played no part in reproduction, Niels Stensen of Denmark in 1667 concluded that they contained ova, like the ovaries of birds, and were therefore involved in the reproductive process, and should be called ovaries. Van Leeuwenhoek's discovery of the mammalian spermatozoon in 1678, and his suggestion in 1683 that life began when a male spermatozoon impregnated an ovum, set men thinking along the right lines, although it was not until the nineteenth century that fertilization was actually observed.

But there is a moral to this story: let us not dismiss Harvey's observations too lightly, for they were in the main correct. It was only in their interpretation that he erred, and it is salutory for us to see how he came to make so many mistakes.

Harvey's downfall really springs from the fact that he adhered too closely to conventional Aristotelean views on reproduction; he freely admits that Aristotle was his General, and that his former teacher, Fabricius, was his Guide.

The Aristotelean view of reproduction was that the male was the giver of 'seed' which developed in the 'soil' of the womb to form an egg, which was therefore a product of conception[4]. Harvey also adhered to this view, as can be seen from the frontispiece of *De generatione*[2], which depicts Jove seated on his throne and holding an opened egg in his hands from which all manner of mammals, birds, reptiles and insects are emanating; inscribed on the egg are the words 'Ex ovo omnia' (Figure 1).

Harvey devoted the greater part of *De generatione* to an account of the formation of the hen's egg and the development of the chick. The hen's egg obviously poses a particular problem if one believes that eggs are only formed as a result of copulation, because it was well known that a hen could lay an egg without ever having been trodden by a cockerel. Aristotle got around the problem by calling them 'wind-eggs', which he thought were produced as a result of a puff of wind blowing up the bird's vagina when her back was turned. Harvey had particular reason for concern about the origin of wind-eggs; his wife kept a tame parrot for many years, to which she was devoted. Such was the bird's excellence in singing and talking that it was naturally assumed to be a male. When it eventually died, Harvey dissected it and found an egg in the uterus, 'corrupt for want of a male' as he put it. He had a similar experience with a cassowary in King James's menagerie. The bird had been obtained in Java and presented to King James by Prince Maurice of Orange. It was thought to be a male, and was housed in a pen next to a pair of ostriches, which frequently copulated; the sight of this apparently stimulated the cassowary to lay an egg, which Harvey dissected and pronounced to be a wind-egg; he therefore predicted that the bird would soon die for want of laying a fertile egg. The bird did indeed die, and when Harvey carried out an autopsy he found a decomposing egg in its uterus, which he thought must have been the cause of death.

These experiences obviously reinforced in his mind the view that a normal egg had to be concocted out of the seed of the male. Although he was fully aware, as was Fabricius, that the yolk of the egg was shed from the hen's ovary and passed into the uterus, he imagined that the male's seed was necessary for the normal formation of the egg. But even here he was perplexed, because he correctly observed that if he shut a hen away from the cockerel, she could still lay a fertile egg 20 days later.

His studies of the embryology of the chick added little to what was already known from the investigations of his predecessors, Ulysses Aldrovandus, Volcher Coiter and Hieronymus Fabricius, although Harvey does deserve credit for being the first to discover the air sacs of birds, and their relationship to the unusual mode of avian respiration. He was clearly anxious to

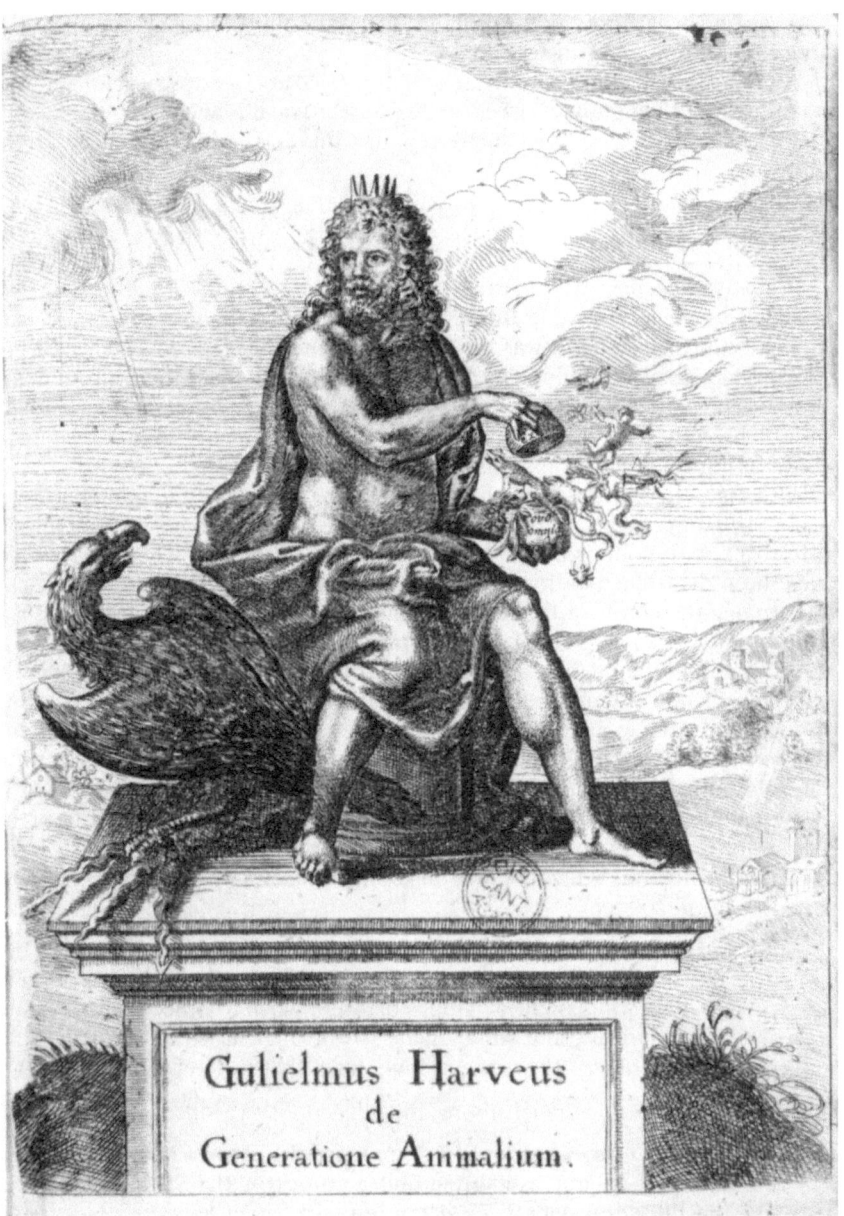

Figure 1 The frontispiece of the 1651 edition of *De Generatione*, showing Jove seated on his throne with an egg in his hands, on which are inscribed the words 'Ex ovo omnia'

355

extend his observations on generation from an oviparous to a viviparous species, and what more natural than that he should turn his attention to the study of reproduction in deer.

Harvey was personal physician to King Charles I, whose custom it was to hunt deer almost every week in his numerous Royal forests, parks and chases. The king was very interested in Harvey's studies on generation, and was

> much delighted in this kind of curiosity, being many times pleased to be an eye witness, and to assert my new inventions. (Ref 3, p. 397)

In many ways deer were ideally suited to Harvey's purpose, since they are seasonal breeders. Red and fallow deer rut in late September and October, and calve in early June. It was the custom to hunt the stags and bucks during the summer, and the hinds and does in the autumn and winter, around the time of conception and early embryonic development. Studying the animals month by month in this fashion therefore gave him unrivalled access to a series of naturally dated mammalian pregnancies.

Although Harvey does not tell us much about the hunt itself, contemporary accounts[5] suggest that the animals would have been hunted on foot or on horseback with hounds until they stood at bay, exhausted, when they would have been dispatched with a thrust of the huntsman's sword. Harvey set out to examine the uterus of the red deer hind and the fallow doe throughout the months of September, October, November and December, in order to discover when he could first discern the products of conception. He clearly expected to find a structure rather like a hen's egg lying free in the uterine lumen soon after copulation in mid-September. One can therefore imagine his confusion when he failed to find anything resembling an embryo until mid-November.

Herein lay the first of his mistakes. Whilst he correctly observed that the rutting behaviour of the stags began in mid-September, he erroneously concluded that this was when copulation took place. A stag's rutting behaviour is plain for all to see:

> At rutting time the males assemble themselves amongst the females, but at other times they feed apart. . . . At that time their lust enrages them so, that they will assault or Doggs or Men, when at other times they are shie and timorous, and suffer themselves to be chased and put to flight upon the alarme of the least barking curre that is. (Ref. 3, pp. 408–9)

But copulation itself is much more difficult to observe since:

> The hind and doe are numbered amongst the chaster rank of animals; because they do not willingly admit coition (for the Stagge and Buck, like the Bull, do celebrate their coition with violence).
>
> The does and hinds are but very seldom compressed, and that too in the night time onely, and in obscure places, such as are purposely made choice of by the males for that performance. (Ref. 3, pp. 409, 410, 411)

Harvey may have seen the occasional copulation since he gives a fairly accurate account of it:

She that is now about the act of rutting, placeth her hinder feet in the furrow or trench provided for the purpose, and (if occasion be) inclining her body doth something depress her haunches: by which means the stag or buck may at one inition (as bulls do) pressing her forward, finish his affaires. (Ref. 3, p. 410)

But unless he had spent many hours in the field, observing deer during the rut, he would not have appreciated that although stags begin to rut in mid-September, it is not until the first two weeks of October that the hinds come into oestrus, and the majority of copulations and conceptions occur[6,7]. (see Figure 2).

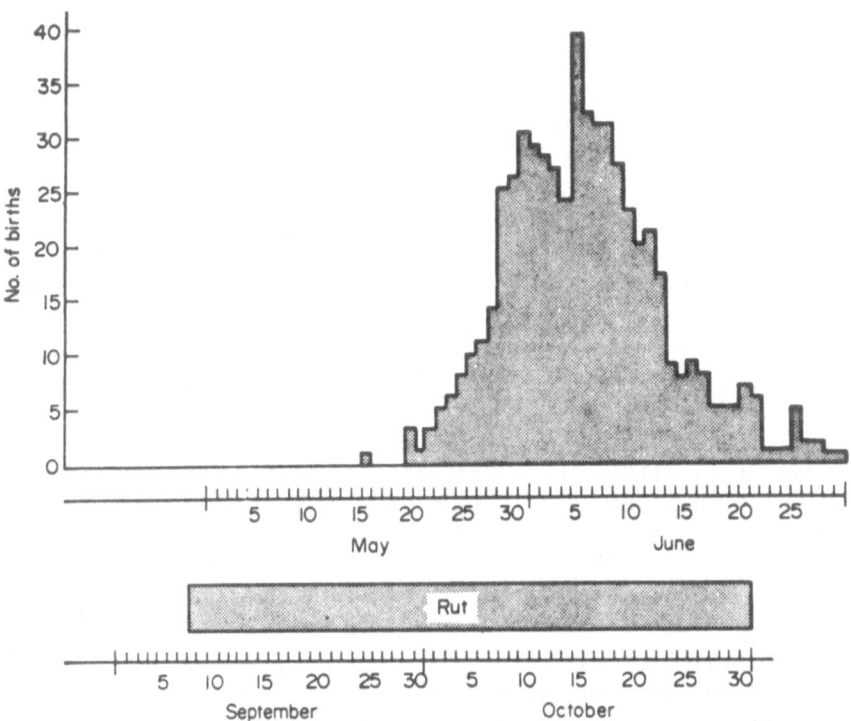

Figure 2 The upper histogram shows the dates of birth of 465 red deer calves caught on the Isle of Rhum, Scotland, between 1960 and 1971. The lower scale, displaced by 233 days (which is the mean length of gestation in red deer), shows the time of conception in relation to the duration of the rut. It can be seen that most conceptions occur in mid to late October, whereas the rut starts in early September. From Ref. 7, p. 476

Harvey's second mistake was to dismiss the ovaries as having nothing to do with reproduction:

And this is my opinion of them, both for sundry reasons elsewhere alledged: as chiefly, because that at the time of coition (when the males testicles are swelled with seed, and full of seminal juice) the horns of the womb indeed are in hindes and does, and all other viviparous animals (wherein they reside) much altered: but the testicles, as they call them, (like things utterly unconcerned in the matter of generation) do neither swell, nor differ any way from the constitution they were of (either before or after coition) affording no testimony at all of their use either in respect of coition, or generation. (Ref. 3, pp. 406–7)

This was less excusable. If he had cut into the substance of the ovaries, he would certainly have noticed the appearance of a corpus luteum following the first ovulation in October[8], and indeed he might even have seen the smaller accessory corpus luteum often formed by ovulation early in gestation in red deer[6]. Furthermore, it had been known since the time of Aristotle that if the ovaries were removed from a sow she was incapable of producing piglets; the operation of spaying female pigs, dogs, and even horses and cattle to prevent them breeding was a common agricultural practice in Harvey's time[4], and John Aubrey[9] tells us that Harvey had a conversation with a sowgelder, although the physiological significance of the way in which the man earned his livelihood seems to have escaped Harvey:

Sowgelder. Ah! my old friend Dr Harvey – I knew him right well – he made me sitt by him 2 or 3 hours together discoursing. Why! had he been stiffe, proud, starcht and retired, as other formall Doctors are, he had known no more than they. From the meanest person in some way or other the learnedst man may learn something. Pride has been on of the greatest stoppers of the Advancement of Learning. (Ref. 9, p. 437)

Harvey's third mistake, which was an understandable one and in part a result of his Aristotelean upbringing, was to expect to find the seed of the male coagulated into a spherical egg lying in the lumen of the uterus immediately after copulation. He was not to know that the stag's ejaculate is only about 2 ml in volume, and is rapidly absorbed by the uterine mucosa, nor that the mammalian egg at ovulation is only 0.1 mm diameter, and hence virtually invisible to the naked eye[10]. Harvey was perhaps led astray by the fact that the human conceptus is indeed egg-like in shape throughout its early stages of growth and development in the uterus (see Figure 3):

Those creatures which beget an Animal within themselves, have upon the first conception something formed in them in manner of an egge. For a moist substance is contained in a Membrane, just as if you should pill off the shell from the Egge: whereupon the depravations of these conceptions are called fluxes. This Conception therefore, as we said before of an Egge, is a true sperme, or seed, embracing in it self the virtue of both sexes, and proportionable to the seed of plants. Aristotle therefore describing the first conceptions of women, saith, they are, as it were, an Egge covered over with a membrane, but the shell taken off: such as Hippocrates records to have dropt from the minstrel, and such as I have often seen fallen from women in the second moneth, which was of the bigness of a pigeons egge, without any foetus at all in it: and sometimes about the bulk of a Pheasants, or Hens egge: and at this time the floating embryo is of the longitude of the naile of the litle-finger. . . .

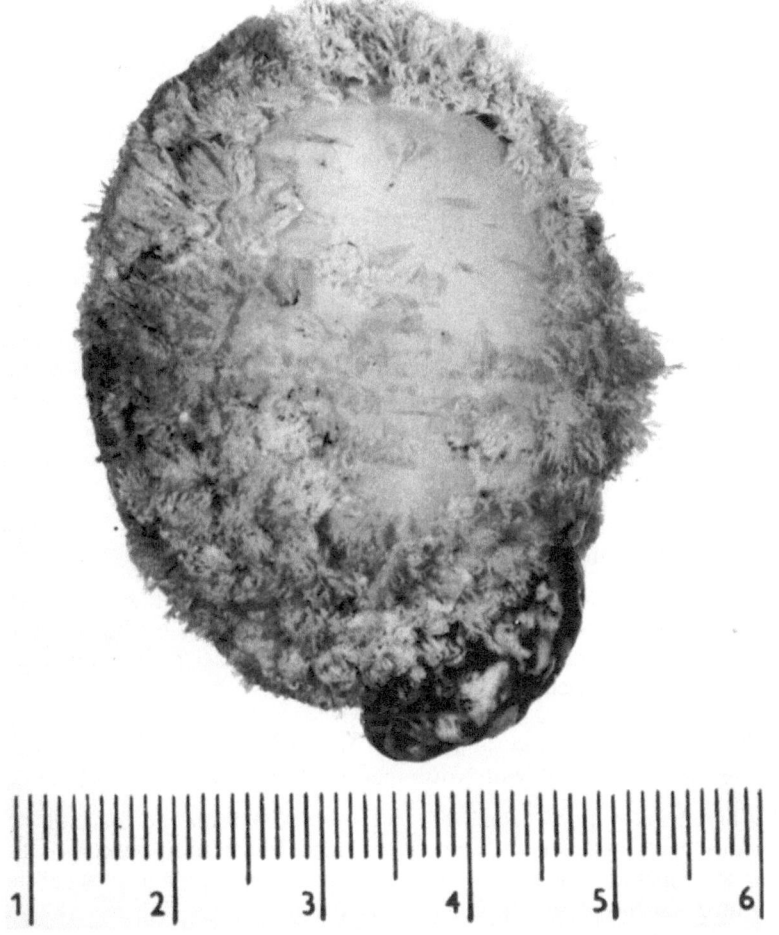

Figure 3 A human conceptus 'about the bulk of a Pheasants, or Hens egg', containing a 1 cm crown–rump length embryo 'the longitude of the naile of the litle finger', with all its membranes intact. It looks remarkably like an egg with the shell peeled off (scale in centimetres)

At the third moneth, this egge exceeds a goose-egge in magnitude, and infolds within it an embryo of the length of two transverse fingers. At the fourth moneth, it is larger than the egge of an ostrich. And thus much have I diligently observed in abortions, having made several dissections of them. (Ref. 3, pp. 420–1)

He was therefore quite unprepared for the unusual shape of the developing deer embryo, which like that of the cow, sheep or pig undergoes a remarkable elongation prior to establishing any placental attachment to the uterus. In cattle, for example, the blastocyst remains about 0.1 mm diameter for the first 10 days after fertilization, and then commences a spectacular elongation so that by 16 days it has become a 6 cm long thin ribbon of tissue. In sheep, the conceptus is 10 cm long, 14 days after ovulation[11].

Harvey almost certainly saw just such an elongating embryo in the uterus of the hind at the very end of October:

> And in some (but that is rare) a certain purulent matter doth stick to the sides, (in manner of sweat) such as is visible in wounds, and ulcers, when they are said to be concocted, and cast forth a white, smooth, and equall matter. When I first discovered this kind of substance, I was in suspence, whether I should conceit it to be the seed of the Male, or some concocted substance arising from it. But because I did observe this matter but seldom, and in few onely, and also seeing twenty days were now past, since any commerce with the male had been celebrated, and likewise for as much as this substance was not thick, clammy, or froathy, (as seed is) but more friable and purulent, inclining to yellow, I concluded that it arrived thither casually rather, or else proceeded from over much sweat, the deere being newly quite spent in the chase. (Ref. 3, pp. 415–16)

He was not able to identify anything resembling a foetus in the uterus until mid-November:

> About the twelfth or fourteenth day of November there is something, which is then first of all to be found in the cavity of the womb of the deere, conducing to the future foetus, and this I truly avouch, and of many years experience.
>
> In hinds also, which go to rut six or seven days before the does, I have still discovered some track of the future conception, about the eighth or nineth day of November. (Ref. 3, p. 419)

When Harvey first recognized the embryo, it took the form of 'certain mucous filaments, like the spiders threads', which soon developed further into a 'wallet . . . filled with a watry, white, stiff, albugineous substance'. Within a few days more, he could observe that:

> This conception now grown, and taken out, is of the figure of a wallet, or double pudding: being besmeared on the outside with a kind of purulent filth; but within it is glibbe, conteining in it a stiff moisture, much like to the more liquid white of an egge.
>
> And in this manner do Hinds and Does, though for a whole moneth together (and more) after their rutting time, no sensible thing at all be contained in their uterus, produce by a kinde of contagion, these conceptions and rudiments in the shape of eggs, . . . which about the eighteenth or one and twentieth day of November (at the farthest) are compleat. (Ref. 3, pp. 420–2).

But Harvey's greatest delight no doubt came from discovering the first signs of the beating heart, or Punctum saliens, of the embryo:

> Having dissected the uterus, I have exposed this Punctum saliens, while it yet continued its palpitation, to the view of our late dread Soveraigne;

which was then so small, that without the advantage of the Sun-beams obliquely illustrating it, he could not have perceived its shivering motion.

The entire colliquamentum being cast into a silver or tinn-bason, which is full of clear warm water, doth very neatly lay open the Punctum saliens to the eye. To which, in the following dayes, a certain gelly, like a little worm, in the form of a magot, is adjoined, (as being the first platform of the future body) divided into two parts; of one part whereof the trunk is constituted, and the head of the other: in the very same manner, as hath been formerly delivered in the history of the hen-egg. (Ref. 3, pp. 423–4)

Allowing for slight differences in the time of conception between different individuals, and the fact that conception in the fallow deer is 1 or 2 weeks later than in the red deer, this descriptive account of the early embryology of deer could hardly be improved upon. How much more graphically Harvey manages to convey the magic and mystery of embryology than any present-day textbook:

A man would admire to see the foetus formed and compleated in the amnion, in so small a time after the first rise and beginning of the blood and Punctum saliens. For about the nineteenth or twentieth day of November, that point makes his first appearance: about the one and twentieth or two and twentieth day, the little unshapen worme or maggot discovers it self: but within six or seven daies after that, the foetus is so compleat, that you may distinguish the male from the female, (by the genital parts) and perceive the feet formed, and the little hoofes cleft, being then like gelly, something inclining to yellow. (Ref. 3, p. 425)

And so we can begin to appreciate how Harvey's meticulous observations, compounded with Aristotelean prejudice, left him with a baffling and insoluble riddle about the origin of life. The evidence of his own eyes showed that the rutting activity of the stags started 'about the midst of September, after the feast of the Holy Cross', and yet he could never see any sign of the seed of the male developing into an egg within the uterus until the middle of November, 2 months later. We can just imagine the scene:

Having likewise plainly shewed that all this while no portion of seed, or conception either was to be found in the womb; and when the King himself had communicated the same as a very wonderful thing to diverse of his followers, a great debate at length arose: The keepers and huntsmen concluded, first, that this did imply, that their conception would be late that year, and thereupon accused the drougth; but afterwards when they understood that the rutting time was past, and gone; and that I stood stiffly upon that, they peremptorily did affirm that I was first mistaken my selfe, and so had drawn the King into my error; and that it could not possibly be, but that something at lest of the conception must needs appear in the uterus: untill at last, being confuted by their own eyes, they sate down in a gaze and gave it over for granted. But all the Kings Physitians persisted stiffly, that it could no waies be, that a conception should go forward unless the males seed did remain in the womb, and that there should be nothing at all residing in the uterus after a fruitfull and effectuall coition; this they ranked amongst their impossibilities. (Ref. 3, pp. 416–17)

So Harvey was forced to conclude:

In bitches, conies, and several other animals, I have certainly discovered, that nothing after coition is to be found in their uterus, for many daies together. In so much that I am very well ascertained that in Viviparous, (as well as in Oviparous creatures) the foetus doth neither proceed from the seed of male and female emitted in coition, nor yet from any commixture of that seed, (as the Physitians will have it) nor yet out of the Menstruous blood, as Aristotle conceits; and likewise that there is not any thing of the conception necessarily in being, presently after coition.
It is also evident, that all females, in the act of coition, do not essund a seed into the uterus; for neither in Hinds, or Does, or several other viviparous animals, is there any track or signe of either seed, or menstruous blood. (Ref. 3, pp. 417–18)

There have been other attempts to explain why it was that Harvey could not recognize an embryo in the uterus until long after mating had taken place. In his detailed analysis of *De Generatione*, Meyer[12] concluded, quite wrongly, that the embryo of the deer was too small for Harvey to see during the first 4 months after copulation. He imagined that in addition to red deer (*Cervus elaphus*) and fallow deer (*Dama dama*), Harvey must have been studying roe deer (*Capreolus capreolus*), a much smaller species that ruts and copulates in the first week of August, following which the blastocyst enters a 5-month period of delayed implantation, remaining barely visible to the naked eye until it begins to elongate in late December or early January[13]. The idea that Harvey had been led astray by studying the delayed-implanting roe deer was also reiterated by Eckstein, Shelesnyak and Amoroso[14]; the only evidence for this suggestion comes from numerous errors in the 1847 Willis translation of *De Generatione*[15] where the original *Dama* of the 1651 Latin text has frequently been mis-translated into English as 'roe' instead of 'doe'. But for anybody conversant with the reproductive biology of red, fallow and roe deer, it is abundantly clear that at no time was Harvey ever describing the roe. Not only are his detailed accounts of the exact timing of the rut and the type of rutting behaviour perfectly consistent with events in the red deer stag and fallow buck, whilst being entirely out of keeping with the roebuck, but more importantly the whole of his account of the early embryology fits perfectly with what we know of the red deer hind and fallow doe, whilst being entirely inappropriate for the roe doe.

No, Harvey merely fell into the trap that still ensnares scientists to this day. His observations were perfectly correct, but he drew the wrong inferences from them. May Harvey's mistakes therefore persuade us that we, too, may often be mistaken. May his wisdom teach us that wisdom was not born with us.

Postscript

In order to commemorate the 400th anniversary of the birth of William Harvey in 1578, we have made a film, entitled 'Harvey's Conception', which uses the original 1653 English text of *De Generatione* as commentary to explain dissections of the uterus of a red deer hind killed on November 1st, when Harvey dismissed the embryo as 'purulent matter', and on November 15th, when the fully formed embryo is clearly visible. The film (16 mm, colour, optical sound, 18 min) is available for distribution from The Film Unit, University of Edinburgh, King's Buildings, Edinburgh, Scotland.

References

1. Harvey, W. (1628). *De motu cordis et saguinis in animalibus.* Frankfurt
2. Harvey, W. (1651). *Exercitationes de generatione animalium. Quibus accedunt quaedam de partu: de membranis ac humoribus uteri: de conceptione.* (Londini)
3. Harvey, W. (1653). *Anatomical exercitations, concerning the generation of living creatures: to which are added particular discourse, of births, and of conceptions, etc.* (London: J. Young for O. Pulleyn)
4. Short, R. V. (1977). The discovery of the ovaries. In S. Zuckerman (ed). *The Ovary*, 2nd edition, Vol. 1. (Academic Press)
5. Turbervile, G. (1576). *The noble art of venerie or hunting.* (London)
6. Guinness, F., Lincoln, G. A. and Short, R. V. (1971). The reproductive cycle of the female red deer, *Cervus elaphus L. J. Reprod. Fertil.*, **27,** 427
7. Lincoln, G. A. and Guinness, F. E. (1973). The sexual significance of the rut in red deer. *J. Reprod. Fertil.* (Suppl.), **19,** 475
8. Lincoln, G. A., Youngson, R. W. and Short, R. V. (1970). The social and sexual behaviour of the red deer stag. *J. Reprod. Fertil.* (Suppl.), **11,** 71
9. Keynes, G. (1966). *The Life of William Harvey.* (Oxford: Clarendon Press)
10. Austin, C. R. (1961). *The mammalian egg.* (Oxford: Blackwell)
11. Betteridge, K. J. (1977). Ed. *Embryo transfer in farm animals.* Monograph 16, Canada Dept. of Agriculture
12. Meyer, A. W. (1936). *An analysis of the* De Generatione Animalium *of William Harvey.* (California: Stanford University Press)
13. Short, R. V. and Hay, M. F. (1966). Delayed implantation in the roe deer, *Capreolus capreolus. Symp. Zool. Soc., London,* **15,** 173
14. Eckstein, P., Shelesnyak, M. C. and Amoroso, E. C. (1959). A survey of the physiology of ovum implantation in mammals. *Mem. Soc. Endocrinol.,* **6,** 3 (Cambridge University Press)
15. Willis, R. (1847). *The Works of William Harvey.* (London: Sydenham Society)

Index